Health Psychology

HEALTH PSYCHOLOGY

EDITORS

Prof. Surila Agarwala

Prof. Ira Das

Dr. Kavita Kumar

ASSOCIATE EDITOR

Dr. Surat Kumar

ALLIED PUBLISHERS PVT. LTD.

New Delhi • Mumbai • Kolkata • Lucknow • Chennai
Nagpur • Bangaluru • Hyderabad • Ahmedabad

ALLIED PUBLISHERS PRIVATE LIMITED

Regd. Off. : 15 J.N. Heredia Marg, Ballard Estate, Mumbai–400001, Ph.: 022-22626476
E-mail: mumbai.books@alliedpublishers.com

12 Prem Nagar, Ashok Marg, Opp. Indira Bhawan, Lucknow–226001, Ph.: 0522-2614253
E-mail: appltdlko@sify.com

Prarthna Flats (2nd Floor), Navrangpura, Ahmedabad–380009, Ph.: 079-26465916
E-mail: ahmbd.books@alliedpublishers.com

3-2-844/6 & 7 Kachiguda Station Road, Hyderabad–500027, Ph.: 040-24619079
E-mail: hyd.books@alliedpublishers.com

5th Main Road, Gandhinagar, Bangaluru–560009, Ph.: 080-22262081
E-mail: bngl.books@alliedpublishers.com

1/13-14 Asaf Ali Road, New Delhi–110002, Ph.: 011-23239001
E-mail: delhi.books@alliedpublishers.com

17 Chittaranjan Avenue, Kolkata–700072, Ph.: 033-22129618
E-mail: cal.books@alliedpublishers.com

81 Hill Road, Ramnagar, Nagpur–440033, Ph.: 0712-2521122
E-mail: ngp.books@alliedpublishers.com

751 Anna Salai, Chennai–600002, Ph.: 044-28523938
E-mail: chennai.books@alliedpublishers.com

Website: www.alliedpublishers.com

ISBN: 978-81-8424-476-2

Published by Sunil Sachdev and printed by Ravi Sachdev at Allied Publishers Pvt. Ltd. (Printing Division), A-104 Mayapuri Phase II, New Delhi-110064

Acknowledgements

We bow in the Lotus Feet of the Supreme Father to have bestowed on us His Immense Blessings to carry out the enormous task of publishing the exposition on Health Psychology.

We are humbly grateful to Prof. V.G. Das, Director, Dayalbagh Educational Institute (D.E.I.), Deemed University, Dayalbagh, Agra for his sustained motivation and encouragement during the compilation of this book on Health Psychology.

The esteemed Faculty members of the Department of Psychology, D.E.I., Deemed University are also extended our heart-felt gratitude for their constant support and best wishes. Our sincere thanks are due to research scholars and all those who have directly or indirectly contributed in the completion of this endeavor.

We are indeed very grateful to all the contributors for rendering their cooperation and timely submission of their research articles. Our sincere thanks are also due to M/s Allied Publishers, New Delhi, especially Mr. Sharad Gupta, Publishing Consultant, for excellent understanding and publishing the work in a timely and professional manner.

Last but not the least, editors also acknowledge the bountiful understanding and unstinted support of their family members throughout this monumental project for completing the strenuous work of compilation of the book on time.

Special thanks to
Prof. S.P. Sinha
Dr. P.K. Mona
Dr. K.J. Sandhu
Dr. Preet Kumari

Preface

"Psychology is the scientific study of human mind and its functions especially those affecting behavior (including human related behavior) in a given context. A human being is a microcosmic system consisting of mutually interacting primary sub-system of spirit-force as its core enveloped by a secondary sub-system of subtle mind entity as its inner periphery and tertiary sub-system of gross physical/material body as its outer periphery with interface at all the above mentioned three levels, viz., spiritual, mental and physical/material with the macrocosmic environment in which it exists as a distinguished denizen of the planet earth. Accordingly, health psychology is a multi-dimensional subject of study... which promises to offer exciting opportunities for scientific studies and deliberations."

This gracious and inspirational message (ISHP, February 2008) by Revered Professor Prem Saran Satsangi Sahab, Chairman, Advisory Committee on Education, Dayalbagh Educational Institutions, Dayalbagh, Agra, can easily and innocently be acknowledged as the sole motivation behind the making of this book.

It is true, that with each passing moment of life, there is a growing concern felt for the health of every human-being on this planet earth. What is aggravating it further is the stress and strain of the modern life style, which in turn is taking a toll of the health of mankind, at large. The scientific and technical advancements are rendering the life's comforts and leisure indispensable, almost *de rigueur*; subsequently, the ever-growing desire for worldly possessions is offering intermittent challenges to one's life, leading to burgeoning stress levels. On such a multi-hued, pulsating and complex canvas, the intervention of contemporary psychological research towards improving the quality of human life is imperative, almost the need of the hour. Relatedly, the role of health psychologists' is also widening, growing multifold, thus, crucial. Today, health psychologists are working with key and multifarious health care professionals: physicians, dentists, nurses, dietitians, social workers, pharmacists, physical and occupational psychologists in order to affect research and impart clinical assessments and treatment services. Health Psychologists are striving to understand how biological, behavioral, and social factors influence health and illness. Many health psychologists are focusing on prevention research and intervention strategies designed to promote health and reduce the risk of diseases. WHO (1948) defined 'health' as "a state of complete physical, mental, and social well-being and not merely the absence of disease or infirmity". In 1986, the Ottawa Charter for Health Promotion of the WHO underscored that health is "a resource for everyday life, not the objective of living. Health is a positive concept emphasizing social and personal resources, as well as physical capacities".

Although health psychology is an off shoot of clinical psychology, yet it can be sub-divided into different areas like clinical health psychology, occupational health psychology, public health psychology, community health psychology, and so on. Health psychology is intertwined with both the theoretical and applied fields. Recent advances in psychological, medical, and physiological research have led to a new level of awareness about health and illness. The conceptualization of the 'Bio-psychosocial model', views health and illness as the product of a combination of factors including biological characteristics (e.g., genetic predisposition), behavioral factors (e.g., lifestyle, stress, health beliefs), and social conditions (e.g., cultural influences, family relationships, social support).

The key to any significant contribution to the vibrant realm of health psychology is highly dependant on its contemporiety. This book is an effort to compile and integrate a number of contemporary issues related to health psychology. Theory, empirical research and contemporary health practices for e.g. therapies have been put together to deal with the intricate issues of health related to every realm of life. The editors have made an effort to offer a peek review of the contemporary research and investigations being carried out in the area of health psychology. Using inter-disciplinary approach, editors have tried to address most of the major current concerns of health issues that every human is facing today.

Psychologists', Medical practitioners, Medicinal chemists', researchers from Humanities from all over the world have contributed to the diverse issues concerning health. In this book selected research papers have been incorporated from the 'International Seminar on Health Psychology, 2008 (ISHP, 2008), held at Department of Psychology, Faculty of Social Sciences, Dayalbagh Educational Institute, Deemed University, Dayalbagh, Agra, India. The book consists of four sections.

I

Section 1 of the book constitutes fifteen scientific papers on clinical health psychology. The topics highlighted in this section comprises of varied themes like subjective well-being and core effects, consciousness, health and well- being, neuroscience, behavior modification techniques, chronic illnesses and others. Robert A. Cummins discusses about Subjective Well-Being (SWB) as an emerging major diagnostic and outcome variable in Psychology and in Medicine. SWB is a sensitive indicator of pathology and of remedial success. SWB mainly comprises 'core affect', which is a psychologically managed, positive mood state, managed around a genetically determined 'set-point', with the aim of keeping people feeling positive. The management system is called Subjective Well-being Homeostasis which keeps the perception of SWB stable, even though the person may be experiencing some stress or anxiety. The author purports that though the measurement of subjective well-being is highly useful for health psychologists, the interpretation of such data requires an understanding of homeostasis.

S.K. Kiran Kumar in his exposition examines the relation between consciousness, health and well-being at individual and collective level and discusses the strategies of intervention. People across the world are often living mindlessly in pursuit of needs and desires which have created not only personal health problems but also have brought about ecological imbalance threatening the well-being of the planet itself. The author stresses that we need to promote health and well-being where not the individual level interventions alone matters, but it is the macro level interventions at national and international level, through raising of consciousness of people at large that can do any good. In the next article, Rupali *et al.,* investigated the time management of non-working married women between the age range of 25–40 years from Agra, India and Minnesota, USA. Interesting results about Subjective Well-Being are indicated in the paper comparing the women of the two countries in view of spending time on entertainment activities and spiritual activities.

One important aspect of scientific inquiry is to provide an objective assessment by utilization of tests, questionnaire, experiments etc. Russell J. Sawa and Jennifer M. Sawa constructed and employed the Family Function Questionnaire Part-1 (FFQI) to explore the possibility of using this self-report questionnaire, in primary care settings. The authors confirm that the FFQI is useful to screen families for family function/ dysfunction, to identify families in need and to help to identify specific problem areas.

C.R. Mukundan in his theoretical disposition reviews the neuro-experiential perspective of brain and mind. He examines the nature and components of human experience. Experience comprises of sensory–perceptual components related to the external world, motor components related to actions and responses, proprioceptive components of internal conditions, and emotions. Learning through experience is therefore, of paramount importance not only for planning and creating future but also for their reality verification. In yet another paper on neuroscience, Vijay Kumar talks about the many fascinating aspects of the human brain. The complexities and intricacies of the brain and its many functions are laid out in his article.

P.K. Mona and Monika Abrol have investigated the coping style, anxiety and depression of coronary heart disease patients treated with medicine alone and those treated surgically. The patients were divided into two groups, i.e. of surgically (coronary artery by-pass grafting) and medically managed CHD patients. The study has great implications in the area of chronic illnesses.

Dealing with the most chronic illness of the present time, the research by Ira Das and Sheenu, relates the activity level of type II diabetic and non-diabetic individuals. The patients were all 1st generation diabetics. The conclusions revealed that rigorous and high physical activity of diabetic group was found to be significantly low in comparison to that of the non-diabetic group, whereas light physical activity was significantly higher for the diabetic group.

The empirical study by Jaishree Sharma and Ravi Sidhu entails a very sensitive issue being faced by the ambitious youth of today. They dealt with the problem of adolescent population diverging towards coaching institutions for competing in professional courses after their XI and XII classes along with the burden of board examinations and stress of adolescent boys and girls and their involvement in recreational activities. The study throws light on the gender differences.

Infant Mortality Rate (IMR) is regarded as an important and sensitive indicator of the health status of a community. Garima Srivastava and Ravi Sidhu describes maternal stress as a cause of health status among neonates. The physical stress had the sharpest effect on anthropometric status of neonates indicating that decrease in anthropometric measurements in neonate is an effect of maternal stress.

Adopting a behavior modification approach, the research by Surila Agarwala and Satya Singh compares the self-esteem among orphan and non-orphan children and the effectiveness of behavior intervention in enhancing self-esteem of children. Results showed effectiveness of behavior intervention in enhancing self-esteem of both orphan and non-orphan children. In another article on intervention strategies, Surila Agarwala and Shraddha Sharma relates the self-esteem among individuals having high depression and low depression. The study suggested that the effectiveness of behavior intervention in reducing depression led to enhancement in self-esteem.

A descriptive, informative and explanatory disposition on behavioral problems and symptoms due to extensive use of internet has been contributed by Saran Kumari Sharma. The compilation is also based on the coping strategies of reduction of this latest clinical disorder with some pleasure deriving skills which are practical and within the reach of everyone. Latest research findings which are included in this paper will facilitate the individual in leading a happy, healthy, peaceful and energetic life. The author has given some humble suggestions for making the atmosphere of schools, colleges and community congenial and relaxing in the interest of progressive global community. In a cross cultural investigation, Gur Pyari Prakash evaluates the different emotional moods amongst Indians and Kenyan college students. Cultural variations were observed in the areas viz. anxiety, depression and guilt amongst Indian and Kenyan students.

Gerontology is a fast growing area in which psychologists are keenly investigating and providing their valuable inputs. In the present scenario we are aware that in old age, health is the primary concern, because the weak social support system contributes very little to improve their health status. On these lines, Seema Kashyap and Ravi Sidhu in their investigation of 300 aged people reported the results of the health status of senescent and senile aged; difference between the genders; economic status and health of aged; the comparison of health between the spouses, and the health of aged of nuclear family vs. joint family. The results have great implications in this field.

II

Section II, constitutes the Occupational Health Psychology (OHP) domain which is a relatively new discipline allied with health psychology. The ancestry of OHP includes health psychology, industrial/organizational psychology, and occupational health. The field is concerned with identifying psychosocial parameters of work-places that give rise to health-related problems in people involving physical health (e.g., cardiovascular disease) or mental health (e.g., depression). OHP is also concerned with the development and implementation of interventions that can prevent or ameliorate work-related health problems. In addition, OHP research has important implications for the economic success of organizations. Other research areas of concern to OHP include unemployment and downsizing, and workplace safety and accident prevention. Research in occupational health psychology indicates that people in jobs that combine little decision latitude with a high psychological workload are at increased risk of cardiovascular disorders. Other OHP research reveals a relation between unemployment and elevations in blood pressure. OHP research also documents a relation between social class and cardiovascular disease. The section comprises of four empirical researches.

In the present global scenario, organizations are facing dynamic and changing environment and require employees who can easily adjust to these changing situations. At the time of hiring, they recruit new employees who are able to fit better with the organizational demands and values. This will definitely lead to higher employees' satisfaction and reduced turnover. The most essential reason for leaving a job is that, the jobs are not compatible with the employees' personalities (Schneider, 1987). It is important that their personalities fit with the organizations culture and value system.

With this perspective Kavita Kumar explores the personality type A/B and the value pattern of engineers' viz. academic and management. It was observed that there is significant difference between the two groups of engineers with regard to their personality type A/B and their value system. A significant difference in the hierarchy of value system between the academic and management engineers was also observed. In an empirical compilation, D. S. Narban attempts to reduce anxiety level of aspirants of campus placement using experiential learning approach. The qualitative inputs substantiated the quantitative results which has great potential of wide applications in Clinical Health Psychology, Organizational Psychology, and Social Psychology.

A scientific and engineering analysis by Sanjay Srivastava *et al.* depicts the designing and implementation of an intelligent system to reduce Occupational Health Hazards (OHHs) of workers of a glass/bangle manufacturing unit at Firozabad, India. Artificial Neural Networks (ANNs) with back-propagation learning as model free estimators to evaluate OHHs of workers for different job combinations were applied. In the next article Gur Pyari Mehra outlines the health and safety issues of workers in an engineering work shop of a Public Sector Company; passing through a transitory phase of closing of its redundant shop floors, collaborating with multinational companies to meet the increasing demand of high targets, international quality standards and customer care. Behavior Based Safety Method was applied which turned out to be extremely successful.

III

Section III of the book outlines the most recent trends that have emerged to treat the illnesses—yoga, spirituality and therapies viz. psychotherapy, gestalt therapy, music therapy, art therapy and others. Here it can be aptly mentioned that Psychology has had its roots in philosophical traditions and spiritual thoughts. But the implications and methods were adjudged non-scientific because they lacked objectivity and proof. However, in recent years, scientists, psychologists and health professionals have already acknowledged and promoted the role of yoga and spirituality in health care. The current literature in psychology and spirituality encourage the use of spirituality in health care. The need of the hour is to address and implement spirituality, yoga and other therapies in health psychology to help people with their mind-body problems. Psychological therapies can improve the quality of life of the patient by helping the patient recover at least some of his psychological well-being. In this section there are ten research papers out of which the last three are demonstrative articles by the therapists themselves.

Seven interdisciplinary scholars lead by Russell J. Sawa, describes the interim findings of an ongoing study on spirituality and healing. The study included interviewing 25 spiritual healers from a wide spectrum of cultures and religions. The methodology involved the application of the philosophy of Bernard Lonergan, a Canadian scholar. The transcripts of the interview are being analyzed line by line to determine what it means. They aim at coming to a common agreement as to what the propositions are; which is indeed a difficult dialectical process. The group is still in the phase of deciding.

The chapter by C. Giri and Rakesh Giri deals with a system encompassing *Charvaka, Mimamsa, Vaisnavism, Nyaya-Vaisheshic, Samkhya-Yoga, Sankar Vedanta* and *Kashmir Shavivism*. It is reviewed in this article that the *Kashmir Shavivism* is the culmination of being free from distinctions of caste, creed, color, profound metaphysical base embodying the oneness of cosmos and the individual self *vis-e-vis* other systems of real healing and psychotherapy. The experts believe that this serves as an example of progressive evolution of Indian mind.

Ratan Saini underscores that the human-being who is the *ansha* of the All-Intelligent Supreme Being, has forgotten the 'True Objective of Life', that is to liberate him from the worldly entanglements to achieve the communion with the Creator of the Universe. The worldly desires and psychological variables like pride, anger, competition, social status etc. offer numerous hindrances in this path. A true Religion teaches that the supreme objective of man's life is to surrender himself to a spiritual Guru who has Himself traversed this path. The wisdom society perpetuates on better worldliness, and 'brotherhood of man and the Fatherhood of God'.

Ganesh Shankar emphasizes that Yoga Psychotherapy is experiencing a strong impetus all over the world, in the backdrop of a large number of emotional disturbances. The treatments of psychiatric illnesses and prophylaxis in psychosocial conflict constellations have generated scope for psychotherapies. Psychotherapy is not only confined to the therapeutic context but is also intertwined with psycho-social conflicts, such as partner conflicts or ethnic conflicts etc.

Renu Josan and Agam Kulshreshtha purport that the psychologists and researchers in mental health have zeroed in on the practice of meditation as an effective therapy. It describes a state of consciousness. The treatise explores how the modern man wallowing in the fiery gulf of anxiety, stress, alienation, insomnia and mental anguish, can redeem himself through the practice of meditation. Sunita Gupta examined how the psycho-physiological responsiveness to meditation affects the recovery of coronary heart disease patients. In her empirical work, Pre-Post design was used for recording psycho-physiological assessments of coronary heart patients. It was observed in the findings that the meditation has relaxing and soothing effect on heart patients.

A study by Surila Agarwala et al. focused on the behavior modification of the posture defects of primary school children. The article provides an overview of the various kinds of defective sitting postures. The awareness is needed among parents and teachers to correct the sitting postures of children for their mental and physical well-being.

The next three contributions are demonstrative monographs submitted by expert therapists in the area of Geastalt therapy, Art therapy and an innovative therapy known as systemic constellation.

Miodrag B. Milovonovic shares his point of view of awareness about yoga and psychotherapy *vis-e-vis* Gestalt therapy. Gestalt therapy, developed by Friedrich Pearls is a Concentration Therapy aiming to achieve the feeling of oneself. A demonstrative session by the author /therapist himself has been included in the paper.

Ralitza M. Vladimirov's 'Expressive Arts Therapy' awakens the spiritual force within the human kind, allowing in, the most natural way of mental, emotional, and spiritual expression achieving stages of awareness and fulfillment. The 5 major forms of art: Music, Dance-Movement, Drama, Art, Poetry offer themselves as universal language by expressing thoughts, emotions and feelings; in turn effecting the physical, mental, emotional and spiritual healing.

Stefan Reiter talks about a relatively new discipline known as 'Systemic constellation' which is based on family therapy. It deals with a system in which, a number of elements are connected to one another in continuously evolving relationships. It is believed that German priest and therapist Bert Hellinger, employing Gestalt Therapy and NLP (neuro-linguistic programming) developed the constellation work. The energies in the constellation field often cause surprising and inexplicable reactions. The author/therapist has shared his own experiences while conducting therapy sessions to suggest the relevance of systemic constellation work.

IV

Section IV constitutes the interdisciplinary research in the field of health psychology. It has an ensemble of articles from Medical practitioners, Biochemists, Medicinal Chemists, Humanities professionals, incorporated to suggest how different disciplines have come together to show their concerns and solutions for the health related issues of the human race. There are 5 research monographs in this section.

Surat Kumar and Kavita Kumar correlate the medicinal chemistry approach to modify the Type A/B behavior by using β-blocker drugs. The chapter describes the synthesis of β-blocker drugs for the management of CNS-CVS disorders. The β-blocking drugs have demonstrated the ability to modify beta adrenergic reactivity, which is perhaps an important physiological characteristic of Type A persons. The central effect of β-blockers influences both physiological responses such as BP, HR, and cardiovascular reactivity, as well as overt behavior.

Rishi Nigam and Parul Rishi studied the dietary patterns and nutritional status of children using physical and bio-chemical parameters. Recommendations for excess fat management, iron deficiency management, total diet management, life style management and dietary behavior management were made.

Pediatricians are facing an ever-growing problem of treating children and adolescents with psychosomatic symptoms. Bindu Dhingra and Anjoo Bhatnagar undertook a retrospective study in the Department of Pediatrics of a tertiary level hospital to describe the clinical profile of psychosomatic symptoms in children and adolescents upto 18 years of age between 2004 and 2007. Stress factors which resulted in the psychosomatic symptomatology were predominantly scholastic problems. R. Bhatnagar *et al.,* investigated the reasons for low level of success of Government run health care programs in the management of Tuberculosis. Lack of knowledge among the patients about the natural course of the disease and the facility of DOTS contributed to its failure. Extensive community meetings and patient-DOT provider meetings are not only essential but mandatory for the continued success of the program.

Prem Kumari Srivastava has made a brilliant attempt to show how literary studies and psycho-analysis intersect and impinge upon each other at several junctures, thereby making literature and psychology a mutually inclusive domains. Tackling anxieties that plague women's health and psyche; her study on Virginia Woolf captures intellectual angst and psychological despair of a woman writer/protagonist, bordering on schizophrenia, relapsing into madness on numerous occasions. Here, woman is the primary signifier and her mental health in terms of the use of past and memory as a means to respond to contemporary reality is at the centre.

Towards the end, we would like to state that apart from the mutative and organic nature of present researches, recent scholarship also stands out primarily because of two key features: contemporary relevance and diverse inter-disciplinary approaches. The aforementioned capsule accounts of the compiled papers in this book offer a glimpse of just that. We sincerely hope that your detailed engagement and serious journey into the various sections of the book will be enriching and enjoyable to say the least!

Dedicated in the loving memory
of

Revered Dr. M.B. Lal Sahab

The Founder Director
of
Dayalbagh Educational Institute
(Deemed University)
Dayalbagh, Agra

Contents

Section–1
Clinical Health Psychology

SECTION–2

Occupational Health Psychology

SECTION–3

Yoga, Meditation and Therapies

Section–4

Inter-Disciplinary Approaches

SECTION–1

Clinical Health Psychology

Health Psychology, Subjective Well-Being and Core Affect

Robert A. Cummins*

ABSTRACT

Subjective Well-being (SWB) is emerging as a major diagnostic and outcome variable in Psychology and in Medicine. It is a sensitive indicator of pathology and of remedial success. However, the effective use of SWB for this purpose depends on understanding its special characteristics. One is the non-linear way SWB behaves in the transition from health to ill-health. The reason for this is that SWB mainly comprises 'core affect', which is a psychologically managed, positive mood state. Core affect is a mixture of trait contentment, happiness and alertness. It is managed around a 'set-point', which is genetically determined, with the aim of keeping people feeling positive. This is why SWB is generally felt as a positive and stable trait. The management system is called Subjective Well-being Homeostasis and the presence of this system explains why SWB data have a non-linear relationship with sources of challenge. Homeostasis keeps the perception of SWB stable, even though the person may be experiencing some stress or anxiety. Thus, importantly, increasing levels of stress will not decrease SWB until the level of challenge exceeds the threshold of the homeostatic system. The presence of this threshold also explains why SWB measurement is such an important diagnostic tool. All homeostatic systems have a limited capacity to absorb challenge and so SWB data that lie below the normal range reveal such failure, which is associated with a felt loss of positive affect and a high probability of depression. Thus, while the measurement of subjective well-being is highly useful for health psychologists, the interpretation of such data requires an understanding of homeostasis.

INTRODUCTION

The Historical Context

Subjective Well-being (SWB) has been a topic of scientific study for over 30 years. However, it is commonly considered that the area was launched into scientific prominence by the publications of Andrews and Withey (1976) and Campbell, Converse, and Rodgers (1976). Both texts demonstrated that SWB data could be reliably measured and that the statistical analyses of such data, using ordinary linear statistics, produced interesting results. Of particular importance, they found their measures of SWB to be remarkably stable. It is this stability and reliability of measurement that has made SWB such an attractive new area for quantitative

---

*School of Psychology, Deakin University, Melbourne, Australia.
E-mail: cummins@deakin.edu.au

investigation. It must also be said that researchers in this area have encountered many problems in their attempts to create a systematic body of knowledge. Two of the most difficult issues are the problems of measurement and terminology (see Diener, 2006 for a review).

The problems with terminology have been horrendous. Even as the early researchers used the term 'happiness' to describe the area of their study, they recognized that the term was ambiguous. For example, Fordyce (1983) grapples with his use of the term describing 'happiness' as 'an emotional sense of well-being—that goes by many names (contentment, fulfilment, self-satisfaction, joy, peace of mind, *etc.*)'. The problem that Fordyce recognized is that, in common English usage, happiness generally refers to a state of mind that has been caused by an acute experience, such as a cup of tea on a hot day. But this is not what the well-being researchers generally intend to measure. They strive to measure a dispositional state of happiness that is much more stable. So in order to make this distinction, 'trait' or 'dispositional' happiness has come to be known as SWB in order to reduce terminological confusion.

Measuring SWB in a consistent manner has posed the other major challenge to research cohesion. There are several reasons for this. The first is that, in the presence of terminological confusion, opinions vary as to what should be measured. The second is that a surprisingly high proportion of researchers find it necessary to invent their own scale. The result is a huge legacy of instruments. The Australian Centre on Quality of Life (ACQOL, 2008) lists many hundreds of scales that purport to measure SWB in one form or another. This has greatly limited progress in understanding SWB since these scales are of very mixed psychometric quality and many of them measure quite different constructs. The unfortunate result is a confused and massive literature that, despite three decades of research, still lacks conceptual cohesion.

However, despite the difficulties of conceptualization and measurement, SWB is gaining prominence as an interesting new facet of the human condition. After all, if people feel that their lives are not worth living, what is the use of life (see Schalock, 1997)? And a fundamental truth is that the objective measures of wealth and health cannot be used as proxy measures of SWB. For example, there is generally a low correlation between objectively measured physical health and SWB (Cummins, Woerner, Tomyn, Gibson and Knapp, 2006) provided that the people concerned have the resources to deal with the consequences of their poor health for daily living.

So the reality is that 'Quality of life' is now understood to be a dual construct comprising both an easily measured objective dimension and a subjective dimension that is more challenging to measure and understand. Moreover, these two forms of measurement are usually quite independent of one another. We propose that the reason for this independence is that SWB is being managed by a psychological system that we call SWB homeostasis (see Cummins, 2003; Cummins, Gullone and Lau, 2002).

Homeostasis involves various mechanisms. Some of these are dispositional and include processes of adaptation, selective-attention, and social comparison. Some of them are resources external to the person, such as money and close relationships, that can be used to shield the person from adversity. These various devices act in concert to maintain the average level of SWB at around 75 percentage of the measurement scale maximum in Western nations (Cummins, Eckersley, Pallant, Van Vugt and Misajon, 2003). That is, when SWB scores are standardized to a 0–100 scale (completely dissatisfied—completely satisfied) people in Australia, on average, feel 75 percent satisfied with their lives.

So, the totality of life quality must be measured in two dimensions. The objective and the subjective measures provide important and different views. Which view is most relevant to policy makers will depend, to some extent, on the population concerned. In the context of North America, authors such as Schalock (1997) consider it is how people feel about their life quality that is the ultimate test of a life worth living. And certainly in circumstances where basic material needs are met, as is most common within that society, authors generally agree that life quality can be most meaningfully assessed by subjective variables (*e.g.,* Cummins, 2000a; Headey, 1981; Spilker, 1990). However, in countries such as India, where it is more common for people to lack the physical resources that they need for normal life quality, measuring their objective circumstances is also crucial to understanding the relative areas of need. Moreover, when the objective circumstances of living are very tough, they defeat the capacity of the homeostatic system and SWB falls below its normal levels. When this occurs, people are at high risk of depression and their functioning is severely impaired. So, understanding the relationship between the objective circumstances of living, most particularly wealth and health, and SWB is crucial for its application within Health Psychology.

SUBJECTIVE WELL-BEING HOMEOSTASIS

The theory of Subjective Well-being Homeostasis proposes that, in a manner analogous to the homeostatic maintenance of body temperature, subjective well-being is actively controlled and maintained (see Cummins and Nistico, 2002, for an extended description). SWB homeostasis is attempting to maintain a normal positive sense of well-being that is a generalized and rather abstract view of the self. It is exemplified by a response to the classic question "How satisfied are you with your life as a whole?" Given the extraordinary generality of this question, the response that people give does not represent a cognitive evaluation of their life. Rather it reflects a deep and stable positive mood state that we call Core Affect (see later). This is a mood state that is dominated by a sense of contentment flavored with a touch of happiness and excitement. It is this general and abstract state of subjective well-being which the homeostatic system seeks to defend. As one consequence, the level of satisfaction people record to this question has the following characteristics:

1. It is normally very stable. While unusually good or bad events will cause it to change in the short term, over a period of time homeostasis will normally return SWB to its previous level (see Hanestad and Albrektsen, 1992; Headey and Wearing, 1989).
2. Each person has a level of Core Affect that is set genetically. This 'set-point' for SWB lies in the 'satisfied' sector of the dissatisfied-satisfied continuum. That is, on a scale where zero represents complete dissatisfaction with life and 100 represents complete satisfaction, people's set-point normally lies within the positive sector of the scale (see Cummins *et al.*, 2002).
3. At a population level within Western nations, the average set-point is 75. In other words, on average, people feel that their general satisfaction with life is about three-quarters of its maximum extent (Cummins, 1995, 1998).

While this generalized sense of well-being is held positive with remarkable tenacity, it is not immutable. A sufficiently adverse environment can defeat the homeostatic system and, when this occurs, the level of subjective well-being falls below its homeostatic range. For example, people who experience strong, chronic pain from arthritis or from the stress of caring for a severely disabled family member at home have low levels of subjective well-being (Cummins, 2001). However, for people who are maintaining a normally functioning homeostatic system, their levels of SWB will show little relationship to normal variations in their chronic circumstances of living.

So, how does homeostasis work to defend SWB against the unusually good and the unusually bad experiences of life? The answer we propose is that there are two levels of defense and we call these defensive systems 'buffers'. One set of buffers is external to the person and the other internal.

Homeostatic Buffers

Interaction with the environment constantly threatens to move well-being up or down in sympathy with momentary positive and negative experience. And to some extent this does occur. However, most people are adept at avoiding strong challenges through the maintenance of established life routines that make their daily experiences predictable and manageable. Under such ordinary life conditions, the level of the mood-state varies by perhaps 10 percentage points or so from one moment to the next, and this is the Set-Point Range. Homeostasis works hardest at the edges of this range to prevent more drastic mood changes which, of course, do occur from time to time. Strong and unexpected positive or negative experience will shift the sense of personal well-being to abnormally higher or lower values, usually for a brief period of time, until adaptation occurs. However, if the negative experience is sufficiently strong and sustained, homeostasis will lack the power to restore equilibrium and SWB will remain below its set-point range. Such homeostatic defeat is marked by a sustained loss of positive mood and a high risk of depression.

So the first line of defense for homeostasis is to avoid, or at least rapidly attenuate, negative environmental interactions. This is the role of the external buffers.

External Buffers

The two most important sources for the defence of our SWB are close relationships and money. Of these two, the most powerful buffer is a relationship with another human being that involves mutual sharing of intimacies and support (Cummins, Walter and Woerner, 2007). Almost universally, the research literature attests to the power of such relationships to moderate the influence of potential stressors on SWB (for reviews see Henderson, 1977; Sarason, Sarason and Pierce, 1990).

Money is also a very important external buffer, but there are misconceptions as to what money can and cannot do in relation to personal wellbeing. For example, it cannot shift the set-point to create a perpetually happier person. Set-points for SWB are proposed to be under genetic control (Cummins *et al.*, 2003), so in this sense money cannot buy happiness. No matter how rich someone is, their average level of SWB cannot be sustained higher than a level that lies towards the top of their set-point range. People adapt readily to luxurious living standards, so genetics trumps wealth after a certain level of income has been achieved. While this opinion flies in the face of those Positive Psychologists who believe that people can be made endlessly happier, it is supported by the findings of a recent report. Cummins *et al.* (2007) studied the cumulative data from the Australian Unity Well-being Index which comprises SWB data from about 30,000 Australians. The purpose of the analysis was to determine the demographic groups with the highest and the lowest wellbeing. It is reported that the maximum average subgroup score is 81.0 points. Thus, this seems to be the maximum SWB that can be maintained as a group average even for people who have close relationships and plenty of money.

The true power of wealth is to protect well-being through its capacity to be used as a highly flexible resource (Cummins, 2000b) that allows people to defend themselves against the negative potential inherent within their environment. Wealthy people pay others to perform tasks they do not wish to do themselves. Poor people, who lack such resources, must fend for themselves to a much greater extent. Poor people, therefore, have a level of SWB that is far more at the mercy of their environment.

Internal Buffers

When we fail to control our external environment and SWB is threatened, our internal buffers come into play. These comprise protective cognitive devices that are designed to minimize the impact of personal failure on our positive feelings about our self. There are many such devices, collectively called Secondary Control techniques (Rothbaum, Weisz and Snyder, 1982) and a detailed discussion of these systems in relation to SWB is provided in Cummins and Nistico (2002) and Cummins, *et al.* (2002).They have the role of protecting our SWB against the conscious reality of life. They do this by altering the way we see ourselves in relation to some challenging agent such that the negative potential in the challenge is deflected away from the core view of self. So the role of these buffers is mainly to minimize the impact of personal failure. The ways of thinking that can achieve this are highly varied. For example, one can find meaning in the event ('God is testing me'), fail to take responsibility for the failure ('it was not my fault') or regard the failure [dropping a vase] as unimportant ('I did not need that old vase anyway').

In summary, the combined external and internal buffers ensure that our well-being is robustly defended. There is, therefore, considerable stability in the SWB of populations and, as has been stated, the mean for Western societies like Australia are consistently at about 75 points on a 0 to 100 scale. But what comprises SWB? Until we can answer this, we do not know what homeostasis is really defending.

WHAT IS HOMEOSTASIS DEFENDING?

Most contemporary theorists regard the measurement of SWB, obtained through a considered verbal or written response, to involve both affective and cognitive processes. This was first recognized by Campbell *et al.* (1976) who suggested that this amalgam should be measured through questions of 'satisfaction'. This form of question has since become standard for SWB measurement. However, relatively little research has been directed to examining the relative contribution of affect and cognition. Certainly the two components are separable (Lucas, Diener and Suh, 1996) but whether, as claimed by Diener, Napa Scollon and Lucas (2004), SWB represents a dominantly cognitive evaluation, is moot. Indeed, to the contrary, more recent research (Davern, Cummins and Stokes, 2007) weighs the balance in favour of affect as the central element, this being characterized by a construct called 'Core Affect' (Russell, 2003).

According to Russell (2003), Core Affect is a neuro-physiological state that is experienced as a feeling. While this feeling can be consciously accessed, it is not tied to any specific object in the manner of an emotional response. Instead it is a mood-state, which refers to how the individual senses himself in an abstract but personal way. It can be conceptualized as a deep form of trait affect, analogous to felt body temperature in that it is always there, can be assessed when attention is drawn to it, extremes are most obvious, and it exists without words to describe it. In conformity with the circumplex model of affect, Core Affect comprises a blend of hedonic (pleasant-unpleasant) and arousal values (activation-deactivation).

As an extension of Russell's conception, we propose that Core Affect is not only the affective constituent of SWB but also the basic steady-state, set-point that homeostasis seeks to defend. Within this conception, Core Affect comprises the most basic experienced feeling, being hard-wired for each individual, comprising the tonic state of affect that provides the activation energy, or motivation, for behavior. We further propose that core affect perfuses all higher process, including personality (for a review of the neurobiology of personality, see Depue and Collins, 1999), memory and momentary experience. Consistent with this fundamental role, we propose that the process of evolution has naturally selected individuals who experience a level of Core Affect corresponding to 70–80 points pleasant or positive. This level, then, constitutes the optimum set-point range for SWB, corresponding to the most adaptive range of core affect described in Cummins' (2000a; 2003) theory of SWB homeostasis.

While Core affect perfuses all cognitive processes to some degree, the ones that are most strongly influenced are those rather abstract notions of the self (*e.g.,* I am a good person). These self-perceptions are held at strength of positivity that approximates core affect.

As measured by Davern *et al.* (2007), Core Affect can be most parsimoniously represented as the combined affects of happiness, contentment, and excitement. These represent the activated and deactivated pleasant quadrants of the affective circumplex (for a review of affect see Cropanzano, Weiss, Hale and Reb, 2003). We tested the relative strength of Core Affect, cognition, and all five factors of personality, as predictors of SWB. The cognitive component of SWB was measured using 7 items derived from Multiple Discrepancies Theory (Michalos, 1985). These items address the perceived gap between what the respondent currently has and general life aspirations, what age-matched others have, the best one has had in the past, expected to have 3 years ago and expects to have after 5 years, deserves and needs.

Consistent with previous research, all three components correlated significantly with SWB and with one another. However, when the variances were controlled by structural equation modelling, it was demonstrated that affect and MDT are the dominant components of SWB. Indeed, after accounting for both of these, personality made only a very small contribution to the explanation of SWB variance. The simplified model from this paper is reproduced in Figure 1. The personality factors are designated as: N—Neuroticism, E—Extraversion, O—Openness, A—Agreeableness, C—Conscientiousness.

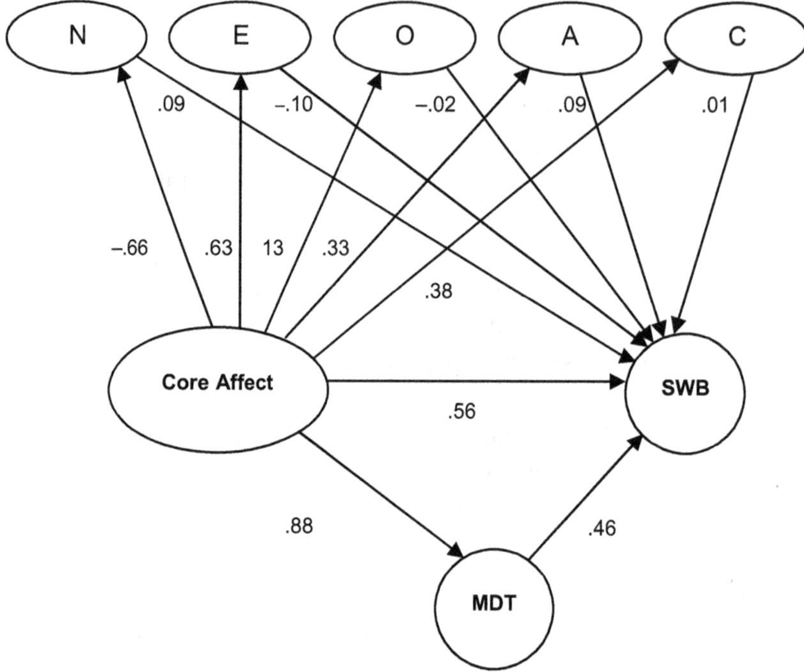

Figure 1: Simplified Affective-Cognitive Model of SWB (from Davern *et al.*, 2007)

It seems clear from this analysis that core affect is the central component of SWB and, we propose, is the driving force behind individual set point levels in SWB homeostasis. This finding has now been replicated using independent data (Blore and Stokes, unpublished).

DIAGNOSTIC RANGES FOR DEPRESSION

From all of the above, SWB can be characterized as a stable positive mood-state that normally operates within a narrow range of values for each individual. The level of this set-point-range is genetically determined and a homeostatic system acts to maintain SWB within this range. However, if the level of challenge to SWB becomes too great, homeostasis fails and SWB drops below the set-point range. We propose that this loss of positive mood is depression. The relationship between SWB and the Depression sub-scale of the Depression, Anxiety and Stress Scale (Lovibond and Lovibond, 1995) is shown in Figure 2.

The data for Figure 2 are taken from Davern (2004). The pattern of these results is consistent with the homeostatic model. The depression scores represent the level of challenge to homeostasis. The seven items that comprise this scale include symptoms of low energy, loss of purpose, low self-esteem, *etc.* Thus, as the level of challenge (depression score) increases from 0 to 8, the value of SWB moves down in a linear fashion to approximate the lower homeostatic threshold of 70 points. Then, over the depression rating of 9 to 12, homeostasis 'holds-the-line' and SWB remains unchanged. However, at a depression score of 13 or greater, homeostasis is overwhelmed, control of SWB passes from the homeostatic system to the challenging agent, and SWB drops markedly.

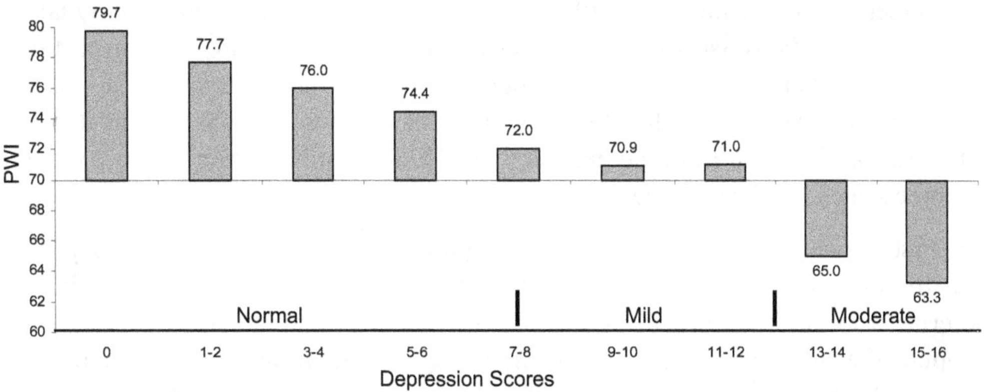

Figure 2: The Relationship between the PWI and the DASS Depression Scale

This pattern is obviously fairly clear-cut using sub-group mean scores and it can be seen that, if homeostatic defeat is taken as the definition for depression, then this conforms to a depression rating of moderate using the DASS. But the matching of PWI and depression scores for individuals is more complex. Since individuals have set-points within the positive range, it is not possible to be precise concerning the diagnostic meaning of an individual SWB score that lies above 50 points. A SWB value of 60 points can represent either a low set-point or a depressed high set-point.

Thus, in interpreting individual scores there are two forces to be considered. First there is the set-point, which lies somewhere in the positive range between 55 and 95 points. Second there is the chronic negative life experience that is challenging homeostatic control. So the combination of these forces allows for the following diagnostic approximations.

(a) If the individual score lies above 70 points the homeostatic system is likely to be functioning normally and the person is not depressed.
(b) If the individual score lies below 50 points the person is highly likely to be depressed. This applies to 4.4% of our general population samples in Australia.
(c) The diagnostic meaning of individual scores between 50 and 70 is uncertain. 70 points represents normal homeostatic control for most people (Cummins, 2003). As scores progressively move lower, the closer that they approximate 50 points, the higher the probability that they represent homeostatic defeat rather than a low set-point.

In summary, the following scheme is a guide to the interpretation of scores: 70 or above points = normal; 51–69 points = either a low set-point or strong homeostatic challenge, even defeat; 50 or less = homeostatic defeat and depression.

MEASURING SUBJECTIVE WELL-BEING

The Directory of Instruments available through the Australian Centre on Quality of Life (ACQOL, 2008) lists over 700 scales that purport to measure some aspect of life quality. Most claim to measure well-being in some form. So how can a researcher make a choice from such a daunting list? The answer is to know what it is that needs to be measured, and so from the perspective of SWB that has given in this paper there are three scales that I recommend.

The first is one of the oldest. It is the single question 'How satisfied are you with your life as a whole?' (Andrews and Withey, 1976). This question perfectly fulfills the criteria for an item measuring SWB to be both personal and abstract. No one can compute the answer to the question in terms of cognition. So it is answered in reference to the ongoing mood state, which normally approximates the set-point core affect (Davern *et al.*, 2007). The drawback to using this question, however, is that it is a single item. As such it is not as reliable as a multi-item scale, so two alternative scales have been devised.

The most widely used index of SWB is the Satisfaction with Life Scale (Diener, Emmons, Larsen and Griffin, 1985). This scale is designed to measure global life satisfaction through five items, each of which involves an overall judgment of life in general. The scores from these items are then summed as a measure of SWB. For a copy of the scale go to: http://s.psych.uiuc.edu/~ediener/hottopic/hottopic.html.

The importance of the SWLS is that it represents an expanded version of 'life as a whole'. The items are not designed to give individual insights into the structure of SWB. This differs from the second scale to be recommended. The Personal Well-being Index (International Well-being Group, 2006) has a quite different design as the 'first-level deconstruction' of life as a whole. It contains eight items, referred to as 'domains', where each item represents a broad, semi-abstract area of life. The theoretical basis for the PWI is that the domains together describe the experience of overall life satisfaction. Empirically they tend to explain about 50–60 percent of the variance in 'life as a whole'. The manual is available from (International Well-being Group, 2006).

The PWI is designed to be a 'work in progress', with the scale evolving as new data show ways for it to be successfully modified. The International Well-being Group oversights this evolution and the eighth domain of Spiritual/Religious satisfaction was added to the scale in 2006.

The disadvantage of the PWI over the SWLS is that, because the domains are slightly more specific in their focus, they are also slightly further-away from the mood state of core affect. The advantage of the PWI is that each of the domains carries its own information concerning a broad aspect of life. Because of this, the scale can be analyzed at either the level of individual domains or at the level of a single combined score. A further advantage of the PWI is that there are parallel versions for adults who have a cognitive or intellectual disability, school children and pre-school children (International Well-being Group, 2006).

SUMMARY

Subjective Well-being (SWB) can be defined as a normally positive state of mind that involves the whole life experience. This implies that it is normal for people to feel positive about themselves. The reason for this is the presence of a psychological/ neurological system that has the task of maintaining normal levels of well-being through the defense of core affect.

Because of this homeostatic system, there is generally a low correlation between medical health and SWB. There is also a non-linear relationship between SWB and levels of stress and anxiety. Therefore none of such variables can be used as proxy measures of SWB, which must be measured directly.

The importance of measuring SWB is that it can indicate when the level of challenge exceeds the threshold of the homeostatic system. This makes SWB measurement an important diagnostic tool, since lower than normal SWB indicates a felt loss of positive affect and a high probability of depression. Thus, while the measurement of subjective well-being is highly useful for health psychologists, the interpretation of such data requires an understanding of homeostasis.

REFERENCES

ACQOL (2008). *Australian Centre on Quality of Life—Directory of Instruments,* http://www.deakin.edu.au/research/acqol/instruments/index.htm

Andrews, F.M. and Withey, S.B. (1976). *Social Indicators of Well-Being: American's Perceptions of Life Quality*. New York: Plenum Press.

Campbell, A., Converse, P.E. and Rodgers, W.L. (1976). *The Quality of American Life: Perceptions, Evaluations, and Satisfactions*. Russell Sage Foundation: New York.

Cropanzano, R., Weiss, H.M., Hale, J.M.S. and Reb, J. (2003). "The structure of affect: Reconsidering the Relationship between Negative and Positive Affectivity." *Journal of Management, 29*(6), 831–858.

Cummins, R.A. (1995). "On the Trail of the Gold Standard for Life Satisfaction." *Social Indicators Research, 35*, 179–200.

Cummins, R.A. (1998). "The Second Approximation to an International Standard of Life Satisfaction. " *Social Indicators Research, 43*, 307–334.

Cummins, R.A. (2000a). "Objective and Subjective Quality of Life: An Interactive Model." *Social Indicators Research, 52*, 55–72.

Cummins, R.A. (2000b). "Personal Income and Subjective Well-Being: A Review." *Journal of Happiness Studies, 1*, 133–158.

Cummins, R.A. (2001). "The Subjective Well-Being of People Caring for a Severely Disabled Family Member at Home: A Review." *Journal of Intellectual and Developmental Disability, 26*, 83–100.

Cummins, R.A. (2003). "Normative Life Satisfaction: Measurement Issues and a Homeostatic Model." *Social Indicators Research, 64*, 225–256.

Cummins, R.A., Eckersley, R., Pallant, J., Van Vugt, J. and Misajon, R. (2003). "Developing a National Index of Subjective Well-Being: The Australian Unity Well-Being Index." *Social Indicators Research, 64*, 159–190.

Cummins, R.A., Gullone, E. and Lau, A.L.D. (2002). "A Model of Subjective Well-Being Homeostasis: The Role of Personality." In E. Gullone and R.A. Cummins (Eds.), *The Universality of Subjective Well-Being Indicators: Social Indicators Research Series* (pp. 7–46). Dordrecht: Kluwer.

Cummins, R.A. and Nistico, H. (2002). "Maintaining Life Satisfaction: The Role of Positive Cognitive Bias." *Journal of Happiness Studies, 3*, 37–69.

Cummins, R.A., Walter, J. and Woerner, J. (2007). *Australian Unity Well-Being Index: Report 16.1 - "The Well-Being of Australians—Groups with the Highest and Lowest Well-Being in Australia"*. Melbourne: Australian Centre on Quality of Life, School of Psychology, Deakin University.

Cummins, R.A., Woerner, J., Tomyn, A., Gibson, A. and Knapp, T. (2006). *Australian Unity Well-Being Index: Report 16.0 - "The Well-Being of Australians—Mortgage Payments and Home Ownership"*, http://www.deakin.edu.au/research/acqol/index_wellbeing/index.htm

Davern, M. (2004). *Subjective Well-being as an Affective Construct. Thesis.* Deakin University, Melbourne.

Davern, M., Cummins, R.A. and Stokes, M. (2007). "Subjective Well-Being as an Affective/ Cognitive Construct." *Journal of Happiness Studies*, 8, 429–449.

Depue, R.A. and Collins, P.F. (1999). "Neurobiology of the Structure of Personality: Dopamine Facilitation of Incentive Motivation and Extraversion." *Behavioral and Brain Sciences,* 22, 491–569.

Diener, E. (2006). "Guidelines for National Indicators of Subjective Well-Being and Ill-Being." *Journal of Happiness Studies, 7*, 397–404.

Diener, E., Emmons, R.A., Larsen, R.J. and Griffin, S. (1985). "The Satisfaction with Life Scale." *Journal of Personality Assessment, 49*, 71–75.

Diener, E.D., Napa Scollon, C.N. and Lucas, R.E. (2004). "The Evolving Concept of Subjective Well-Being: The Multifaceted Nature of Happiness." In P.T. Costa and I.C. Siegler (Eds.), *Recent Advances in Psychology and Aging*. Amsterdam: Elsevier Science BV.

Fordyce, M.W. (1983). "A Program to Increase Happiness: Further Studies." *Journal of Counseling Psychology,* 30, 483–498.

Hanestad, B.R. and Albrektsen, G. (1992). "The Stability of Quality of Life Experience in People with Type 1 Diabetes Over a Period of a Year." *Journal of Advanced Nursing,* 17, 777–784.

Headey, B. (1981). "The Quality of Life in Australia." *Social Indicators Research,* 9, 155–181.

Headey, B. and Wearing, A. (1989). "Personality, Life Events and Subjective Well-Being: Toward a Dynamic Equilibrium Model." *Journal of Personality and Social Psychology,* 57, 731–739.

Henderson, S. (1977). "The Social Network, Support and Neurosis. The Function of Attachment in Adult Life." *British Journal of Psychiatry,* 131, 185–191.

International Well-Being Group (2006). *Personal Well-Being Index,* http://www.deakin.edu.au/research/acqol/instruments/wellbeing_index.htm

Lau, A.L.D., Cummins, R.A. and McPherson, W. (2005). "An Investigation into the Cross-Cultural Equivalence of the Personal Well-Being Index." *Social Indicators Research,* 72, 403–430.

Lee, J.W., Jones, P.S., Mineyama, Y. and Zhang, X.E. (2002). "Cultural Differences in Responses to a Likert Scale." *Research in Nursing and Health,* 25, 295–306.

Lovibond, S.H. and Lovibond, P.F. (1995). *Manual for the Depression Anxiety Stress Scales.* Sydney: Psychology Foundation.

Lucas, R.E., Diener, E. and Suh, E. (1996). "Discriminant Validity of Well-Being Measures." *Journal of Personality and Social Psychology,* 71, 616–628.

Michalos, A.C. (1985). "Multiple Discrepancies Theory (MDT)." *Social Indicators Research,* 16, 347–413.

Rothbaum, F., Weisz, J.R. and Snyder, S.S. (1982). "Changing the World and Changing the Self: A Two-Process Model of Perceived Control." *Journal of Personality and Social Psychology,* 42, 5–37.

Russell, J.A. (2003). "Core Affect and the Psychological Construction of Emotion." *Psychological Review,* 110(1), 145–172.

Sarason, B.R., Sarason, I.G. and Pierce, G.R. (1990). *Social Support: An Interactional View.* New York: John Wiley and Sons.

Schalock, R.L. (1997). "The Conceptualization and Measurement of Quality of Life: Current Status and Future Considerations." *Journal of Developmental Disabilities,* 5, 1–21.

Spilker, B. (1990). "Introduction. In B. Spilker (Ed.)", *Quality of Life Assessments in Clinical Trials* (pp. 3–9). New York: Raven Press.

Stening, B.W. and Everett, J.E. (1984). "Response Styles in a Cross-Cultural Managerial Study." *Journal of Social Psychology,* 122, 151–156.

United Nations (2006). *Table 15: Inequality in Income or Expenditure (PDF). Human Development Report 2006, 335. United Nations Development Programme,* http://hdr.undp.org/hdr2006/pdfs/report/HDR06-complete.pdf#page=335.

World Bank (1997). *World Values Surveys; GNP/Capita Purchasing Power Estimates from World Bank, World Development Report, 1997,* http://margaux.grandvinum.se/SebTest/wvs/articles/folder_published/article_base_56.

Consciousness, Health and Well-Being

S.K. Kiran Kumar*

ABSTRACT

In today's world health and well-being, *ārogya* and *swāsthya,* have become a source of primary concern and also expenditure. We see mushrooming of many clinics, nursing homes, hospitals, *etc.*, all in the name of health care facilities. We have many companies offering health insurance. Even ancient Yoga is pressed into service for promoting health and well-being. But have these developments really enhanced the *ārogya* and *swāsthya* of masses? This is a debatable point because more and more research shows, as one author had put it, "most modern maladies are of the mind" and people across the world are often living mindlessly in pursuit of needs and desires which have created not only personal health problems, it also has brought about ecological imbalance threatening the well-being of the planet itself. In this juncture if we need to promote health and well-being it is not the individual level interventions alone matters, but it is the macro level interventions at national and international level, through raising of consciousness of people at large that can do any good. The paper will focus on examining the relation between consciousness, health and well-being at individual and collective level and strategies of intervention.

INTRODUCTION

In today's world health and well-being, *ārogya* and *swāsthya,* have become a source of primary concern and also expenditure. There is an old saying in Sanskrit, *vaidyarāja namahsthubhyam yamarāja sahodaraha yamastu hartih prānan vaidyah prānan dhanāni ca !* - "Oh doctor, respects to you, the brother of the Lord of death (Yamarāja); while the Lord of death snatches only life, the doctor, both life and money!" This saying seems to be very appropriate in modern day context all over the world. It has become so unbearable for a person of average means to meet the expenditure; people all over the world have started exploring how to get cheap health care. It is instructive to learn something about how this works out from a news paper article published in the United States titled "Man turns to India for cheap care for parents" by Laurie Goering in the *Chicago Tribune* of 8 August 2007. Goering observes that "with the cost of nursing homes, home nurses and medications painfully high in the United States, the elderly and their caregivers have long looked abroad for better solutions. Many families now drive regularly to Mexico or Canada to buy cheaper drugs, or hire recent immigrants—some of them undocumented—to help them look after frail parents. A growing number of aging couples have bought retirement homes in

*Department of Psychology, University of Mysore, Karnataka, India.
E-mail: kiku@sancharnet.in

Mexico, where help is cheap and Medicare-funded health care just a quick drive across the border".

But one enterprising US citizen hit upon the idea of "outsourcing his parents to India" for cheap health care. The story goes that one Mr. Steve Herzfeld drove home from North Carolina to Florida to take care of his mother who broke her hip in 2004. After three years of caring both aged parents, father suffering from Alzheimer's disease and mother from advanced Parkinson's disease, like any other care giver he experienced the stress associated and wanted to find some health care facility for them. He found that the cheapest one would cost $6,600-a-month, which would quickly bankrupt his parents. His father did not want to accept the financial help offered by his uncle, nor was he. He also felt that nursing homes are, "a hell of a way to end your life," and said "I wouldn't want someone to do that to me." So when a businessman friend suggested that Herzfeld consider a move to India he thought it is the best idea and moved along with his parents. Herzfeld, had previously spent five years in India, and "admired India's long time, though recently slipping, respect for the elderly". Now, as "care manager rather than the actual worker" has time for things such as strolls in the botanical gardens with his father. "He said, "I wouldn't say it's a solution for everybody, but I consider it the best solution to our problem,". To cut the story short, now every time Herzfeld looks at the bills—less than $2,000 a month for food, rent, utilities, medications, phones and 24-hour staffing—Herzfeld thinks he's done the right thing for his parents and himself. The family keeps in touch with relatives and friends back home *via* e-mail and Internet videophone. The question that comes to my mind is, is health care cheap for Indians as well?

There is another aspect in Herzfeld story to which we can now turn our attention. As Herzfeld found India has a tradition for respecting the elderly, which is slipping. Not only that his aged parents got that respect in India, their health care included the following aspects as well: "his mother gets daily massages, physical therapy and 24-hour help getting to the bathroom; his father has a full-time personal assistant and *a cook who has won him over to a vegetarian diet healthy enough that he no longer needs his cholesterol medication*; his mother has a nurse, on duty all day, *braids flowers into the old woman's gray hair, massages her legs and arms, holds her hand while she watches television and feeds her meals*". These are few illustrations, to show health care is not just paying some $. It is something more than that. It is a contrast to the individualistic life style of the West. The following incidence illustrates it well. "Just hours after arriving in India, Herzfeld's jet-lagged father tried to chase his new Indian personal aide out of the bathroom—the youth had been instructed to help him with the toilet—and fell, cracking his head on the bathtub. The family spent the first night in the hospital as Ernest was stitched up".

Herzfeld's story illustrates two important points about health care: one is the economics of it; and the other psycho-social. We can first look into the economics of health care. The expenditure incurred by a person for health care include (a) diagnostic expenditure—amount spent on blood and urine examination, X-ray, EEG, ECG, PET Scan, MRI, and so on; (b) expenditure for treatment—cost of medicines, injections, and surgery; (c) expenditure related to service provided by health professionals—doctors, nurses, physiotherapists, and so on; (d) and expenditure related to creation and maintenance of infrastructure—clinics, nursing homes, administrative staff, record maintenance, and so on. Since now a days it is not necessarily the doctor who establishes the health care facility, but some persons with capital health care has become an industry involving profit motivation. Thus, we see mushrooming of many clinics, nursing homes, hospitals, *etc*., all in the name of health care facilities. We have many companies offering health insurance. Even ancient Yoga is pressed into service for promoting health and well-being. But have these developments really enhanced the *ārogya* and *swāsthya* of masses? This is a debatable point because more and more research shows, as one author had put it, "most modern maladies are of the mind" and people across the world are often living mindlessly in pursuit of needs and desires which has created not only personal health problems, it also has brought about ecological imbalance threatening the well-being of the planet itself. In this juncture if we need to promote health and well-being it is not the individual level interventions alone matters, but it is the macro level interventions at national and international level, through raising of consciousness of people at large that can do any good.

Modern health care industry is rooted in what is known as biomedical model. Biomedical model asks the following questions—What causes illness? What is responsible for illness? How should illness be treated? Who is responsible for treatment? The answers are: (1) Chemical imbalances, bacteria, viruses, and general pre-disposition causes illness; (2) external forces, not individuals who are responsible for illness; (3) Vaccination, surgery, chemo-therapy, radiotherapy, *etc*., which change the physical state of the body is the mode of treatment; (4) It is the medical profession who is responsible for the treatment. These questions and related answers govern the health care system and the related expenditure.

Biomedical model is founded on a philosophy where the questions—what is the relationship between health and illness? What is the relationship between the mind and the body? What is the role of psychology in health and illness?—are answered in the following way: (a) health and illness are qualitatively different, either/or, not a continuum; (b) body and mind function independently; (c) and illness may have psychological consequences, but not psychological causes. In view of the above paradigm many health care endeavors may be best described as illness care, because psychology has no role in it. This brings us to the psycho-social aspect of health care.

A contemporary model that addresses this is well known as bio-psycho-social model and health psychology has emerged within this model. "Health psychology sets out to provide an integrated model of the individual by establishing a holistic approach to health. Therefore, it challenges the traditional medical model of the mind-body split and provides theories and research to support the notion of a mind and body that are one", (Ogden, 2000). Within bio-psycho-social model researchers have tried to understand the meaning of health and illness using a phenomenological approach, by asking people what they mean by that. Here is one set of findings reported by Lau (1995) (Box 1 and 2).

Box 1

What does it mean to be Healthy?

- *Physiological/physical, e.g.,* good condition, have energy
- *Psychological, e.g.,* happy, energetic, feel good psychologically
- *Behavioral, e.g.,* eat, sleep properly
- *Future consequences, e.g.,* live longer
- *The absence of, e.g.,* not sick, no disease, no symptoms.

Box 2

What does it mean to be Ill?

- Not feeling normal, *e.g.,* "I don't feel right"
- Specific symptoms, *e.g.,* physiological/psychological
- Specific illness, *e.g.,* cancer, cold, depression
- Consequence of illness, *e.g.,* "I can't do what I usually do"
- Time line, *e.g.,* how long the symptoms lost
- The absence of health, *e.g.,* not being healthy

In addition to understanding health and illness, researchers have also tried to describe what health behavior is. Kasl and Cobb (1966) distinguish between health behavior, illness behavior and sick role behavior. Health behavior was a behavior aimed to prevent disease (*e.g.,* eating a healthy diet). Illness behavior was a behavior aimed to seek remedy (*e.g.,* going to the doctor). Sick role behavior was any activity aimed to get well (*e.g.,* taking prescribed medication, resting).

Matarazzo (1984) distinguishes between health impairing habits and health protective behaviors. Health impairing habits, which he called behavior pathogens (*e.g.,* smoking, eating a high fat diet) and Health protective behaviors, which he called as "behavioral immunogens" (*e.g.,* attending a health check).

Health psychology describes variables such as "beliefs (risk perceptions, outcome expectancies, costs and benefits, intentions, implementation intentions)," "emotions (fear, depression, anxiety)", and "behaviors (smoking, drinking, eating, screening) as separate and discrete." (Ogden, 2000, p. 336). According to Ogden the approach of bio-psycho-social model and of health psychology is like "Dividing up the soup". As Ogden states, first it identifies variables and "It then develops models and theories to examine how these variables inter-relate. For example, it asks, "What beliefs predict smoking?", "What emotions relate to screening? Therefore, it separates out "the soup" into discrete entities and then tries to put them back together'. (p. 336).

The current approaches within bio-psycho-social model to health care can be represented with the following diagram, which is still very much grounded in a mechanistic worldview. The biological, psychological, and social factors are seen as three interrelated wheels and the treatment is to fix them (see Figure 1).

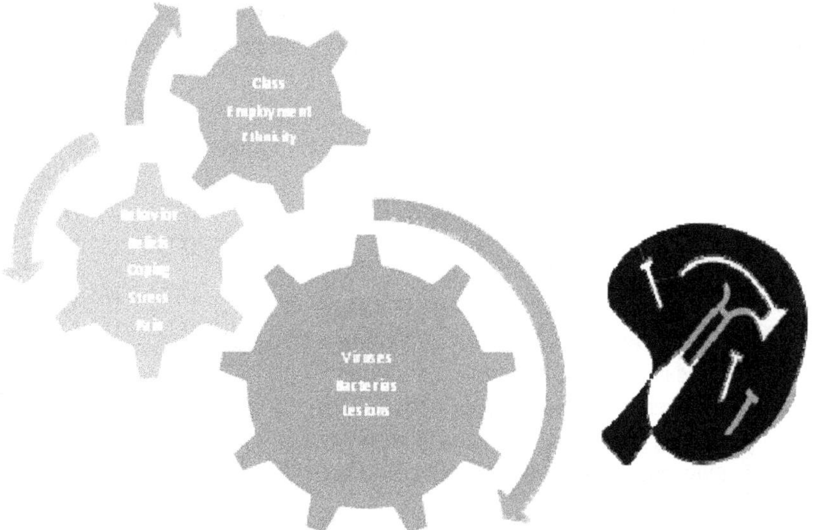

Figure 1: A Mechanical View of Bio-psycho-social Model

The current bio-psycho-social model raises some issues. Ogden has formulated these issues as follows (Box 3).

Box 3

- "However, does this approach really represent an integrated individual?"
- "Although all these perspectives and the research that has been carried out in their support indicate that the mind and the body interact, they are still defined as separate."
- "The mind reflects the individuals' psychological states (*i.e.,* their beliefs, cognitions, perceptions), which influence but are separate to their bodies (*i.e.,* the illness, the body, the body's systems)." (2000, p. 336)

Further Ogden observes that *"Psychology" is the culprit* for the present state of affairs because:

Box 4

- "Perhaps these different beliefs, emotions, and behaviors were not separate until psychology came along."
- "Is there really a difference between all the different beliefs? Is the thought "I am depressed" a cognition or an emotion? When I am sitting quietly thinking, am I behaving?"
- "HP assumes differences and then looks for association. However, perhaps without the original separation there would be nothing to separate." (p. 336)

In view of the limitations of bio-psycho-social model many alternative approaches to health care all carrying the nomenclature "holistic approach" have emerged in the past few decades. Many different holistic approaches have been discussed in literature and I have provided a schematic representation of them.

ALTERNATIVE APPROACHES—HOLISTIC MODELS

1. Family Systems

Family systems approach view the sociological, psychological, and biological aspects as subsystems interacting, with social factors influencing psychological characteristics, which in turn affect biology result in health or illness (Figure 2).

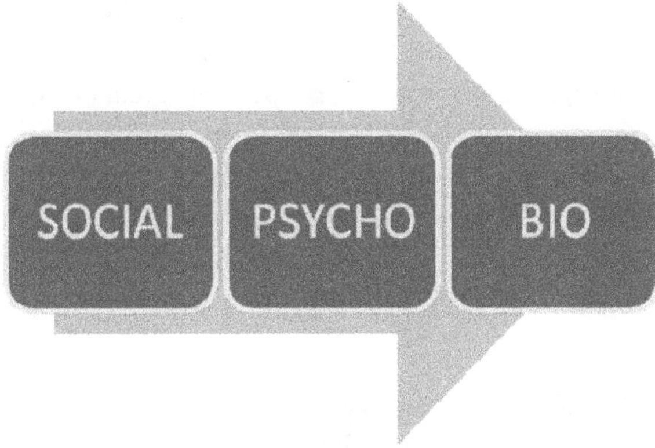

Figure 2: A Linear View of the Family Systems Holistic Approach

2. Four Factors

Another holistic model that is a little more comprehensive is the one which includes ecological dimension in addition to the other three. The emphasis here is not only to take into account one's social environment, but even the conditions of our physical environment that may affect our health and illness.

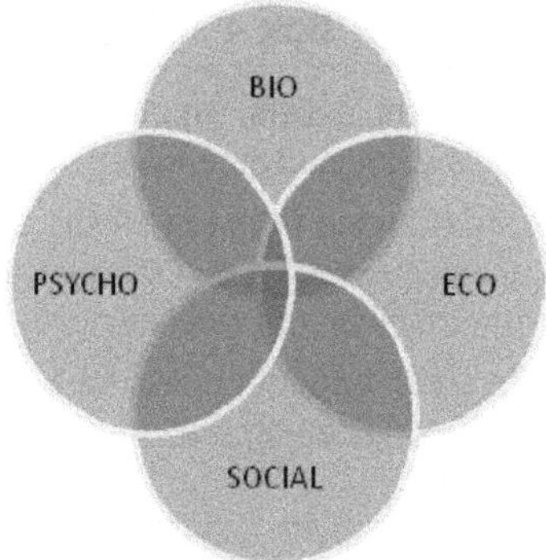

Figue 3: Holistic Model with Four Factors

3. Five Factors

While the other models include what is tangible, this model includes an intangible dimension called spirituality. Spirituality expresses in human behavior in three distinct ways: as religious faith with an intrinsic motivation (intrinsic religiosity); as expanded awareness that include paranormal phenomena; and as virtues such as compassion, altruism, forgiveness, love, and so on. In recent years, there have been many researches which take into account the religious behavior of people in determining recovery from illness on the one hand, and in maintaining health. Different types of healing procedures that are rooted in expanded awareness include prayer for healing, pranic healing, Reiki, distance healing, and so on. The third aspect of spirituality related to virtuous behavior is being used in psychotherapeutic practices informed by humanistic, transpersonal, and more recently positive psychological frameworks. The above models of holistic approach have been by and large guided by theories developed in Western tradition. Two other holistic approaches, which are rooted in Indian indigenous concepts, may also be considered here.

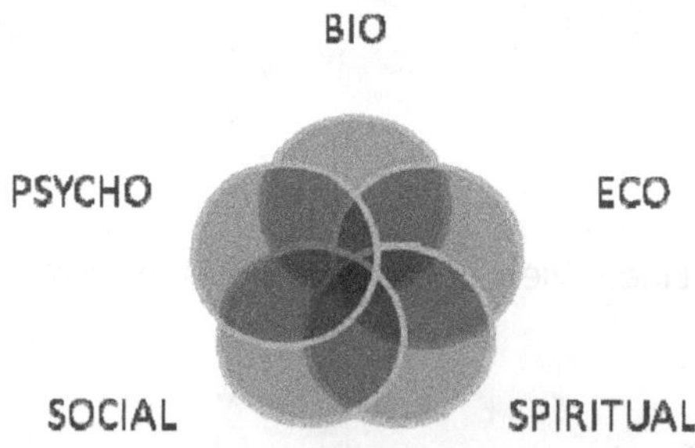

Figure 4: Holistic Model with Five Factors

4. Panchakosha

It is in the Taittiriya Upanishad, that we come across a detailed description of the dimensions of human personality using the metaphor of *kosha,* which means sheath. They are: *annamaya kosha, prānamaya kosha, manomaya kosha, vijñānamaya kosha,* and *ānandamaya kosha*. The physical (anna), vital (prāna), mental (mano), intuitive (vijñāna) and pure awareness (ānanda) are represented as concentric dimensions, which is again a metaphor. Each person has the locus of identity primarily rooted in one of the dimensions and all behavior centers around that. Most human beings identify primarily with the first three sheaths and the waking, dream and sleep states are limited by the activity of these three. Illness, health and well-being are related to the activities of these three koshas. Biomedical, bio-psycho-social and holistic approaches—models 1 and 2—may be conveniently grouped together as addressing these three koshas. It is the holistic model 3 that take into account the fourth kosha, *viz.*, intuitive dimension, which is the first stage of spiritual development.

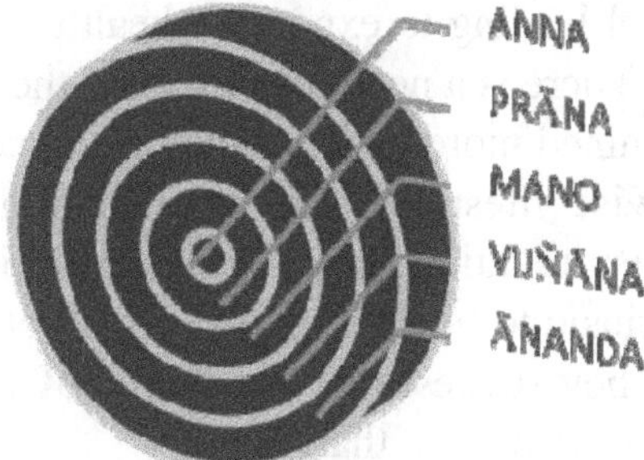

Figure 5: Holistic Model of Panchakosha

5. Expanded Consciousness

Beyond vijñānamaya kosha is ānandamaya kosha. In English, it may be roughly translated as pure consciousness. In Indian tradition its nature is described as *sat-chit-ānanda* in Vedic tradition. To experience that is to have an expanded range of awareness, and also being not affected by the phenomena associated with other koshas. To be in that state is what is called an enlightened state, liberated state, an integrated state and so on.

It is the state of ultimate well-being, which is qualitatively different from what is ordinarily experienced. It is a state of well-being, despite disease, ill health, poverty, or any other condition normally associated with suffering in an ordinary human being. It is regarded as a state of inner peace, and tranquility. In the diagram below you see that it is represented as a homogenous field and Buddha in the centre represent that state of ultimate well-being.

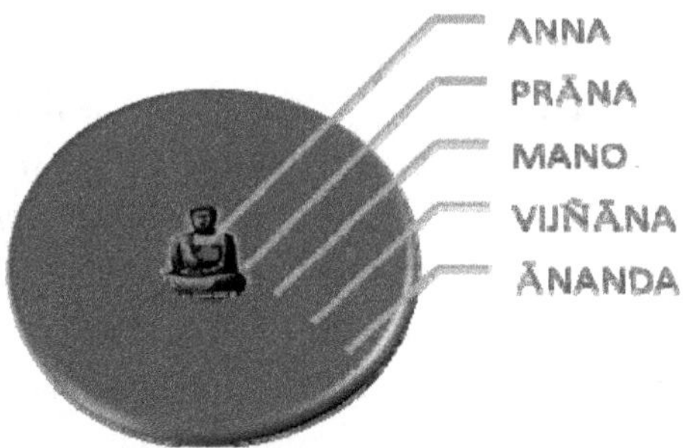

Figure 6: Holistic Model of Panchakosha—An Integrated State

CONCLUSION

Contemporarily the models of understanding and intervening with illness and health have been gradually incorporating the physical, psychological, social, ecological, and spiritual dimensions. But a majority of the approaches have still remained operating within the biomedical model leading to expensive health care for an average citizen, irrespective of the country. There is a need to appreciate the fact that most illnesses of contemporary era are determined more by psychological factors and also by ecological conditions created by unwise lifestyles. The appreciation of the role of spiritual aspects is not adequate. Indian tradition goes a step forward in asserting that ultimately a state of well-being is intrinsic to human nature and is not contingent on any of the factors mentioned above. They suggest that the source of well-being is within every individual and one only need to tap into that.

REFERENCES

Kasl, S.V. and Cobb, S. (1966). "Health Behavior, Illness Behavior, and Sick Role Behavior." *Archives of Environmental Health*, 12, 531–41.

Lau, R.R. (1995). "Cognitive Representations of Health and Illness." In D. Gochman (Ed.), *Handbook of Health Behavior Research,* Vol. 1. New York: Plenum Press.

Matarazzo, J.D. (1984). "Behavioral Health: A 1990 Challenge for the Health Sciences Profession." In J.D. Matarazzo, N.E. Miller, S.M. Weiss, J.A. Herd and S.M. Weiss (Eds.)., *Behavioral Health: A Handbook of Health Enhancement and Disease Prevention.* New York: John Wiley, 3–40.

Ogden, Jane (2000). *Health Psychology—A Text Book*, Buckingham: Open University Press, 336.

Taittiriya Upanishad, Brahmananda Valli.

Time Management of Married Women with Better Well-Being

Rupali Das[1], Monica Sengar[2] and Ira Das*[3]

ABSTRACT

An Expost-facto research was done to study the time management of non-working married women between the age range of 25–40 years. The sample of 115 women consisted of 80 women from Agra, India and 35 women from Minnesota USA. PGI Psychological Well-being scale by Moudgil, Verma, Kaur and Pal and Time Management Scale (prepared by the investigator herself) were administered on the women in the sample. The sample was dichotomized into two groups on the basis of median of well being scores. No significant difference was found between women with high well being and those with low well being as far as the time spent on Family Centered activities and Personal Routine activities are concerned. However among women living in India, those with high well being spent significantly more time on entertainment activities than those with low well being. On the other hand, women in India with low well being spent significantly greater time on spiritual activities as compared to their high well being counter parts. This shows that women with better well being tend more towards enjoying worldly pleasures and do not care for spiritual activities. For women living in USA, no significant difference was found in the time spent on entertainment activities whether belonging to high well being or low well being group, both spending equal time on entertainment. Both these high and low well being groups of women living in USA also spent equally little time on spiritual activities. In case of all the women in the sample maximum time is spent on personal routine activities (45%), 2nd highest on family centered (32.5%), 3rd highest entertainment activities (17.5%) and least on spiritual activities (5%).

INTRODUCTION

Subjective well-being is the ultimate goal that all married women are striving to achieve. Sellers, Sherill, Ward and David, 2006; Berkel, 2005; Bergman and Daukantaite, 2006; Noor and Naraini, 2006. As a result of varied inherited potentialities and varying environmental facilities women achieve different levels of educational, social and economic status in society. Although nature has gifted varying levels of abilities and opportunities to different women, the time gifted to each individual woman for a single day is the same *i.e.,* 24 hours a day. Each woman tries to spend these limited 24 hours in such a way so as to have maximum satisfaction from life. It depends upon their needs and values, how they spend their valuable yet limited time each day.

---

* Corresponding author.

[1] 7320, Gallager Dr., Apt. 219, Minneapolis, MN, USA.

[2, 3] Department of Psychology, Faculty of Social Sciences, Dayalbagh Educational Institute, (Deemed University) Dayalbagh, Agra, India.

Apart from the routine activities, there are certain activities for which some particular type of women would definitely spare some time according to their needs and values. The investigators therefore classified the total time of 24 hours a day into four categories, in developing a time management scale. These are: (1) Time spent on Routine Personal activities; (2) Time spent on family oriented activities; (3) Time spent on entertainment activities; (4) Time spent on spiritual activities. Today young adult educated married woman has multiple duties, as she has to play the role of a wife, a mother, a counselor and a responsible member of her own family, as well as her husband's family and social group. She has to divide her time in such a manner, that she can adjust with others and still remain physically, mentally and emotionally balanced. Then only she can have the feeling of subjective well-being. The investigators were therefore curious to know how the women with high subjective well-being manage to spend their time daily. It was hypothesized that women with better subjective well-being would differ in their time management from those women who have low subjective well-being *i.e.,* Time management is defined as proper allocation of time for different tasks, prioritizing so as to have most effective use of time.

MEASURES

Part–A

Time Management Scale for Married Women prepared by the investigator herself. It has four sections related to four types of activities *i.e.,* (1) Personal routine activities, (2) Family oriented activities, (3) Spiritual activities and (4) Entertainment activities. Out of the total time of 24 hours a day, a woman respondent had to give information about the time spent by her on these four categories of activities daily. It was assumed that higher the time spent on a particular activity, higher is the priority level given to that activity in life.

Scoring of Time Management Scale: The investigator calculated the midpoint of the slot at which the respondent had made a (✓) mark *e.g.,* if she had tick (✓) marked the option 30 min to 1 hour, she was given 45 minutes, which is the most representative time of that interval. In this way, the investigator found the middle time for all the responses and added these time amounts to get the total time spent on each of the four categories of activities by each respondent.

Part–B

Well-being Scale: Subjective well-being of women in the sample was measured by PGI Well-being Scale by Moudgil, Verma, Kaur and Pal which is in Hindi. It has 20 items. The items were translated into English and its Hindi-English version reliability was established.

Reliability: The inter rater reliability was found to be .86, Hindi-English Reliability was 1.0 and test retest reliability is .86 for the test.

Validity: Criterion related validity coefficient of well-being scale against criterion of neuroticism was found to be $r = -.75$ which is highly significant. This indicates that as the neuroticism decreases feeling of well-being increases.

All the respondents were asked a question, what they would like to become if they had to take birth again, to which majority of respondents with high well-being replied that they would like to be what they are today, or 'my own self'. This indicates high validity of the scale.

SAMPLE

The sample consisted of 80 Indian women residing in Agra, India and 35 Indian women residing in Minnesota USA. All women in the sample were married non-working and within the age range of 25 years to 40 years. All of them were of middle socio-economic status and were atleast graduate.

DATA ANALYSIS AND RESULTS

On the basis of the median of their well-being scores women in the sample were dichotomized into two groups: (1) Better well-being (with scores higher than the median), and (2) Low well-being group (with scores lower than the median). Time spent by these groups was then compared, on all the four categories of activities (as measured by Time Management Scale).

RESULTS

Table 1 indicates the time spent on family oriented activities by women of Agra group with Better well-being and Lower well-being. Though the Mean time spent by Women with better well-being is less *i.e.,* 377.55 minutes in comparison to 383 minutes spent by average women with low well-being, the differences is not significant even at .05 level (t = .198, df = 78). This indicates that time spent on family oriented activities is not related to well-being of women. Both the groups of women spent almost equal time (about 6 hours) on activities related to household works and for the benefit of the family.

Table 5 also indicates the time spent on family oriented activities by women of Minnesota group with better well-being and lower well-being. Women residing in USA also do not show any significant difference in time spent on family oriented activity by better well-being and lower well-being groups, the means being 323.74 and 316.84 minutes respectively. As compared to Agra group, Minnesota group of women spend significantly less time on family oriented activities probably due to the use of modern technological devices.

Table 2 and Table 6 show the mean time spent by women with better well-being and lower well-being in case of women residing in Agra and those residing in USA, respectively. The difference between the means are not significant in case of both the samples of women indicating that women of all groups spend at least sometime on routine personal activities such as sleeping, eating personal hygiene *etc.* so the value of t is not significant even at .05 level.

Table 3 and Table 7 indicate the significance of difference in time spent on entertainment activities by women with better well-being and those with lower well-being. Table 3 indicates that the difference is highly significant ($t = 3.68$ $p < .01$) in case of women residing in Agra, but Table 7 indicates that the difference is not significant ($t = .73$, $p > .05$) in case of women residing in Minnesota. These results indicate that in India only women with better well-being spend more time on entertainment activities, but in case of women residing in USA, all the women (with better well-being or low well-being) spend their time on entertainment activities. This shows that Indian women in USA spend more of their time on entertainments irrespective of their feelings of well-being.

Table 4 and Table 8 indicate the significance of difference in time spent on spiritual activities by women with better well-being and those with lower well-being. As is clear from Table 4 Indian women living in Agra India and having better well-being spend significantly less time on spiritual activities ($t = 2.64$, $p < .01$) in comparison to their counterparts with low subjective well-being. Table 8, on the other hand informs that women residing in USA spend less time on spiritual activities by women with high well-being.

Table 1: Significance of Difference between Mean Time Spent on Family Oriented Activities, by Agra Group

Groups	*Mean*	*N*	*df*	*Variance*	*t*	*Significance Level*
Better well-being	377.55	40	78	12442.61	.198	p > .05
Low well-being	382	40		7838		

Table 2: Significance of Difference between Mean Time (in minutes) Spent on Personal Routine Activities, by Agra Group

Groups	*Mean*	*N*	*df*	*Variance*	*t*	*Significance Level*
Better well-being	533.5	40	78	7752.82	1.50	p > .05
Low well-being	569	40		14264.55		

Table 3: Significance of Difference between Mean Time (in minutes) Spent on Entertainment Activities, by Agra Group

Groups	*Mean*	*N*	*df*	*Variance*	*t*	*Significance Level*
Better well-being	247.65	40	78	6471	3.677	$p < .01$
Low well-being	173	40		9565		

Table 4: Significance of Difference between Mean Time Spent on Spiritual Activities, by Agra Group

Groups	*Mean*	*N*	*df*	*Variance*	*t*	*Significance Level*
Better well-being	31.0	40	78	526.06	2.64	$p < .01$
Low well-being	43.2	40		326		

Table 5: Significance of Difference between Mean Time Spent on Family Oriented Activities, by Minnesota Group

Groups	*N*	*df*	*Mean*	*SD*	SE_D	*t*	*Significance Level*
Better well-being	15	33	323.74	71.98	27.1	.254	$p > .05$
Low well-being	20		316.84	88.21			

Table 6: Significance of Difference between Mean Time Spent on Personal Routine Activities, by Minnesota Group

Groups	*N*	*df*	*Mean*	*SD*	SE_D	*t*	*Significance Level*
Better well-being	15	33	567.53	81.47	27	.33	$p > .05$
Low well-being	20		558.60	75.77			

Table 7: Significance of Difference between Mean Time Spent on Family Oriented Activities, by Minnesota Group

Groups	*N*	*df*	*Mean*	*SD*	SE_D	*t*	*Significance Level*
Better well-being	15	33	320.47	104.52	37.48	.73	$p > .05$
Low well-being	20		293.15	116.32			

Table 8: Significance of Difference between Mean Time Spent on Spiritual Activities, by Minnesota Group

Groups	*N*	*df*	*Mean*	*SD*	SE_D	*t*	*Significance Level*
Better well-being	15	33	33.93	28	8.50	.69	$p > .05$
Low well-being	20		28	20			

The investigators therefore conclude that women with better well-being tend to spend more of their time on entertainment activities whether residing in India or USA. Women with low well-being, on the other hand, spend more of their time on spiritual activities and less time on entertainment as compared to women with better well-being, if they are living in India. However, women with low well-being, residing in USA, still spend almost equal time on entertainment and spiritual activities when compared to their better well-being counterparts. The investigators therefore conclude that women living in India tend more towards spirituality if they are not feeling well and are unhappy, but women living in USA do not tend towards spirituality if they are not feeling well. For those living in USA, well-being is not related to spiritual activities. They are involved in entertainments irrespective of their well-being.

Table 9 indicates the coefficient of correlation between well-being scores and time spent on different activities by women living in USA which are mostly low and not significant. Among the family oriented activities (category f), item 1 and 4 have negative correlation indicating that more is the time spent on cleaning the house and washing utensils, lower is the subjective well-being in women. Among Personal Routine activities (category p) item has negative correlation indicating that increase in time spent on relaxation and rest (not sleep) decreases well-being of women. Item 19 has high positive correlation (r = .345) indicating that time spent on health care, makeup and visiting beauty parlour is positively correlated to well-being of women residing in USA. Among entertainment activities (category e) watching TV serials (item 10) has negative correlation with well-being, but time spent on hobbies, window-shopping and attending parties have positive (though low) correlation with well-being. Among spiritual activities (category s), time spent on Meditation (item 20) alone has positive correlation with well-being. Time spent on all other items, such as prayer, religious activities, reading holy books and charitable activities have almost zero correlation with well-being scores.

Table 9: Coefficient of Correlation of Well-being with Time Spent on Different Activities

Item No.	*Category*	*r*	*Item No.*	*Category*	*r*	*Item No.*	*Category*	*r*
1.	f	.26	10.	e	–.336	19.	p	.345
2.	f	.016	11.	e	.166	20.	s	.269
3.	f	.075	12.	e	.279	21.	e	.265
4.	f	–.24	13.	e	–.046	22.	s	.073
5.	f	.008	14.	p	.01	23.	s	.076
6.	p	–.033	15.	e	.224	24.	p	–.283
7.	p	.047	16.	e	.17	25.	p	.046
8.	p	–.13	17.	f	.178			
9.	s	–.04	18.	s	–.055			

In case of all the women in the sample maximum time is spent on personal routine activities (45%), 2nd highest on family centered (32.5%), 3rd highest entertainment activities (17.5%) and least on spiritual activities (5%).

REFERENCES

Bergman R. and Daukantaite (2006). "The Importance of Social Circumstances for Swedish Women's Subjective Well-Being." *International Journal of Social Welfare. 15(11), 27–36, Psychological Abstract,* 93(8), 2006.

Berkel, L.V. (2005). "Relation Variable and Life Satisfaction in African American and Asian American College Women." *Journal of College Counselling, Psychological Abstract,* 92(9), 2005.

Kiran Kumar, S.K. (2006). "Happiness and Well-Being in Indian Tradition." *Psychological Studies,* 51, 105.112.

Latha and Yuvraj, T. (2007). "Spirituality: An Exploration of Factor Structure." *Psychological Studies,* 53(3), 223–227, 2007.

Mudgil, Verma, Kaur and Pal (1986). "PGI Well-Being Scale." PGI, Chandigarh.

Noor and Naraini (2006). "Malaysian Women's State of Well-Being: Empirical Validation of a Conceptual Model." *Journal of Social Psychology 146(1) 95–115, Psychological Abstract,* 93(5), 2006.

Sellers, S. and Ward, D. (2006). "Dimensions of Depression: A Qualitative Study of Well-Being among Black African Immigrant Women." *Psychological Abstract,* March 2006 5(1), 45–66.

The Family Function Questionnaire—Part I: Assessment of a Primary Care Screening Tool

Russell J. Sawa*[1] and Jennifer M. Sawa[2]

ABSTRACT

This paper examines a self-report questionnaire, which has been used in primary care settings. The thrust of its development is for use in the primary care setting. In the present study, data from 223 families were used to establish the validity of the questionnaire, which was successfully accomplished. Factor analysis was used to determine the underlying constructs, and five distinct constructs were found. A Logistic Regression analysis was then applied to determine the predictive value of these constructs. Two constructs, cohesiveness and connectedness proved to be highly successful predictors of family function. These constructs are evaluated with 12 questions, nearly half of the original 25 questions in the original FFQ1 form. The three other constructs, rules, conflict, and problems, were not.

INTRODUCTION

In primary care it is almost always the individual who is seen clinically. Yet, primary care espouses the context of the family in the treatment of patients (Starfield, 1994, 1998). Whereas in other areas of clinical practice the purpose of assessment "involves the collection of information to diagnose and treat presenting problems and evaluate the success of the intervention" (Grotevant, 1989), in primary care the purpose of an assessment is mainly to identify patients who may need help. This help could be education by the doctor, or setting aside time to see the patient together with their spouse or entire family, or, more commonly, referring them to a specialist in counseling. A rapid assessment in the medical office is ideal. It is also ideal if the assessment is highly correlated with a theoretical model that can be taught to clinicians (Miller, 1989).

The theoretical basis of the Family Function Questionnaire—I (FFQ1) is The Primary Care Family Assessment Model (PCFA) (Russell J. Sawa, 1985), which was developed from the McMaster Model (Epstein, Bishop and Levin, 1978). The PCFA has been used to teach student physicians, practicing physicians, and student social workers at a Masters level (R.J. Sawa, Falk, Henderson and Pablo, 1985). The assessment questionnaire was designed for obtaining information from family members to help the clinician formulate hypotheses prior to seeing the family. This

---

*Corresponding author.

[1,2]University of Calgary, Calgary, Alta, Canada. E-mail: [1]sawa@ucalgary.ca

questionnaire has been used clinically for more than a quarter century (Russell J. Sawa, 1985). It is based on an epistemology which is reality based (R.J. Sawa and Meynell, 2000) as appropriate for primary care clinicians (Russell J Sawa, 1986; Russell J. Sawa, 1988, 1998, 1992).

The goal of this study is to simplify theory and practice, so that the FFQ1 can be used by busy clinicians such as doctors, nurses and social workers who do not have the luxury of long visits. The expectation is that clinicians will be able to identify those who need help and either refer them, counsel them, or work with them briefly over time in the context of primary care. The reworking of the constructs is based on thirty years of clinical experience, and the analyses are discussed in this paper.

This paper explores the FFQ1 in terms of how well the questionnaire fits with theory (through factor analysis), and how well the questionnaire can predict families that warrant further assessment/treatment (through regression analyses).

FAMILY ASSESSMENT AND SELF-REPORT MEASURES: A BRIEF REVIEW OF THE LITERATURE

Ransom (1992) points out that the distinction between "individual oriented primary care" *vs.* "family-centered primary care" may be misplaced (p. 77). He believes, and we agree, that "The greater contrast is between disease-or procedure-focused and person-focused approaches, instead of between individual and family approaches" (Ransom, 1992). As he points out, if individual refers to a person, then "taking the person seriously and fully necessarily means including significant other people and relationships in that person's life" (p. 77). This lays the foundation for inquiring about the patient's family during a medical encounter. Ransom further argues that it is important to move from a strictly variable centered approach to a person centered one. Cook (2005) points out the importance of recognizing who the unit of measurement is, the individual, a dyad, or the whole family. The family is the unit of measurement "whenever an item is constructed that has the characteristics of the family as a whole as its target. For example, the item 'People in my family look out for each other' has the family as the unit of measurement (Cook, 2005). Cook also comments on the advantages in terms of time and resources, of a self-report approach over observational approaches.

The PCFA was developed from the McMaster Model. The McMaster Model, and our standard of comparison, the Family APGAR (G. Smilkstein, 1978), are both based on structural-functional theory (Neabel, 2000). Structural-functional theory emphasizes the interdependence or relationships between family members. The Family APGAR provides a valid standard to compare the FFQ1 to, as it possesses good homogeneity, reliability, and stability.

As Neabel *et al.* (2000) discuss, it is essential that an assessment tool be reliable and valid. Reliable scales have 3 characteristics: Homogeneity, Stability, and Equivalence. Generally the coefficient value should be at least 7.0 or higher for an instrument to be considered reliable, as does both the McMaster Model and the Family APGAR. An instrument is valid if it obtains the data that it is supposed to obtain, and both of these models are found to be valid.

The Family APGAR is a five item measure of perceived family support, and it highly correlates with therapists' ratings of family distress (Gardner, 2001). There are also reports questioning both the usefulness and validity of the Family APGAR, to the extent that it was judged as not useable for measurement of family dysfunction. We, as does the literature generally (Good, 1979) (Good, Smilkstein, Good, Shaffer and Arrons, 1979; (Smilkstein, G., Ashworth, C. and Montaro, I, 1982) Smilkstein, Ashworth and Montano, 1982), do not agree with this assessment. It has been found to be internally consistent (Neabel *et al.*, 2000, p. 200).

THE FAMILY FUNCTION QUESTIONNAIRE—PART 1 IN LIGHT OF THE LITERATURE

The FFQ1 has been used in clinical settings to help screen families for family function/dysfunction, thus identifying families that may be in need, and helping to identify specific problem areas. The device gathers information at the family, marital, and individual level, and this analysis of multiple systemic sources is important in the measuring of family assessments (Cook, 2005). We examined the internal structure of the FFQ1 *via* factor analysis, with encouraging results, as will be discussed below.

Grotevant (1989) asserts that it is theory that should drive the decisions of how assessments are to be made, and the FFQ1 follows this logic, in that the assessment developed from the theory of the PCFA, which we assume, like the McMaster Model examines organization and structural patterns within the family. As such, it is part of what is called 'structural-functional' theory of the family. This theory views the family as a social system with a strong focus on family functioning (Neabel *et al.*, 2000).

The literature on family assessment also addresses the importance of examining the internal structure of measures (Miller, Bishop, Epstein and Keitner, 1990), and the FFQ1 examines the internal structure of the measure *via* factor analysis, with encouraging results, as will be discussed below. The Family Assessment Device (FAD) has also demonstrated factor loadings that align with theory. Both the FAD and FFQ1 are based on the McMaster Model. In contrast to the FAD, The FFQ1 also has the benefit of being a shorter questionnaire that may be easier for families to use, and may be more simple for clinicians to score.

The potential usefulness of the FFQ1 is clear when faced with the reality that clinicians are facing more diverse and restrictive realities in the assessment of families (Miller and Goddard, 1989). The FFQ1 is a measure that is easy to understand, and is designed for not only parents to complete, but for children as well. This is a very useful trait of the measure, as there is a need to develop family assessment scales that can be used by children and adolescents (Kaufman, Tarnowski, Simonian and Graves, 1991). Though the FFQ1 has been designed for children as well as adults, the exact reading level required to complete this questionnaire could be assessed. However, the use of this questionnaire for children is promising, as many have completed the FFQ1 over the years. The questions in FFQ1 appear to be easier to understand than those of the Family APGAR. Words that are present in the APGAR such as "life-style" and "sorrow" may be difficult for young children to understand.

In addition, some of the benefits inherent in the use of the FFQ1 stem from the simple fact that it is a self-report measure. Observational approaches to family assessment may take a substantial amount of time and effort (Cook, 2005). Observational methods must occur in specific contexts where family members can interact in ways that will give the observer information that is needed. Such an approach is unfeasible for the primary care clinician.

The FFQ1 not only provides information on where families may be having difficulty, but also sheds light on the areas that are strengths. For instance, the results may indicate that a family is skilled at sharing problems and feelings with one another. By providing such information, clinicians may help families capitalize on their strengths (Hodges, 2004). The FFQ1 also provides the benefit of families being able to identify specific problems that they think are of particular importance. For example, question 26 asks, "What do you think your family's main problems (if any) are?". Though this question does not contribute to the family's overall score, and is not included in the analyses, it is an open question and thus gives family members the opportunity to express their opinion of what is important to them.

HISTORICAL DEVELOPMENT OF FFQ1

The FFQ1 is based on theory, as Grotevant suggests (Grotevant, 1989). The initial research was published as the Silent Majority, a study of university students at McGill University which compared the mental health of students with the functioning of their families (Westley, 1969). The McMaster Model was built on this theoretical base (Epstein, 1978). The principal author of this article studied family therapy under two of the authors of the McMaster Model in 1978 (Epstein and Bishop), while the model was being developed at McMaster University, before going into medical practice. While in practice and teaching he created a model, the Primary Care Family

Assessment Model (PCFA), which was designed to be more appropriate for primary care physicians (Russell J. Sawa, 1985). The assessment involved individual questionnaires (My Family Questionnaire, FFQ1 and FFQ2) and an interview with the whole family (for more information on the My Family Questionnaire and the FFQ2, which are not examined in this paper, see Sawa, 1985). The factor analysis, to be discussed below, was exploratory, as the researcher wished to know which principles the 25 questions fell under; whether there was anything new apart from the theory of the PCFA.

METHOD

Participants

The participants in this study were patients who were seen by family physicians in an academic family practice unit, both in teaching and non-teaching situations and the community. Informed consent was obtained, and approval from the Faculty of Medicine's ethics committee. For the factor analysis, 233 couples participated. For the regression analysis, data from 97 couples were used, as these couples had completed both the APGAR and the FFFQ1.

Measures

The Family Function Questionnaire—Part I is a measure in the self-report format based on questions derived from the Primary Care Family Assessment Model (Russell J. Sawa, 1985). The measure consists of 25 yes/no questions (see appendix A). Additional information is obtained by including a comments section and open-ended questions asking the respondent to describe his/her family's main problems.

The strategy for scale development was based primarily on the clinical and theoretic experience of the instrument designer. The test was conceived of after several years of experience with the PCFA model. The questionnaire was experimented with briefly in the clinical setting before its final form was derived and it has not been changed since its creation in 1980. For the FFQ1, yes and no answers to the 25 questions could indicate either functionality or dysfunctionality depending on the question; consequently, the questions were first scaled unidirectional in terms of family functionality such that dysfunctionality = 0, and functionality = 1. Thus, total questionnaire scores ranged from 0 to 25, with higher scores indicating functionality.

Procedure

The FFQ1 and the Family APGAR were filled out individually by all family members, including children usually at age 12 and above, prior to being seen. In the teaching setting, a team of students and their supervisor read the forms before seeing the family, and then generated hypotheses about the functioning of the family prior to seeing them. An assessment of the whole family was then conducted while the entire team observed the interview, conducted by the supervisor or student resident being supervised. Families were then referred for counselling, if appropriate, by a family therapist who worked in the family practice unit. For statistical analyses, we averaged scores of husbands and wives.

RESULTS

Factor Analysis

For the questionnaire, the 25 variables had an internal consistency of 0.63. This level was deemed adequate for this study as determined by Cronbach's Alpha. This is an indication that the FFQ1 is a measure with adequate reliability. Cronbach's Alpha ranged from .547 to .652.

Out of the 253 correlations in the correlation matrix that the factor analysis was based on, approximately 23% were medium to high correlations.

The factor analysis model used was a principal-components analysis with Varimax Rotation, which resulted in the possible use of one to seven factors. Seven factors had eigenvalues of 1.00 or greater; five factors were finally adopted. Even though these five factors did not fit exactly in the four dimensions of the PFCA model, they coincided clearly with the theoretical logic based on family functioning. How they differ will be explored in the discussion section. Table 1 illustrates the five separate factors and the principles behind these factors as they relate to family functioning.

Overall, the five factors accounted for 56% of the common variance, and the eigenvalues ranged from 4.23 on factor one, to 1.49 on factor five. Ultimately, 23 variables can be expressed in the following five factors: Cohesiveness, Conflict, Rules, Connectedness, and Problems. Variables 20 and 21 were removed, as they did not suitably load on any factor. Factor loadings are illustrated in Table 2.

Happy family, talking about problems, sharing feelings, clear speaking, happy with tasks, showing feelings, care of interests/activities, showing affection, and someone to share worries with at home were all significantly loaded onto Factor 1, Cohesiveness. This factor refers to the kinds of relationship bonds within the family. These bonds may be viewed as degrees of closeness. The bonds within families range from intimate, close, positive, distant, conflictual, and too close. Factor 1 accounted for 18.38% of the variance of the results.

Table 1: Description of the Five Factors

Factor	*Description*
Cohesiveness	Refers to the kinds of relationship bonds, which are found in the family. These bonds can be viewed as degrees of closeness. The bonds may be intimate (adult to adult), close (as appropriate to parent and child, but not equal as that between adults), positive (bonds not as strong as intimate or close, yet still close bonds between members of the nuclear family), distant (relationships which are not close), conflictual and too close (as in enmeshment).
Conflict	The factor conflict is derived from the ordinary meaning of the word. Conflict arises from difference. If there is no room for difference in the family, then the results are irritation and fighting. This causes distress, and may be the main reason couples and families come to a counsellor or physician for help.
Rules	The term 'rules' is also defined by the ordinary meaning of the word. Rules need not be explicit in a highly functioning family, but often need to be worked out in lower functioning families with children. When children do not have appropriate rules, especially in troubled families, this may be a reflection of an inadequate alliance of the parents. This is further reflected in deficient communication between the parents themselves and their children.
Connectedness	Connectedness refers to the health of the bonds within the family and between the family and the larger system. This system includes the family of origin, friends, as well as the spiritual or meaning dimension within a family.
Problems	Problems refer to problems that a family is unable to solve, which are characteristic of families who are in distress. At times, the problems are due to individual developmental difficulties in spouses, and are exhibited by repetitive patterns, which in turn cause negative emotions between spouses. Problems also result from poor communication, which inhibits functional problem-solving strategies.

Factor 2 had significant loadings of the prefer less arguing, prefer less yelling, anger frightening and family counselling questions. Factor 2, Conflict, arises from differences within the family. If there is no room for difference in the family, irritation and fighting result, which causes distress and may be the main reason families come to a counsellor or physician for help. Factor 2 accounted for 13.20% of the variance in the data.

Factor 3 accounted for 9.47% of the total variance in the data, and contained significant loadings with the questions pertaining to expectations at home, rules present, clear rules, and reasonable rules. This factor, labeled as Rules is defined in the ordinary meaning of the word. Rules are understood regulations within a family that regulates the behaviour of family members. They need not be explicit in highly functioning families, yet often need to be worked out in lower functioning families with children. When children do not have appropriate rules, especially in troubled families, this is often a reflection of the inadequate alliance of the parents, and is further a reflection of deficient communication between the parents and children.

Table 2: Varimax-Rotated Factor Loading Matrix for Principal-Component Analysis of the Family Function Questionnaire—Part I

Question	*Factor*				
	1	*2*	*3*	*4*	*5*
Question 1	.525*	–.388	.070	.110	.318
Question 2	–.195	.438	–.091	–.003	–.611*
Question 3	.007	.121	–.078	.001	.733*
Question 4	.778*	–.116	.167	.136	–.028
Question 5	.780*	–.006	.144	.113	–.064
Question 6	.607*	–.148	.176	–.073	.280
Question 7	.421	–.152	.454*	.180	.001
Question 8	.367*	–.120	.113	.477	–.028
Question 9	–.102	.870*	.021	–.141	.067
Question 10	.328	–.238	.067	.504*	–.046
Question 11	–.097	–.045	.140	.718*	.163
Question 12	.043	.065	.789*	.115	–.031
Question 13	.295	–.089	.709*	–.055	.176
Question 14	.311	–.032	.695*	.053	–.086
Question 15	.647*	–.089	.347	–.190	.139
Question 16	–.098	.883*	–.010	–.150	.056
Question 17	–.264	.649*	–.071	–.177	–.076
Question 18	.573*	–.179	.016	.294	.084
Question 19	.631*	–.194	.096	.081	.146
Question 22	.613*	–.159	.209	.204	–.007
Question 23	.113	.022	–.138	.463*	–.218
Question 24	–.288	.624*	–.056	.095	–.219
Question 25	–.081	.279	–.153	–.530	–.412*
Eigenvalue	4.23	3.04	2.17	1.85	1.49
Percentage of Variance	18.38	13.20	9.46	8.03	6.48

Extraction Method: Principle Component Analyses.

Rotation Method: Varimax Rotation with Kaiser Normalization.

Note: Factor names: 1 = Cohesion; 2 = Conflict; 3 = Rules; 4 = Connectedness; 5 = Problems.

* Factor loadings of ≥ .4 were considered in the creation and naming of the factors. For Questions 8 and 25, there were medium to high loadings with two questions. We chose items that best fit the theory.

Factor 4 had significant loadings with the questions addressing freedom for outside activities/friends, school/work, and someone outside family to share worries with. This factor, labeled Connectedness accounts for 8.03% of the overall variance in the data. Connectedness refers to the health of the bonds within the family, and between the family and the larger system. The larger system includes the family or origin, friends, and the spiritual or meaning dimension within the family.

Lastly, Factor 5, Problems, had significant loadings on the questions relating to family as whole have problems, one member of family having problems, and money as a problem. This factor relates to the idea that families and couples who are in distress have problems that they are unable to solve. This is sometimes due to the individual developmental difficulties in the spouses, and is exhibited by repetitive patterns, which cause negative emotions between the spouses. Effective problem solving involves identifying the problem, communicating the problem to the appropriate family member, seeking solutions, and checking to see if solutions are successful. These steps are usually not conscious, and effective families go through these steps intuitively. Overall, Factor 5 accounted for 6.48% of the variance in the data. Table 3 illustrates which questions load on which factor, with the corresponding question numbers.

Table 3: Description of the Five Factors, with Significantly Loaded Questions

Factor	*Questions*
Cohesiveness	1. Do you have a happy family? 4. Are you able to talk about your problems in the family? 5. Are you able to share your feelings with family members? 6. Do people speak clearly at home? 8. Are you happy with your tasks at home? 15. Are people able to show their feelings at home? 18. Do other family members care about your interests and activities? 19. Is it easy to show affection at home? 22. Do you have someone at home you can share your worries with?
Conflict	9. Would you prefer that there were less arguing at home? 16. Would you prefer that there were less yelling at home? 17. Do you sometimes find the anger at home frightening? 24. Do you think your family could use some counselling?
Rules	7. Do you know what is expected of you at home? 12. Are there rules at home? 13. Are the rules clear? 14. Are the rules reasonable?
Connectedness	10. Is there enough freedom for outside friends and activities? 11. Are things going well at school or work? 23. Do you have someone outside the home you can share your worries with?
Problems	2. Do you feel that your family as a whole has a problem? 3. Do you feel that only one member of your family has a problem? 25. Do you think money is a problem in the family?

REGRESSION ANALYSIS

In order to identify whether or not the five factors could predict dysfunction, a logistic regression analysis using the Enter Method was conducted with the APGAR. The APGAR scores were divided along the lines of highly functional families, as opposed to severely and moderately dysfunctional families. The following was discovered: The constant –8.981, while the five factors had slopes ranging from |0.06| to |4.276|. Cohesiveness and Connectedness had significant slopes. Table 4 illustrates the findings.

Table 4: Statistic Regression for the Five Factors

	B	*Probability*
Factor 1: Cohesiveness	4.276	.000
Factor 2: Conflict	.387	.506
Factor 3: Rules	–.060	.929
Factor 4: Connectedness	1.449	.027
Factor 5: Problems	–.181	.807
Constant	–8.981	.000

In following the regression equation $Y = a + bX$, where Y refers to family function, b refers to the slope, a refers to the intercept, and X is a particular factor score, the equation to predict family function is as follow:

Y = –8.981 + 4.276 Factor 1 + 0.387 Factor 2 – 0.060 Factor 3 + 1.449 Factor 4 – 0.181 Factor 5

As illustrated by the table, not all of the five factors were equal in terms of how well they can predict family function. Despite the encouraging results of the factor analysis, where all of the constructs were independent from one another with significant loadings, not all of the five factors have been demonstrated as significant predictors of family function. However, Cohesiveness is a significant predictor of family function ($p < .001$), as is Connectedness ($p < .05$). A stepwise Logistic regression, using the Likelihood-Ratio model was also run with only Cohesiveness and Connectedness taken into the model. These two factors seem to be very strong in predicting dysfunction.

DISCUSSION

The PCFA is composed of four dimensions, connectedness (outside the family) developmental stage accomplishment, internal function, and health and coping (Sawa, 1985). Each of these offers a view of family function, and could be used to assess a family in a way that leads to relevant interventions. The first dimension, connectedness, is primarily assessed by My Family questionnaire, and FFQ2. FFQ1 was expected to primarily relate to the internal function of the family. Surprisingly, upon factor analysis, five distinct constructs emerged. They were then named cohesiveness, connectedness, rules, conflict and problems. While cohesiveness does describe internal family function, with rules being a part of internal function, connectedness was also picked up in several of the questions. Yet, two new constructs emerged, that of conflict and problems. The questions relating to the last two were devised intuitively as being important in family function when the questions were initially written. They do however relate to the fourth dimension health and coping, upon reflection, as conflict and inability to solve problems affect both coping with stress and health of family members. Yet both conflict and problems did appear as distinct constructs, each with factor loadings of their own.

Cohesiveness relates to the internal family function in the PCFA. This includes the love and commitment of spouses, the communication, sexual relations, emotional relations, and rules and roles within the family. In the FFQ1, we find the ability to talk and share feelings, speaking clearly expectations and happiness with tasks, and happiness in the family are a very similar construct. Rules (internal function in the PCFA) are a subset of cohesiveness in the FFQ1, yet now considered a separate and distinct construct from the factor analysis. This is fleshed out with the questions "Do you know what is expected of you at home?", "Are there rules?", "Are the rules clear?" and "Are the rules reasonable?"

The factor analysis did provide five, clean constructs that are independent of one another, and each provide an avenue into an area of family function. This supports the belief of the FFQ1 being a well-constructed assessment device, and that through its use, clinicians can gain an understanding of how a family is functioning, and whether or not they need help.

The five factors that emerged from our analyses, each represents distinct areas of family function. Each of them is also correlated with an existing assessment tool, the Family APGAR. The Family APGAR was designed for use in primary care and has been validated and deemed reliable. The questions are found to correlate well with family function as distinguished from family dysfunction. Each of these factors has within it specific questions which individually distinguish function from dysfunction.

The theoretical model, the PFA, from which these five factors in the FFQ1 are derived is a very teachable model, and has been successfully used in teaching family medicine residents (Sawa, 1985). The advantage of this questionnaire is that it relates directly with a primary care assessment model, the PCFA. Another advantage of this questionnaire is that it also provides a window into educational strategies for the primary care clinician, because it identifies specific problem areas in the family as well as screening for patients who could profit from a family intervention.

Two questions from the FFQ1 were eliminated because they did not suitably load onto any of the five factors. Question 20 asks, "Would you prefer that the family did more things together?" and Question 21 asks, "Do mom and dad spend enough time alone together? (Husband and wife if no children)". It is possible that these questions identify function more globally and influence all the factors. This lack of loading was an unexpected finding.

The logistic regression analysis gave mixed results. Rules, conflict and problems proved to be poor predictors of family functioning. However, cohesiveness and connectedness were demonstrated as being strong predictors. Upon reflection, this is not surprising. The theoretical basis of the PCFA is functional, and cohesiveness (Olson, 1988) and connectedness (Bowen, 1982) are central to the function of families, and the cornerstone of some models of family function. Problems, conflict and rules are important but not central to an understanding of the function of a family as a system.

LIMITATIONS

We fall prey to the limitation which Ransom pointed out, namely treating persons as if they were numbers, and taking averages where necessary, such as with husbands and wives, in order to work with our data. We also excluded the data from children in our present analysis, as we were unsure how to deal with their differences from adults and from each other (boy *vs.* girls).

CONCLUSION

The factor analysis provided encouraging results for the FFQ1, as five separate and unique constructs were identified that coincided with theory on family functioning. However, not all factors are significant predictors of family function. Cohesiveness and Connectedness are significant predictors of family functioning, and provide insight into how the FFQ1 could be reworked in the future. While Problems, Rules, and Conflict do provide information useful to clinicians about the functioning of a family, and what kind of intervention and treatment may be helpful, it is only Cohesiveness and Connectedness that should be considered when screening a family for their level of functioning. The next steps would be to examine the FFQ1 closely in light of these results, perhaps using only Cohesiveness and Connectedness for scoring and therefore to predict family functioning. However, we are closer to finding an instrument that may prove invaluable in identifying families who are in need.

FUTURE RESEARCH POSSIBILITIES

Though the results of the analyses on the FFQ1 are encouraging, there is still work to be done. Firstly, the fact that only two of the factors predict family function needs to be addressed, and decisions need to be made on how the questionnaire should be modified. The fact that the questionnaire has been used for over a quarter of a century speaks to the reliability of this instrument. Nevertheless, when the questionnaire has been reworked, further tests of reliability and validity need to be addressed. Normative samples should be found, and further testing should be conducted with random sampling. It would also be interesting to examine how family functioning differs across cultures. Differences between husbands and wives, as well as between children and adults should also be explored in future research.

REFERENCES

Bowen, M. (1982). *Family Therapy in Clinical Practice.* New York: Jason Aronson.

Cook, W.L. (2005). "The SRM Approach to Family Assessment." *European Journal of Psychological Assessment*, 21(4), 216–225.

Epstein, N.B., Bishop, D.S. and Levin, S. (1978). "The McMaster Model of Family Functioning." *Journal of Marital and Family Counseling,* 4, 19–31.

Gardner, W., Nutting, P.A., Kelly, J.K., Kellepher, J., Werner, J.J., Farley, T., Stewart, L., Hartsell, M. and Orzano, A.J. (2001). "Does the Family APGAR Effectively Measure Family Functioning?" *The Journal of Family Practice,* 50(1), 19–25.

Good, M.J., Smilkstein, G., Good, B.J., Shafer, T. and Arons, T. (1979). "The Family APGAR Index: A Study of Construct Validity." *Journal of Family Practice*, 8, 577–582.

Grotevant, H.D. (1989). "The Role of Theory in Guiding Family Assessment." *Journal of Family Psychology*, 3, 2.

Miller, B.C. (1989). "Selective Views of Family Assessment: A Commentary." *Journal of Family Practice*, 3(2), 215–221.

Neabel, B., Fothergill-Bourbonnais, F. and Dunning, J. (2000). "Family Assessment Tools: A Review of the Literature from 1978–1997." *Heart and Lung*, 29(3), 196–209.

Olson, D., Russell, C. and Sprenkle, D.H. (1988). *The Circumplex Model: Systemic Assessment and Treatment of Families.* Binghamton, N.Y.: Haworth.

Ransom, D. (1992). "New Directions in the Methodology of Family-Centered Health Care Research." In R.J. Sawa (Ed.), *Family Health Care.* Newbury Park, CA: Sage.

Sawa, R.J. (1985). *Family Dynamics for Physicians: Guidelines to Assessment and Treatment.* Lewiston, Ont.: Edwin Mellen Press.

Sawa, R.J. (1986). "Assessing Interviewing Skills: The Simulated Office Oral." *Journal of Family Practice,* 23(6), 567–571.

Sawa, R.J. (1988). "Incorporating the Family into Medical Care." *Canadian Family Physician*, 34, 87–93.

Sawa, R.J. (1998). *Family Therapy and Family Medicine: An Interdisciplinary Epistemology.* Unpublisheddoctoral Dissertation, University of Calgary, Calgary.

Sawa, R.J. (Ed.). (1992). *Family Health Care.* Newbury Park, CA: Sage.

Sawa, R.J., Falk, W.A., Henderson, E.A. and Pablo, R.Y. (1985). "Family Practice Impact of a Curriculum in Family Dynamics." *Family Systems Medicine*, 3(11), 50–59.

Sawa, R.J. and Meynell, H.A. (2000). "On Insight, Objectivity and the Pathology of Families. Method." *Journal of Lonergan Studies*, 18, 145–160.

Smilkstein, G. (1978). "The Family APGAR: A Proposal for a Family Function Test and Its Use by Physicians." *Journal of Family Practice,* 6, 1231–1235.

Smilkstein, G., Ashworth, C. and Montaro, I. (1982). "Validity and Reliability of the Family APGAR as a Test of Family Function." *Journal of Family Practice*, 15, 303–311.

Starfield, B. (1994). Primary Care: *Is it Essential? Lancet,* 344, 1129–1133.

Starfield, B. (1998). *Primary Care: Balancing Health Needs, Services and Technology.* New York: Oxford University Press.

Westley, W.A.E., N.B. (1969). *The Silent Majority.* San Francisco: Jossey-Bass.

Neural Correlates of Experience

C.R. Mukundan*

ABSTRACT

This paper attempts to briefly examine the nature and components of human experience. Experience comprises of sensory-perceptual components related to the external world, motor components related to actions and responses, proprioceptive components of internal conditions, and emotions. Awareness may often accompany them together or at close proximity along with their verbal transcoding. Neuro-imaging studies have revealed the nature of neural participation in the brain during real and imagined presence of these components. It has been found that emotions and associated responses could be initiated even without normal sensation and awareness of external stimuli. The profile of activation of the neural structures in the brain during real and imagined sensory and motor events is akin to each other, which make us wonder how the brain may differentiate between real and imagined worlds and actions. Primary sensory areas are activated in real and sensory events, and primary motor cortex is activated in real and imagined motor activities. The only means for the brain to differentiate such imagined events from real events is through reality verification. Experiencing is the personalized and subjective method of reality verification, despite the fact interpretation of experience may depend on the knowledge base and the needs of an individual. Though experience itself may have real components, its interpretation may be erroneous, unless great care is taken in identification and elucidation of the real components and their relationships. Such interpretations are bound to change according to the changes in the available knowledge base. Thinking is a motor act and part of speech, which helps to verbally represent the components of experience and the relationship among them in parts and total. The process further leads to verbal awareness, which in turn allows introspection and ability to plan, predict, anticipate, and change interpretations and course of actions. Learning through experience is therefore, of paramount importance not only for planning and creating future but also for their reality verification.

INTRODUCTION

Experience has never been treated as a regular area of study in psychology, as areas of perception, motor functions, cognition, behavior and emotions are considered. Experience is a word translated from the German word "*Erfahrung*" meaning coherency of experiences in life. It is further evolved to include a state of the individual, which helps to acquire knowledge and skills. A core feature of experience is its participatory quality; one can acquire personal skills only through the experience one acquires during participation in an activity. Experience of participation may be in the form of

*Department of Clinical Psychology, National Institute of Mental Health and Neuro-Sciences, Bangalore, India. E-mail: crmukundan@gmail.com

a personal accomplishment or achievement. Experience may be associated with innumerable activities such as swimming, playing as well as listening to music, driving, running sailing, gardening, trekking, thinking, reading, dancing, playing, watching movie acting, praying, making a movie, writing, sex, travelling, skating, painting, sky diving, gambling, meditation, sculpturing, riding, eating, oration, etc. Personal experience does not automatically generate knowledge; it may have to be inferred. Experiential knowledge may always require further independent verification. One acquires this through repeated practice or experience. Experience can also be merely an emotional state of the mind. Love, compassion, and empathy, which are not part of survival emotions such as fear, anger, rage, aggressiveness, and flight, are also experiential. A state of spiritual realization is also called experiential; feeling of well-being is experiential. The altered mental state of a person under the effect of a drug or intoxicating substance may be said to be experiential, though the contents may not be reality verifiable.

Experiencing is considered to mean living through, achieving, coming into contact, suffering, undergoing, being subjected to, encountering, participating, happening, or occurrence in life. There is no activity, occupation, or aspect of living, which is devoid of experiencing. The entire thrill, pleasure, and aim of living for everyone are drawn from experience. The most important aspect of experiencing is that it is personal and the self of the experiencing person is the only experiencing agent. The "self" is the experiencing agency, which renders experiencing a personal and private affair, the nature of which can only be inferred by others. Further the self interprets, assigns meaning and significance to the state of experience and to the components contributing to experience. This renders experience non-predictive and non-deductive, as the knowledge base used may be different from person to person and it may not have any scientific validity. The interpretive schema may often be self-created and hence vary from person to person. The intensity and quality of experience may vary from person to person based on the contextual interpretations, the emotions aroused in the person, and the intensity of the sensory-motor participation. However, all those factors that contribute to and influence the state of experiencing are within the brain of the experiencing individual.

Events in the body that contribute to experiencing are sensory events leading to perception, motor events related to responses and actions, proprioceptive conditions and their perceptions, and emotions (Mukundan 2007). They may contribute singularly or in combination; presence of emotion plays the most important role as it makes an experience significant and memorable to the experiencing person. For example, one can look at the rising sun; and the sensory inputs and the associated encoding can produce an intense experience in one, whereas the same sensory input may produce no such experience in another. The meaning assigned to the sensory and motor components determines the emotions aroused and the significance of the experience to the person. It is now well established that emotional arousal and responses such as fear can occur even without perception of the sensory event and its awareness (LeDoux 1996, 2003; de Gelder *et al.,* 1999; Vuilleumier *et al.,* 2003, 2002; Bishop *et al.,* 2004; Pessoa 2005). This is called pre-attentive emotion. The emotional response in the preattentive emotion and the associated responses are considered memory and not perception evoked. All intentional processing is suggested to start at an unconscious level before the individual becomes conscious of the processing and it becomes intentional (Libet 2001, 1999, 1985). He opinioned that one is not conscious of any of the mental activities when they are initiated in the brain and one may become conscious of the processing including intentions only when the neural processing associated with the mental activity persists for sufficiently long time.

The excitement and fulfillment one may experience in a simple perceptual situation may not be the same as the emotional response of defensive or survival value seen in pre-attentive emotion. Emotion has a much larger spectrum of manifestation (Mukundan, 2007) than the survival related responses, which we have readily adapted from the animal world. Emotional states related to non-survival needs are generally ignored in scientific investigations, though they play crucial roles in shaping human behavior and forming their destiny. Experiences of compassion and empathy, love, well-being, beauty, music, *etc.* may be considered such emotional states, which we consider unique to human beings. Beauty and music are mental states requiring sensory inputs, beauty being defined through visual, and music being defined through auditory inputs. All these mental states may be generated in the presence of real stimuli as well as in the presence of mental imageries. The recreated mental imageries may further be willfully recreated and maintained internally. They may have high contextual specificity, and which may be self-specific. The significance of what one perceives, what it may mean to each person may vary from person to person and hence they may have varying effects in producing emotions and controlling behavior. Remembrance of experiences constitutes recreation of such mental imageries, both in sensory and motor modalities. The mental recreation of the original sensory and motor components of experience brings back the memory in a real-like manner and not merely as an idea.

Reality is a word that we use to refer to what truly exists in the universe. We believe that reality is what exists even without our knowledge and understanding. However, we use the word reality also to refer to the brain-mind made world also. This reality is a creation of the mind based on what it understands of the real universe and what it wants it to be, and what it creates from it. It is this reality what the mind considers its destiny and what it wants to change and shape for greater accomplishments. The mind extracts the principles of the real universe and uses them cleverly to define and create its own reality. As it is a mind made reality, its rules are also made in the mind.

The definitions of this reality and what they mean depends on how one has designed to relate to them and in what context the relationships are made and maintained. It also depends on the emotions and aspirations of persons as individuals and as groups. There is no escape from this reality, which we have made for ourselves, and the whole span of life of a person is shaped by the reality one has chosen to define for the self. There is no doubt that the universe has only one reality as matter exits in whatever forms, whether we know about it or not. However, the second reality defined by the mind has become several folds more important for each of us. Civilization, culture, societies, governments, families, ambitions, achievements, creativity are defined as part of this reality, and hence they have become the core of human beings and their existence. The second level of self-defined reality is made possible because of the unique property of the human brain, which we may call the brain-mind. Man's happiness, achievements and fulfillment depends on the realization of the dreams, which they try to give shape and materialize. It is in this context human emotions and relationships become nonlinear and beyond rational explanations. Human behavior ceases to be decided so much by 'fear and flee' or 'rage and aggression' rules, commonly seen in the animal world. Suffering and penance are sought out, happiness is found in sharing suffering, and the happiness of another may become more precious than own. Life is spent in self-designed assignments, which takes each through adventure, suffering, achievements, fulfillments, and happiness.

Large spectrum of human behavior is initiated and controlled from within though this may be a functional extension of 'conditioned behavior' during the early development of the human brain. External control of behavior is the essence of conditioning principles whereas complex motor programming is a capability to generate behavior from within (Goldberg, 1985). As external stimuli serve as the source and target for the generation of conditioned responses, one learns to generate actions from within, navigate and arrive at pre-defined goals though complex motor programming. As part of complex motor programming, man learns to define purpose for life, define goals to achieve, make action plans, and execute them strategically by changing both goals and strategies using anticipated and actual effects of actions. It is the development of complex motor programming ability that gave the human mind a dimension beyond being stimulus-dependent and input-driven. A most important requirement for the creation of new realities by the self involves learning complex skills, which must be accomplished through vigorous practice involving experiential learning. For example, one has to learn for a decade or two before he or she can give a stage performance of dance or drama, to become a professional using expertise in life-physical sciences, business management, *etc*.

Development of awareness of the self and its activities has resulted in otherwise unknown functional capabilities in nature. Awareness of intentions, actions plans, predicted outcome has helped to alter intentions as well as re-plan the entire action plans already in process. The conscious could select and control the outcome of the volitional process—the intended action, by vetoing it, or blocking the performance of the act (Libet, 1985). The neural system of the human brain possess the unique capability to generate actions from within and simultaneously monitor and change the output in terms of anticipations and actual effects. This is most explicitly seen with regard to language—speech function, which has an exceptional functional status, as we tend to verbalize or transcode not only own actions and conditions but also everything that is perceived. Large areas of the brain commonly process the lexical, semantic, and contextual meanings of the speech received and speech produced as either inner speech (thinking) or explicit speech. The listening centers of the brain learn to monitor not only inputs from the outside, but also what its own talking centers generate in terms of thoughts and speech and thereby know not only their presence but also their contents (Mukundan, 1999, 1998). Through verbalization in the form of thoughts or explicit speech of the cognitive processes, one learns to know or become aware of the multifaceted cognitive processing that takes place in the brain. Such monitoring coupled with the monitoring of sensory and motor events develop and grow into a large reference system, which we call the self (Mukundan, 2007). One may concurrently engage in verbalization as cognitive processes or actions take place, or monitor them. Verbalization of this type may depend on the habitual training rather than a rule. As one may verbalizes every facet of own actions, responses, and emotions, one has the opportunity to become aware of the thoughts and what they refer to. When this happens simultaneously, awareness is affirmed by the actual happenings or experiences. When verbalization takes place later, the awareness may be supported by the sensory–motor mental imageries of the associated processes. Verbalization and consequential awareness help to use thoughts as a means for controlling the self, as thoughts can be generated to design and reflect strategic and rational plans, which can be in turn used for the control of own emotions and self-generated behavior. Complex motor programming involves strategy for converting volitional energy into specific intentions, planning, setting goals, anticipating consequences, using strategic controls as per predictions, initiating and executing actions according to predefined plans. One learns to alter even goals and actions plans strategically as per the anticipated and actual effects during the course of executing sequence of actions, which are expected to take the person to the final goal. Such acts have a high experiential value as participation of the individual is intentional and active and as per interpretation used by the self. Experiences generated from such complex motor programming form the core of all endeavors in life of a person leading to achievements, accomplishments, growth, as well as contributing to subjective states of well-being and happiness.

Experiencing is therefore an integral aspect of interaction with the reality designed and built by the self and the reality of the universe that exists even without the understanding and knowledge of the self. It is constituted by the sensory-perceptual events, the pro-prioceptive perceptions, the responses and the actions, and the emotions of initiated in the brain. It is a combination of the associated neural activities and their interpretations within the context they take place. Perception of internal bodily conditions and changes are also important components of experience. Perception of autonomic conditions and changes, such as palpitation, respiratory changes, tension in the stomach muscles and other areas are important pro-prioceptive signals, which make a person experience internal states associated with emotion, tension, anxiety and relaxation. These changes may said to be accompaniments of emotional states, and the change in their rate and patterns may be stress induced in a person. All perceptions are accompanied by activation of the respective primary sensory areas and related association areas and all motor activities are associated with specific motor areas in the primary motor cortex and other motor association areas in the premotor cortex. The role of supplementary motor cortex in voluntary activity has been demonstrated in several studies (Goldberg, 1985).

Our chief interest in the present presentation is in the type of activation of the brain shown during remembrance and intentional imagination of perceptual and motor activities. In the visual mode, remembrance may involve recreation of visual mental imageries of visual entities comprising of persons, objects, places, *etc*. During the recreation of visual mental imageries, the primary visual cortex is activated as if the area is receiving visual sensory information as in real visual perception (Kosslyn *et al.,* 2005, 1999a, 1999b, 1997, Kozhevnikov *et al.,* 2005; Beck *et al.,* 2001; Klein *et al.,* 2004, 2000; Ganis *et al.,* 2004; Sparing *et al.,* 2002). These studies have shown that along with the activation of the primary cortical areas, the other visual association areas are also activated during the recreation of mental imageries as in real perception. In normal perception, the activation of the primary cortical area is part of the sensory registration required for further perceptual processing. The fact that the same areas of the brain are activated during the remembrance or recreation of associated mental imageries show that there is no significant difference between the two processes in terms of the activation of the brain. Both real and imagined perceptions can give rise to associated emotions in the individual and the experience of imagined perception could be almost as exciting as that of real perception. Ability to recreate the mental imageries and associated emotions renders the remembrance almost like real, providing the notion of affirmation and acceptance of their reality. For the individual who has recreated the mental imagery, it is reliving a past visual experience. The visual mental imageries may be recreated initially using their verbally transcoded details or by directly recalling the original visual components from memory and reconstituting the mental imagery from them (Kosslyn *et al.,* 2005). Original signals of shape, color, and spatial relations may be verbally encoded by the perceiver and used during remembrance (Kozhevnikov *et al.,* 2005). Reconstitution of mental imageries requires extensive engagement of the different neural structures of the brain. Use of verbally transcoded information for reconstituting visual mental imageries involve the engagement of fronto-parietal areas, right dorsolateral-parietal area, the midbrain, left insular, and right inferior temporal areas (Ganis *et al.,* 2004; Beck *et al.,* 2001; Mellet *et al.,* 2000).

Studies have shown that brain activation pattern similar to sensory mental imageries is found with regard to motor mental imageries also. Mental motor imageries are equally important components of remembrance, which help to reconstitute remembrance of the original experience. The activation of the brain involving the primary motor area and the supplementary motor cortex was demonstrated in the phantom limb phenomenon and in lost limb conditions (Melzack 1990; Ramachandran, Hirstein 1991; Dettmers *et al.,* 2001; Lacourse *et al.,* 2005; Pineda 2005; Maruno *et al.,* 2000; Abbruzzese *et al.,* 1999; Maruff *et al.,* 1999; Porro *et al.,* 1996). The recreation of the motor mental imageries of the proprioceptive signals helps an individual re-experience the bodily sensations related to motor participation. In remembrance of actions, limb positions and their movements are recalled by recreating their motor mental imageries. Activation of motor cortex and premotor areas, including parietal lobes were found in imagined body movements or mental rotation of body parts (Amick *et al.* 2006; de Fiorio *et al.,* 2006; Nyberg *et al.,* 2006; de Lange *et al.,* 2005; Rodriguez *et al.,* 2004; Solodkin *et al.,* 2004; Ross *et al.,* 2003; Rosen *et al.,* 2001). The findings indicate that the major part of the motor system of the brain respond almost in the same manner in actual and imagined movements of body parts. Though imagined movements are exclusive mental activities, the brain responds as though actual movements are indeed taking place.

Emotions of pain, happiness, and other states have been always considered real whenever they are experienced by a person, whether the emotion is evoked in the presence of actual or imagined threat or situation. Hypnotically induced and anticipated pain is found to produce activation of the same areas in the brain that respond to actual pain, which include prefrontal cortex, anterior cingulated cortex, medial frontal cortex and somatosensory associations areas (Rainville *et al.,* 2005, Raij *et al.,* 2005; Ploghaus *et al.,* 2003; Wager *et al.,* 2004; Eisenberger *et al.,* 2003; Porro *et al.,* 2003). Most of the emotional dispositions in the daily life of an individual are produced by imagined and anticipated events and situations rather than actual events and situations. The emotions aroused during such anticipated and imagined conditions play a very important role in determining the well-being and happiness of an individual. What is striking and requiring serious consideration is the fact that imagined perception, movements and emotions are as real as the real ones as far as important brain responses are concerned. In terms of pleasure and pain, feelings of threat and security, the imagined conditions are therefore, as real to the brain as that of real conditions. The emotional state of a person plays crucial role in determining performance, efficiency, and ability to achieve goals in life. An imagined state is a virtual reality as far as the brain is concerned. A sustained imagined emotional pre-disposition, which may take place in the absence of a real threat and exigency in life, may be accompanied by associated brain responses, rendering the pre-disposition a real threat to the well-being and achievements of the individual. A focused effort for changing the imaged mental disposition must help to reduce its intensity and thereby release the brain from the associated responses.

A question of paramount importance is one related to the true difference between the imagined state and what may the real state. It is easily understood that the visual and auditory hallucinations of a schizophrenic patient are indeed a mental phenomenon with accompanying brain responses in the absence of related external stimulus inputs, occurring because the patient is not able to realize that it is a process taking place only within the brain and there is no corresponding external condition or stimulus. The difference between the door seen as a visual hallucination by a patient with schizophrenia and that seen by a normal person is that that one cannot walk through the imaginary door seen by the mentally disturbed patient, whereas one can walk through the door seen by the so-called normal person. Walking out through the door is an experience, which has sensory and motor components, and the experience helps to verify the reality of the perception of the door. One may see a red rose and one may not know if it is real, an illusion, or an idea. If only one can extend the hand and touch the red rose, pick it up with the fingers, one knows it is a real rose. The act of extending the hand and picking up the flower with the fingers are important requirements for the reality verification of the perception of the red rose. The act of picking up the flower and holding it in the hand is an experience. The sensory-motor contact, the thoughts, and feelings of closely holding and possessing it are significant components that constitute the specific experience. The meaning and the significance of the experience is indeed assigned based on the context in which it occurs. The context may be unique to an individual, known only to the individual self. The context may be determined by the personal significance and the emotions derived from the associated experience. All experiences have a time and space reference as long as they are associated with reality contacts. The context is what we call the source memory, which includes the time and space references of the episode or experience (Cycowicz *et al.,* 2001; Troyer *et al.*, 1999; Craik *et al.,* 1996; Johnson *et al.,* 1993).

Accessing source memory is very critical for the recall of experiences or autobiographical episodes, which facilitate the retrieval of the right episode.

Experiencing allows direct but personal verification of every perception, wherever and whenever possible. The reality of perception can be also verified through experimentation, which can be repeated to determine the reliability of the findings. The setting or rising sun in the horizon is an exciting experience for many; an experience which one cannot verify though contact and possession. However, experiencing is the only way one can personally establish contact with the reality and personally verify the reality. Most import aspect of an experience is what the person makes it to be. Understanding of the nature of contact with the reality and the verification process used indeed depend on the knowledge base available to an individual. Accuracy of an experiential verification is therefore a function of the knowledge base and the analytical strategies used by the experiencing individual. The significance of the experience may change from person to person depending on the meanings assigned by each to the sensory-motor components. That experience involves a sensory-motor contact with reality is the unmistakable part and the only mechanism through which one can establish a relationship with reality. However, there is choice to assign meaning to the experience and thereby define the reality itself. The components taking part in the process of experiencing is the total individual and the experiences are always referred to the self of the individual represented by the specific body and mind. This makes experiencing a unique process of self-verification. Another self can have the same sensory-motor participation and experience the same independently, but not share with another self.

When both sensory and motor events are imaginary, both perceptual and motor contacts with reality are absent. If one imagines that reality is also verified, it may indeed represent a psychotic condition of the person. It is a pathological condition, as it takes away the opportunity one has for establishing contact with reality, whatever may be the relative nature of that reality. Not seeking contact with reality and experiencing the reality is nonliving. One can define what one wants to seek in life, whether it is achievable or non-achievable. One can formulate and define a purpose for living, one can set goals in life, and one can self-maneuver for learning the skills required for achieving the goal, and then achieve the goals. That one can define a purpose for life and transform life into a saga of efforts for achieving those goals, while experiencing and expressing that idea in every sequence of actions and thoughts and even become a living symbol of the idea for the rest of world, appear to be highest form and level of experiencing and living.

REFERENCES

Amick, M.M., Schendan, H.E., Ganis, G. and Cronin-Golomb, A. (2006). "Frontostriatal Circuits are Necessary for Visuomotor Transformation: Mental Rotation in Parkinson's Disease." *Neuropsychologia*, 44, 339–49.

Bishop, S.J., Duncan, J. and Lawrence, A.D. (2004). "State Anxiety Modulation of the Amygdala Response to Unattended Threat-Related Stimuli." *J. Neurosci.*, 24, 10364–68.

Craik, F.I., Govoni, R., Naveh-Benjamin, M., Anderson, N.D. (1996). "The Effects of Divided Attention on Encoding and Retrieval Processes in Human Memory." *Journal of Experimental Psychology: General*, 125, 159–80.

Cycowicz, Y.M., Friedman, D., Snodgrass, J.G. and Duff, M. (2001). "Recognition and Source Memory for Pictures in Children and Adults." *Neuropsychologia*, 39(3), 255–67.

de Fiorio, M., Tinazzi, M. and Aglioti, S.M. (2006). "Selective Impairment of Hand Mental Rotation in Patients with Focal Hand Dystonia." *Brain*, 129, 47–54.

de Gelder, B., Vroomen, J., Pourtois, G. and Weiskrantz, L. (1999). "Non-conscious Recognition of affect in the Absence of Striate Cortex." *Neuroreport*, 10, 3759–63.

de Lange, F.P., Hagoort, P. and Toni, I. (2005). "Neural Topography and Content of Movement Representations." *J. Cogn. Neurosci.*, 17, 97–112.

Dettmers, C., Adler, T., Rzanny, R., van Schayck, R., Gaser, C., Weiss, T., Miltner, W.H., Bruckner, L. and Weiller, C. (2001). "Increased Excitability in the Primary Motor Cortex and Supplementary Motor Area in Patients with Phantom Limb Pain after Upper Limb Amputation." *Neurosci. Lett.*, 307, 109–12.

Ehrsson, H.H., Geyer, S. and Naito E. (2003). "Imagery of Voluntary Movement of Fingers, Toes, and Tongue Activates Corresponding Body-part-Specific Motor Representations." *J. Neurophysiol,* 90, 3304–16.

Eisenberger, N.I., Lieberman, M.D. and Williams, K.D. (2003). "Does Rejection Hurt? An FMRI Study of Social Exclusion." *Science*, 302, 290–92.

Ganis, G., Thompson, W.L. and Kosslyn, S.M. (2004). "Brain Areas Underlying Visual Mental Imagery and Visual Perception: An fMRI Study." *Brain Res Cogn Brain Res.*, 20, 226–41.

Goldberg G, Mayer NH, Toglia JU. (1981). "Medial Frontal Cortex Infarction and Alien Hand Sign." *Arch Neurol.* 38(11), 683–86.

Goldberg, E. (2001). *The Executive Brain: Frontal Lobes and the Civilized Mind.* New York, NY: Oxford University Press.

Goldberg, G. (1985). "Supplementary Motor Area Structure and Function: Review and Hypotheses." *The Behavior and Brain Sciences,* 567–15.

Goldenberg, G. (1992). "Loss of Visual Imagery and Loss of Visual Knowledge", *Neuro-Psychologia*, 30, 1081–99.

Johnson, M.K., Hashtroudi, S. and Lindsay, D.S. (1993). "Source Monitoring." *Psychological Bulletin*, 114, 3–28.

Kimura, Y., Yoshino, A., Takahashi, Y. and Nomura, S. (2004). "Interhemispheric Difference in Emotional Response without Awareness." *Physiol. Behav.*, 82, 727–31.

Klein, I., Dubois, J., Mangin, J.F., Kherif, F., Flandin, G., Poline, J.B., Denis, M., Kosslyn, S.M. and Le Bihan, D. (2004). "Retinotopic Organization of Visual Mental Images as Revealed by Functional Magnetic Resonance Imaging." *Brain Res. Cogn. Brain Res.*, 22, 26–31.

Klein, I., Paradis, A.L., Poline, J.B., Kosslyn, S.M., Le Bihan, D. (2000). "Transient Activity in the Human Calcarine Cortex During Visual-mental Imagery: An Event-related fMRI Study." *J. Cogn. Neurosci.*, 12 Suppl. 2, 15–23.

Kosslyn, S.M., Pascual-Leone, A., Felician, O., Camposano, S., Keenan, J.P., Thompson, W.L., Ganis, G. and Sukel, K.E. (1999b). Alpert, N.M. "The Role of Area 17 in Visual Imagery: Convergent Evidence from PET and rTMS." *Science*, 284, 167–70.

Kosslyn, S.M., Sukel, K.E. and Bly, B.M. (1999a). "Squinting with the Mind's Eye: Effects of Stimulus Resolution on Imaginal and Perceptual Comparisons." *Mem Cognit*, 27, 276–87.

Kosslyn, S.M., Thompson, W.L. and Alpert, N.M. (1997). "Neural Systems Shared by Visual Imagery and Visual Perception: A Positron Emission Tomography Study." *Neuroimage*, 6, 320–34.

Kosslyn, S.M., Thompson, W.L., Sukel, K.E. and Alpert, N.M. (2005). "Two Types of Image Generation: Evidence from PET." *Cogn. affect Behav Neurosci.*, 5, 41–53.

Kozhevnikov, M., Kosslyn, S. and Shephard, J. (2005). "Spatial Versus Object Visualizers: A New Characterization of Visual Cognitive Style." *Mem. Cognit.*, 33, 710–26.

Lacourse, M.G., Orr, E.L., Cramer, S.C. and Cohen, M.J. (2005). "Brain Activation during Execution and Motor Imagery of Novel and Skilled Sequential Hand Movements." *Neuroimage,* 27, 505–19.

LeDoux, J. (1996). "Emotional Networks and Motor Control: A Fearful View." *Prog. Brain Res.*, 107, 437–46.

LeDoux, J. (2003). "The Emotional Brain, Fear and the Amygdala." Cell Mol. Neurobiol., 23, 727–38.

Libet, B. (1985). "Unconscious Cerebral Initiative and the Role of Conscious Will in Voluntary Action, *The Behavioral and Brain Sciences*", 8, 529–539; With Open Peer Commentary, 539–558; and Libet's Reply, Theory and Evidence Relating Cerebral Processes to Conscious Will, 558–566.

Libet, B. (1999). "Do we have Free Will?" *Journal of Consciousness Studies*, 6, 47–57.

Libet, B. (2001). "Consciousness, Free Action and the Brain." *Journal of Consciousness Studies*, 8, 59–65.

Maruno, N., Kaminaga, T., Mikami, M. and Furui, S. (2000). "Activation of Supplementary Motor Area during Imaginary Movement of Phantom Toes." *Neurorehabil. Neural Repair,* 14, 345–49.

McGonigle, D.J., Hanninen, R., Salenius, S., Hari, R., Frackowiak, R.S. and Frith, C.D. (2002). "Whose Arm is it Anyway?" *An fMRI Case Study of Supernumerary Phantom Limb. Brain,* 125, 1265–74.

Melzack, R. (1990). "Phantom Limbs and the Concept of a Neuromatrix." *Trends Neurosci,* 13, 88–92.

Melzack, R. (1992). "Phantom limbs." *Sci. Am.*, 266, 120–26.

Mukundan, C.R. (1998). "From Perception to Thinking—Verbal Adaptation in Human Brain." In: Isaac, J.R. and Purendu, H. (Eds.) *Proceedings of International Conference on Cognitive Systems,* New Delhi, Allied Publishers, XXXIX–XIII.

Mukundan, C.R. (1999). "Power of Words: Neuro-Cognitive Approach for Understanding Brain Mechanisms of Awareness." In: Sangeetha Menon, M.G. Narasimhan *et al.* (Eds.) *Scientific and Philosophical Studies on Consciousness.* National Institute of Advanced Studies, Bangalore, India. 127–136.

Mukundan, C.R. (2007). *Brain Experience: Neuroexperiential Perspectives of Brain-Mind.* Atlantic Publishers, New Delhi.

Ohman, A., Esteves, F. and Soares, J.J.F. (1995). "Preparedness and Preattentive Associative Learning: Electrodermal Conditioning to Masked Stimuli." *Journal of Psychophysiology*, 9, 99–108.

Peper, M., Karcher, S., Wohlfarth, R., Reinshagen, G. and LeDoux, J.E. (2001). "Aversive Learning in Patients with Unilateral Lesions of the Amygdala and Hippocampus." *Biol. Psychol.*, 58, 1–23.

Pessoa, L. (2005). "To What Extent are Emotional Visual Stimuli Processed without Attention and Awareness?" *Current Opinion in Neurobiology,* 15, 188–96.

Peter M. Senge (1990). "The Fifth Discipline: The Art and Practice of The Learning Organization." *Currency Doubleday*, New York.

Ploghaus, A., Becerra, L., Borras, C. and Borsook, D. (2003). "Neural Circuitry Underlying Pain Modulation: Expectation, Hypnosis, Placebo." *Trends Cogn. Sci., 7*, 197–200.

Porro, C.A., Cettolo, V., Francescato, M.P. and Baraldi, P. (2003). "Functional Activity Mapping of the Mesial Hemispheric Wall during Anticipation of Pain." *Neuroimage*, 19, 1738–47.

Raij, T.T., Numminen, J., Närvänen, S., Hiltunen, J. and Hari, R. (2005). "Brain Correlates of Subjective Reality of Physically and Psychologically Induced Pain." *Proceedings of the National Academy of Sciences of the United States of America,* 102, 2147–51.

Rainville, P., Bao, Q.V. and Chretien, P. (2005). "Pain-related Emotions Modulate Experimental Pain Perception and Autonomic Responses." *Pain*, 118, 306–18.

Ramachandran, V.S. and Hirstein, W. (1991). "The Perception of Phantom Limbs. D.O. Hebb Lectures." *Brain*, 121, 1603–30.

Rodriguez, M., Muniz, R., Gonzalez, B. and Sabate, M. (2004). "Hand Movement Distribution in the Motor Cortex: The Influence of a Concurrent Task and Motor Imagery." *Neuroimage*, 22, 1480–91.

Rosen, G., Hugdahl, K., Ersland, L., Lundervold, A., Smievoll, A.I., Barndon, R., Sundberg, H., Thomsen, T., Roscher, B.E., Tjolsen, A. and Engelsen, B. (2001). "Different Brain Areas Activated during Imagery of Painful and Non-painful 'Finger Movements' in a Subject with an Amputated Arm." *Neurocase*, 7, 255–60.

Ross, J.S., Tkach, J., Ruggieri, P.M., Lieber, M. and Lapresto, E. (2003). "The Mind's Eye: Functional MR Imaging Evaluation of Golf Motor Imagery." *AJNR Am. J. Neuroradiol.,* 24, 1036–44.

Solodkin, A., Hlustik, P., Chen, E.E. and Small, S.L. (2004). "Fine Modulation in Network Activation during Motor Execution and Motor Imagery." *Cereb Cortex*, 14, 1246–55.

Sparing, R., Mottaghy, F.M., Ganis, G., Thompson, W.L, Topper, R., Kosslyn, S.M. and Pascual-Leone, A. (2002). "Visual Cortex Excitability Increases during Visual Mental Imagery—A TMS Study in Healthy Human Subjects." *Brain Res,* 938, 92–97.

Troyer, A.K., Winocur, G., Craik, F.I. and Moscovitch, M. (1999). "Source Memory and Divided Attention: Reciprocal Costs to Primary and Secondary Tasks", *Neuropsychology*. 13(4), 467–74.

Vuilleumier, P., Armony, J.L., Clarke, K., Husain, M. Driver, J. and Dolan, R.J. (2002). "Neural Response to Emotional Faces with and Without Awareness: Event-related fMRI in a Parietal Patient with Visual Extinction and Spatial Neglect." *Neuropsychologia*, 40, 2156–66.

Vuilleumier, P., Armony, J.L., Driver, J. and Dolan, R.J. (2003). "Distinct Spatial Frequency Sensitivities for Processing Faces and Emotional Expressions." *Nature Neuroscience*, 6, 624–31.

Wager, T.D., Rilling, J.K., Smith, E.E., Sokolik, A., Casey, K.L., Davidson, R.J., Kosslyn, S.M., Rose, R.M. and Cohen, J.D. (2004). "Placebo—Induced Changes in fMRI in the Anticipation and Experience of Pain." *Science*, 5661, 1162– 67.

Williams, L.M., Liddell, B.J., Rathjen, J., Brown, K.J., Gray, J., Phillips, M., Young, A. and Gordon, E. (2004). "Mapping the Time Course of Nonconscious and Conscious Perception of Fear: An Integration of Central and Peripheral Measures." *Hum Brain Mapp,* 21, 64–74.

Glimpses of Some Provocative Concepts in Neuroscience

Vijai Kumar*

BASIC FACTS

The human brain consists of three parts: 1. Cerebral hemispheres; 2. Cerebellum; 3. Brain stem. Brain stem is a remnant of the retinal brain. The cerebrum is divided into four lobes: frontal, parietal, occipital and temporal. Inside the cerebrum, not visible on the surface, is the limbic brain which is the remnant of the mammalian brain.

The surface of the cerebral hemisphere is covered with 1,600 sq. centimeters, 2–3 mm thick cortex called neocortex. There are 6–10 billion neurons in the cortex. Most scientists agree that the unique abilities of the human brain are directly attributable to the cerebral cortex. The neocortex contains six layers of neurons.

The localization of function and specialization of neocortex is over a two-dimensional cortical space and not layer by layer in the third-dimension as well. Cortical neurons lying in the same vertical dimension respond to the same kind of stimulus as the neurons above and below, being functionally identical.

Total number of cells in human body is 50 trillion and number of neurons is more than 100 billion. The elementary signaling units of brain are the nerve cells-neurons.

By the age 20, 5000 neurons die everyday and our brain loses $1/30^{th}$ ounce of its weight every year. At the age of 90 we are still left with > 99 billion neurons. Each neuron summates the information coming to it both spatially and temporally. It responds by exciting or inhibiting other neurons. The impulses travel along the neurons in one direction only. Neuron code defines how individual neurons receive and transmit neuron impulses.

The neurons communicate with each other at synapses where they come as close as a few billionths of an inch apart but these do not touch each other, there always being a gap—the synaptic gap. Number of brain synapses is massive—if counted one per second it will take 35 million years to count all.

FUNCTIONS OF BRAIN

The brain is a complex biological organ of great computational capability which allows cognition. It is the most complex processor of information in the universe. The

*Advisor, Medical Education and Health Care Practices, Dayalbagh, Agra, India.

brain is responsible not only for simple motor behavior such as running and eating but also for complex acts such as thinking, language, music and art. It regulates our thoughts and actions. Brain constructs our sensory experiences and controls our actions. Each mental function of the brain is carried out by specialized neural circuits—the neural assemblies. The on-off electrical nature of neural activity leads to computer brain analogy. In both cases we are talking of temporal and/or spatial patterns of electrical impulses, which allow both systems to compute.

HIPPOCAMPUS AND MEMORIES

Hippocampus, a part of the limbic brain, is required for forming new memories but people can still retrieve old memories even after it is injured. Rather than storing information the hippocampus is believed to create memories by linking together far flung parts of the brain.

SOME INTERESTING AND PROVOCATIVE CONCEPTS

Moving up the ladder of evolution there is massive increase in the number and complexity of connections among the neurons of animal brain.

Absolute brain size would normally suggest a correlation between greater intelligence or complexity of behavior and absolute body weight but this is apparently not the case of either within or between species. Big animals are not necessarily smart ones. If brain weight was an index of intelligence, whales' world out smart men and black snake would be one up on frog! Neither brain weight nor brain-weight body weight ratio gives man his proper distinction in animal hierarchy. The ratio of motor and sensory traffic that passes through medulla on one hand and the number of neurons in cerebral cortex is a good index of hierarchy of intelligence. People are fascinated with the idea of our cerebral hemispheres being really two brains. The right is one more creative in most people, the left one more logical. But the hemispheres of a normal brain hardly exist in splendid isolation. Between them, runs an "enormous interbrain connector" called the corpus callosum. It is packed with around 200 million nerve fibers. In patients whose corpus callosum has been severed to control epileptic attacks, a lack of normal communication between hemispheres has been observed. For example, something sensed in one hemisphere, as well as certain thoughts and memories, may not register in the other. The corpus callosum is the main connecting link between the left and right hemisphere.

Studies on commissurotomy patients have shown that self-conscious experiences arise only in relationship to activities in the dominant hemisphere usually the left. Liaison brain thus represents all those areas of cerebral cortex which are capable of direct liaison with the self-conscious mind or the "second world". In commissurotomy patients this is restricted to the dominant hemisphere, especially the language areas. However, there may well be some liaison areas in the minor hemisphere too.

The set of fundamental rules concerning storage and transmission of information from site to site in brain is called the brain code. It is concerned with the mechanism by which large groups of neurons transmit images, thoughts and feelings which are the fundamental units of our psychological life.

Mental activity is unconsciously motivated. Today's neuroscientific findings confirm what Frued said in early 1900's. It is becoming increasingly clear that a good deal of our mental activity is unconsciously motivated.

Neuroscientists have identified unconscious memory systems that mediate emotional learning. The existence of a neural pathway that by-passes hippocampus, which generates conscious memories, and connects perceptual information with primitive brain that generates fear response, has been demonstrated. The core brain stem and limbic system corresponds to Freud's id. The ventral (inferior) frontal cortex controls selective inhibition = Ego. The dorsal frontal region controls self-conscious thought = Ego. Posterior cortex represents outside world = Super ego.

It has been hypothesized that the brain uses structures designed to map both the organism and external objects to create a fresh, second-order representation. This representation indicates that the organism, as mapped in the brain, is involved in interacting with an object, also mapped in the brain.

Many neuroscientists believe that there is no mind without brain. Mind is brain. Mind and brain are inseparable.

The scientific teachings of our faith exalted however describe mind as a separate entity from the physical brain.

Whatever mental function we consider it is possible to identify distinct parts of the brain that contribute to the production of that function by working in concert. A close correspondence exists between the appearance of mental state or behavior and the activity of the selected brain regions. And that correspondence can be established between a macroscopically identifiable region and function for example, the primary visual context and vision, a language related area and speech *etc*.

ELECTROMAGNETIC STIMULATION OF BRAIN

Electrical activity can be induced in specific brain areas with pulse magnetic fields. It has been tested in depressed patient and has given good results. It is also being tried to rouse people from fatigue or to teach them new skills.

Persinger's "God Helmet", in which temporal lobe is thus stimulated is a variant of the same technique.

Newer theories also hypothesize that brain and self-conscious mind are independent entities. The dualistic hypotheses.

I humbly thank Most Revered Professor P.S. Satsangi Sahab for granting me the inspiration and strength in pursuit of truth and knowledge which has enabled me to compile the above concepts.

Coping Strategies of Coronary Heart Disease Patients Treated with Medicines Only and Treated with Surgery

P.K. Mona[1] and Monika Abrol[2]

ABSTRACT

The present study tries to investigate the coping style, anxiety and depression with the severity of coronary heart disease. The severity is divided into two groups, *i.e.,* of surgically (coronary artery by-pass grafting) and medically managed CHD patients. *Ex-post facto* research design was used. Sample for the present study consisted of 50 coronary heart disease male patients, randomly selected from Escort Heart Institute, Delhi, age range from 35 to 50 years who have participated in the various Coronary Care Units (CCU) on the recommendation of their cardiologists. Out of 50, 25 were medically treated and the rest 25 were surgically managed patients. Coping Response Inventory by Moss (1993), PAI Depression Scale by Krug and Laughlin (1984), and The Strait Trait Anxiety Inventory by Spielberger (1977) were used to compare the coping styles of both the groups. Results indicate that the significant difference exists in the anxiety and depression level of both the groups but no significant difference has been found between the severity of coronary heart disease and the coping styles.

INTRODUCTION

Human life can be viewed conceptually as having two principal characteristics, quality and quantity (Ware, 1997). Disorders of health can adversely affect both of these features. Over the last 200 years, advances in medical technology have dramatically altered the prevailing view of what health is. Initially conceived as freedom from death (when mortality rates were high and life expectancy was short) and subsequently as freedom from disease, health is now defined in terms of positive concepts such as functional excellence or happiness and well being. Advances in medical technology have provided cures for many acute diseases, particularly infectious diseases that were previously fatal. Medicine proved to be dramatic cure and controlled palliation of these disorders over the last 50 years, but in many cases cure is still not possible. The term happiness and well-being are used for good health, a reflection of mental state and directly related to it. Therefore psychology becomes the second crutch along with medicine for quick recovery from any disease.

* Corresponding author.

[1,2] Department of Psychology, Dayalbagh Educational Institute, Deemed University, Dayalbagh, Agra, UP, India. E-mail: [2]monika_6aug@yahoo.co.in

Within psychology, health psychology is the field devoted to understanding psychological influences on how people stay healthy, why they become ill and how they respond when they do get ill. The basic idea of health psychologists is that the mind and body together determine health and illness, and this idea logically implies a model for studying these issues. This model is called the Bio-psychosocial Model. This model maintains that health and illness are caused by multiple factors and produce multiple effects. From this viewpoint, health becomes something that one achieves through attention to biological, psychological and social needs rather than something that is taken for granted. Dunbar's (1943) and Alexander's (1950) work helped shape the emerging field of psychosomatic medicine by offering profiles of particular disorders believed to be psychosomatic in origin—that is, bodily disorders caused by emotional conflict, cardiovascular disorder is one of them.

Cardiovascular Disorders (CVD) are medical problems involving the heart and blood circulation system, such as 'essential hypertension' and 'coronary heart disease'. 'Essential hypertension' refers to elevation of blood pressure that has no identified cause. Coronary Heart Disease (CHD) takes two important forms, angina pectoris and myocardial infarction. This silent illness is to be the single best prediction of both heart attack and stroke.

One possible result of restriction of blood supply to the myocardium is 'angina pectoris', a disorder with symptoms of crushing pain in the chest and difficulty in breathing. Angina is usually precipitated by exercise or stress because these conditions increase demand to the heart. With oxygen restriction, the reserve capacity of the cardiovascular system is reduced, and heart disease becomes evident. The uncomfortable symptoms of angina rarely last more than a few minutes, but angina is a sign of obstruction in the coronary arteries.

'Myocardial infraction' is the medical term for the condition commonly referred to as a heart attack. During myocardial infarction, the damage may be as extensive as to completely disrupt the heartbeat. The signals for a myocardial infarction include a feeling of weakness or dizziness combined with nausea, cold sweating, difficulty in breathing and sensation of crushing pain in the chest and arms, jaw or back. Rapid loss of consciousness or death may occur.

The link between the heart and emotions has been described for thousands of years in religious writings and ancient's medical texts. William Harvey more than 300 years ago helped usher in many current ideas on the connections between the brain and the heart with the statement, "Every affection of the mind that is attended with either pain or pleasure hope or fear, is the cause of an agitation whose influence extends to the heart".

Since it is known that no individual can remain in a continuous state of tension, some strategy is always adopted by a person undergoing stress to deal with stress. These strategies are called 'Coping Strategies'. The coping activities are consciously directed behaviors intended to modify, and to terminate, symptoms. It is true that the emotions and physiological arousal created by stressful situations are highly uncomfortable, and this discomfort motivates the individual to do something to alleviate it. The process by which a person attempts to manage stressful demands is called 'Coping Strategies'.

Two general types of coping strategies can be distinguished: Problem-Solving Efforts and Emotion Focused Coping (Folkman, Schaefer and Lazarus 1979; Leventhal and Nerenz 1982). 'Problem-solving Efforts' are attempts to do some thing constructive about the stressful condition that are harming, threatening or challenging an individual. 'Emotion-Focused Coping' involves efforts to regulate the emotional consequences of the stressful event.

The epidemiological research shows that the conditions of the human living in modern world continuously generate stressful situations in which a wide range of neuro-endocrine, autonomic and immune parameters, elevated blood pressure and chronic troubling emotions are deeply involved.

Most of the so-called civilized persons are in hurry, worry, tension, irregular habit indulgences, abuse of drink-drug-smoke *etc.* These are indirectly contributing to the heavy toll of increased morbidity and mortality, CHD is one of them, it affects all aspects of a patient's life. Immediately after, a coronary heart disease is diagnosed, patients are often in a state of crises marked by physical, social and psychological disequilibrium. They opt different type of coping strategies. Negative emotions may take place. Anger or depression, and anxiety can be thought of as part of the coping process just as are actions that are voluntarily undertaken to confront the event. Patients opt different types of coping strategies according to the severity of heart disease. The present study is aimed to compare the coping strategies of medically treated and surgically managed coronary heart disease patients.

METHODOLOGY

Problem

To compare the coping strategies of medically treated and surgically managed coronary heart disease patients.

Objectives

- To find out the difference in the severity of coronary heart disease and coping styles.

- To find out the difference in the severity of coronary heart disease and level of anxiety.
- To find out the difference in the severity of coronary heart disease and depression.

Design

Ex-post facto research design was used in the present study.

Sample

The sample for the present study consisted of fifty coronary heart disease male patients, age-range from 35 to 50 years who have participated in the various Coronary Care Units (CCU) on recommendation of their respected cardiologists. These patients were randomly selected from Escort Heart Institute, Delhi. Out of 50, 25 were medically treated and the rest 25 were surgically managed. Only By-Pass surgery cases were taken. Both the patients groups were matched in terms of duration of illness, socio-economic status, educational level and marital status. Study was restricted only to married couples who were both alive.

Tool Used

Three psychological tests were used to compare the coping strategies of surgically managed and medically treated coronary heart disease patient.

- IPAT Depression scale-Krug and Laughlin (1984)
- State-Trait Anxiety Inventory by Spielberger (1977)
- Coping Response Inventory (CRI)-Moos (1993).

Statistical Analysis

t-test was used to compare the coping strategies of medically treated and surgically managed CHD patients.

RESULT, DISCUSSION AND CONCLUSION

The present study is aimed to compare the coping strategies of medically treated and surgically managed coronary heart disease. t-test has been used to compare the coping strategies of the two groups, and results are presented in Tables 1, 2 and 3; Graphs 1, 2 and 3.

Table 1: Comparison of the Coping Styles of Medical and Surgical CHD Patients

S. No.	*Coping Styles*	*Medically Treated*		*Surgically Managed*		*t-values*
		Mean	*SDs*	*Mean*	*SDs*	
1.	Logical Analysis	46.36	9.31	47.31	10.62	0.33*
2.	Positive Reappraisal	55.44	10.11	54.63	11.12	0.27*
3.	Guidance & Support	48.08	8.65	50.62	10.51	0.93*
4.	Problem Solving	46.28	9.32	47.91	10.8	0.57*
5.	Cognitive Avoidance	49.44	9.88	50.32	10.1	0.11*
6.	Acceptance/Resignation	49.56	10.61	46.21	11.3	1.08*
7.	Alternative Reward	48.76	10.82	49.32	10.8	0.18*
8.	Emotional Discharge	51.36	11.32	53.81	10.6	0.79*

*Non-significant at .05 level.

Table 2: Comparison of the State—Trait Anxiety of the Medical and Surgical CHD Patients

S. No.	*Anxiety Type*	*Medically Treated*		*Surgically Managed*		*t-values*
		Means	*SDs*	*Means*	*SDs*	
1.	State Anxiety	50.3	8.97	57.9	10.32	2.78*
2.	Trait Anxiety	52.6	9.32	60.4	9.8	2.88*

*Significant at .01 level.

Table 3: Comparison of the Depression scores in Medical and Surgical CHD Patients

S. No.	*Depression Scale*	*Medically Treated*		*Surgically Managed*		*t-value*
		Means	*SD*	*Means*	*SD*	
1.	Depression Scale	70.2	11.9	82.6	12.6	3.58*

*Significant at .01 level.

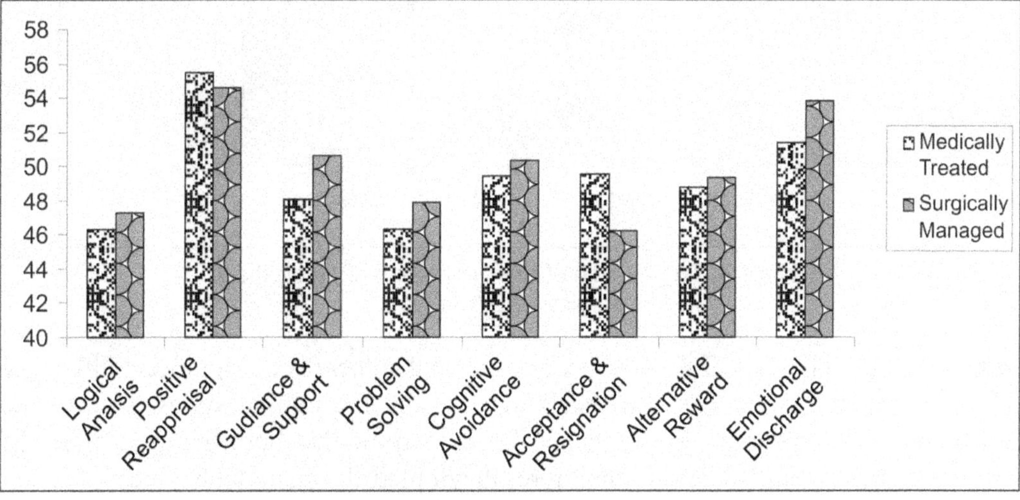

Graph 1: Comparison of the Coping Styles of Medical and Surgical CHD Patients

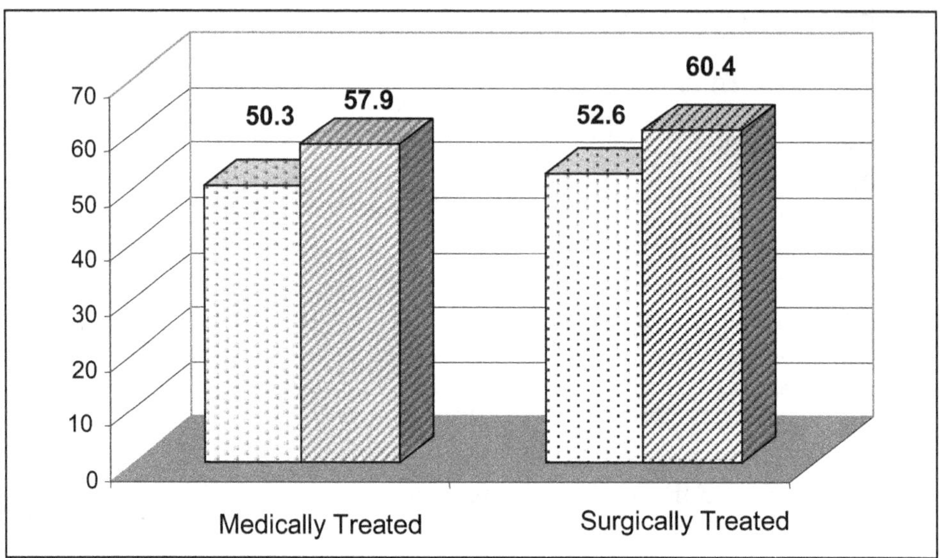

Graph 2: Comparison of the State-Trait Anxiety of the Medical and Surgical CHD Patients

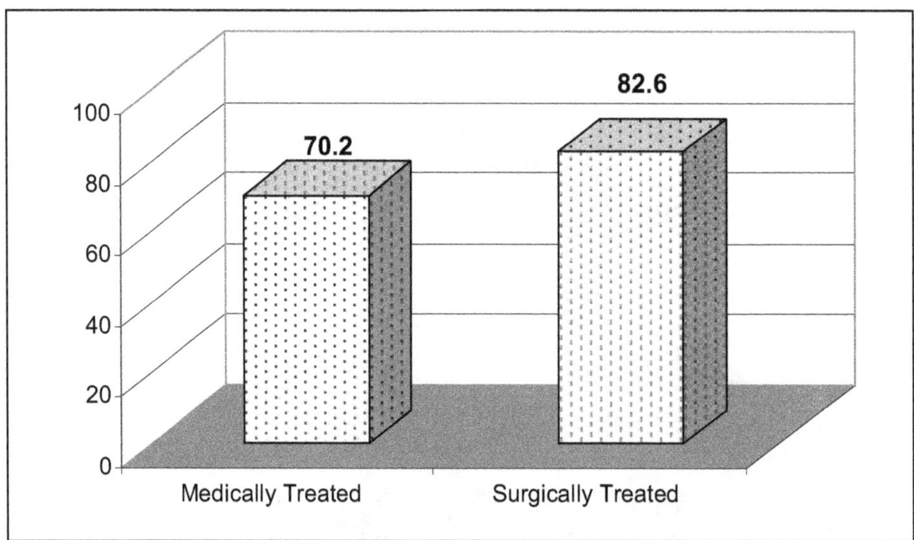

Graph 3: Comparison of the Depression of Medical and Surgical CHD Patients

From the results shown in Table 1 it becomes clear that there is no significant difference between the severity of coronary heart disease and the coping styles. One of the probable causes behind the insignificant results may be that both the groups are the sufferer of the same disease and therefore, they opted the same techniques of facing this mortific disease in spite of differences in their severity.

Although the values are not found statistically significant yet the results show certain trends such as the acceptance/resignation and positive reappraisal coping scores are slightly higher in the medically treated CHD patients. They understand that the heart ailment will always be associated with them for the whole life. They have to depend on the medicine; therefore they accept these kinds of coping strategies.

The 'Logical analysis', 'guidance and support', 'problem-solving', 'cognitive-avoidance' 'alternative-rewards', and 'emotional discharge', coping strategies were accepted more by surgically treated CHD patients. The cause might be that those CHD patients who have suffered from by-pass grafting, experienced more painful time, more complications were also in their life, more restrictions and of course more expenditure than the other group. Therefore they try to get involved in substitute activities and create new source of satisfaction.

The results also show that both the groups scored high in the emotional discharge coping style. They evaporate their stress by expressing negative feeling, such as shouting, crying showing anger hostility *etc*. They become dependent on their cardiologist and the family members.

Table 2 shows the significant difference between the severity of the coronary heart disease and the level of anxiety. The surgical patients were found high on state and trait anxiety both. This may be the result of the host of problems they have been exposed to, such as pain, financial burden, need for caring in getting operation conducted and the fear of impending death. Secondly surgery is the last curing method of the CHD patients.

From Table 3 it is clear that there is significant difference between the severity of CHD and depression. Depression is significantly related to the surgically managed CHD patients. It is one of the major psychological dimensions which is more or less associated with any dreaded disease. The surgical patients have to spend most of the hours either at home or in the hospital wards. The loneliness is one of the major cause contributing to depression. Secondly, due to the severity they develop of cardiophobia, they remain depressed and disturbed.

Throughout the 20th century, Cardiovascular Disease (CVD), including various types of heart disease, was the leading cause of death and disability in this country. It is a general observation that once the patient is diagnosed for cardiac surgery, intense feelings of disorganization, anxiety, fear and other negative emotions may take place.

In such cases patients tend to adopt a number of coping strategies to deal with their illness, including attempts to focus on the positive aspect of the disease. Besides focusing on the positive, the patients who experienced the least emotional distress tend to seek 'social support' and to try to distance themselves emotionally from their illness. Those who experienced more emotional distress tend to cope by using strategies of 'cognitive' or 'behavioral avoidance', such as wishing that the situation would go away or avoiding the situation by misusing drugs, alcohol or food.

Those cardiac patients who react negatively against this mortific disease, psychological intervention may be helpful. 'Psychological counseling' can ameliorate the experience of hospitalization, counteract some of the anxiety of being monitored while intensive care, and increase the patient's confidence in the hospital equipment and personnel. A program of in-hospital counseling tested the effectiveness of counseling for heart attack survivors and spouses.

'Emotional' and 'Social' support provided by spouses can be important for cardiac patients, especially for surgically managed groups; social support lessens the experience of both stress and distress and that social support was more important in the first 6 months after hospitalization than in the next 6 months. Cardiac rehabilitation programs attempt to help heart patients increase their level of physical, social and psychological functioning. These programs typically include regimens for life style changes as well as interventions aimed at reducing the harmful psychological effects of coronary heart disease on patients and their families. Good clinical management may be the key to success.

REFERENCES

Alexander, F. (1950). *Psychosomatic Medicine.* New York: Norton.

Dunbar, F. (1943). *Psychosomatic Diagnosis.* New York: Hoeber.

Folkman, S., Schaefer, C. and Lazarus, R.S. (1979). "Cognative Processes as Mediators of Stress and Coping." In V. Hamilton and Warburton, D.M. (Eds.), *Human Stress and Cognition: An Information Processing Approach,* London, England: Wiley.

Krug, S.E. and Laughlin, J.E. (1984). *Personal Assessment Inventory (PAI) Depression Scale,* New Delhi: Psychological Center.

Leventhal, H. and Nerenz, D.R. (1982). "A Model for Stress Research and Some Implications for the Control of Stress Disorders." In D. Meichenbaum and M. Jaremko (Eds.), *Stress and Prevention and Management: A Cognitive Behavioral Approach*, New York: Plenum.

Moos, R. (1993). *Coping Response Inventory-Adult from Manual.* Odessa, FL. Psychological Assessment Resources.

Spielberger, C.D., Gorscuch, R.L. and Lushene, R. (1977). *Manual for the State-Trait Anxiety Inventory* (Self Evaluation Questionnaire). Pallootto Cadif. Consultant Psychological Press.

Ware, J.E. (1997). "Standards for Validating Health Measures, Definition and Content." *Journal of Chronic Disorder,* 40, 473–480.

Physical Activity of Diabetics and Non-Diabetics

Ira Das*[1] and Sheenu Chaudhary[2]

ABSTRACT

A two matched group design was used to compare the activity level of type II diabetic (*N* = 23) and non-diabetic (*N* = 23) individuals. The patients included in the sample were all 1st generation diabetics. Age range of subjects was between 40 to 75 years. The tool used was Physical Activity Scale prepared by the investigator herself. It has four categories of activities (i) Inactivity (ii) Light Physical Activity (iii) High Physical Activity (iv) Rigorous Physical Activity. Result showed a significant difference in the mean scores of 'Rigorous Physical Activity' between diabetic and non-diabetic individuals ($t = 2.59$ $p < 0.01$). A significant difference was also found in the mean scores of 'High Physical Activity' of diabetic and non-diabetic individuals ($t = 2.002$ $p < 0.05$). The significant difference found in the mean 'Inactivity' scores of diabetic and non-diabetic individuals ($t = 2.10$ $p < 0.05$) indicated that diabetics spend more time on inactivity than the non-diabetics. No significant difference was found in the mean scores of 'Light Physical Activity' between diabetic and non-diabetic individuals ($t = 1.43$ $p > 0.05$). Thus physical activity of diabetic group was found to be significantly low in comparison to that of the non-diabetic group.

INTRODUCTION

Diabetes is a clinical syndrome characterized by hyperglycemia due to deficiency or diminished effectiveness of insulin, a disturbed chemical balance in the body. The word diabetes comes from a Greek expression meaning, "Siphon" and refers to the increased urination and thirst, which often occur in newly diagnosed or uncontrolled cases. These symptoms are due to the high sugar (glucose) content in the urine and blood. Diabetes is a chronic condition of impaired carbohydrate, protein and fat metabolism that results from insufficient secretion of insulin or from insulin resistance. The cells of the body need energy to function, and the primary source of energy is glucose, a simple sugar that results from the digestion of foods containing carbohydrates.

Insulin is a hormone, produced by the beta cells of the pancreas that acts essentially as a key to permit glucose to enter the cells. When there is not enough insulin produced or when insulin resistance develops (that is, the glucose can no longer be used by the cells) glucose stays in the blood instead of entering the cells, resulting in a condition

*Corresponding author.

[1, 2]Department of Psychology, Dayalbagh Educational Institute, Deemed University, Dayalbagh, Agra, UP, India. E-mail: [2]sheenuchoudhary14@gmail.com

called hyperglycemia. The body attempts to rid itself of this excess glucose, yet the cells are not receiving the glucose they need and send signals to the hypothalamus that more food is needed.

The reason that diabetes is such a major public health problem stems less from the consequences of insufficient insulin production *per se.* than from the complications that may develop. Diabetes is associated with a thickening of the arteries due to the build up of wastes in the blood. As a consequence, diabetic patients show high rate of coronary heart disease. Diabetes is a leading cause of blindness among adults, and it accounts for 50% of all the patients who require renal dialysis for kidney failure. Diabetes may also be associated with nervous system damage, including pain and loss of sensation. As a consequence of these complications, diabetics have a shorter life expectancy than do non-diabetic individuals. Diabetes may also exacerbate other difficulties in psychological functioning, contributing to eating disorders (Carroll, Tiggermann and Wade, 1999) and sexual dysfunction in both men and women (Spector, Leiblum, Carey and Rosen, 1993; Weinhardt and Carey, 1996), as well as depression (Talbot, Nouwen, Gingras, Belanger and Audet, 1999), among other problems. Diabetes may produce central nervous system impairment that interferes with memory (Taylor and Rachman, 1988), especially among the elderly (Mooradian, Perryman, Fitten, Kavonian and Morley, 1988).

There are two major types of diabetes mellitus, (i) Insulin-Dependent Diabetes Mellitus (IDDM) or Type I diabetes and (ii) Non-Insulin Dependent Diabetes Mellitus (NIDDM) or Type II diabetes. They differ in origin, pathology, role of genetics in their development, age of onset, and treatment. Type I (or insulin-dependent diabetes mellitus IDDM) diabetes usually develops relatively early in life, earlier for girls than for boys, between the ages of 5 years and 6 years or later between 10 years and 13 years. Type I diabetes is characterized by the abrupt onset of symptoms, which result from lack of insulin production by the beta cells of the pancreas. Type II (or non-insulin-dependent diabetes mellitus NIDDM) diabetes is milder than the insulin dependent type. Type II diabetes is typically a disorder of middle and old age striking those primarily over the age of 40. As obesity is a major contributor it has become more prevalent, especially at earlier ages. This type of diabetes is increasing at astronomical rates.

According to Mohan, Sandeep, Deepa, Shah and Varghese (2007), India leads the world with largest number of diabetic patients earning the dubious distinction of being termed the 'diabetes capital of the world'. Type II diabetes is the commonest form of diabetes constituting 90% of the diabetes population. The global prevalence of diabetes is estimated to increase from 4% in 1995 to 5.4% by the year 2025. The World Health Organization has predicted that the major burden will occur in the developing countries. There will be a 42% increases from 51 to 72 million in the developed countries and 170% increase from 84 to 228 million, in the developing countries. The countries with the largest number of diabetic people are, and will be the year 2025, India, China and United States (King, Herman, and Aubert, 1998).

IMPACT OF PHYSICAL ACTIVITY

Regular physical activity, fitness, and exercise are critically important for the health and well-being of people of all ages. Research has demonstrated that virtually all individuals can benefit from regular physical activity, whether they participate in vigorous exercise or some type of moderate health-enhancing physical activity. Even among frail and very old adults, mobility and functioning can be improved through physical activity.

According to Ramchandran *et al.* (2001) the rise in abdominal obesity are related to low physical activity in women; the percentage with moderate to heavy physical activity being reduced by half in 2000 A.D.

A study by Mohan *et al.* (2001) in Chennai showed that the total activity level considering the activity at work and during leisure time was very low especially in women. The activity score was inversely related to the affluence or wealth score and low activity score showed adverse effects on glucose intolerance. The affluence was calculated using a wealth score system and a significant correlation was seen between increasing wealth score and decreasing total activity. Sedentary life style was one of the significant factors associated with diabetes in this population (Ramchandran, Snehalattha and Vijay, 2002).

A preventive study done in India based on Diabetes Prevention Programme has documented the importance of physical activity in the prevention of diabetes (Ramchandran, Mary, *et al.,* 2006). According to Mohan, *et al.* (2003), prevalence of diabetics was almost three times higher in individuals with light physical activity compared to those doing heavy physical activity.

The understanding of health benefits of physical activity has rapidly increased in recent years. Especially during last two decades it has been proved by Oldridge (1984), Ward and Morgan (1984), and Dishman, *et al.* (1985), that adherence to physical activity is poor even in supervised program for physical activity. To result in true health benefits, it need to be practiced on a permanent basis (Wankel, 1984). Data on the determination of physical activity have been obtained mostly from correlation studies of high intensity activity within supervised settings. Most of the intervention trials performed have also focused on high intensity activity with, as a rule, only a few months follow-up. Specific data on the unsupervised long term maintenance of health related physical activity is thus scarce.

Physical activity is defined 'as any body movement produced by the skeletal muscles and resulting in an increase in energy expenditure' (Bouchard, 1990). This definition is a purely physiological one stripping the activity of its motive and meaning to the individuals, its unique position in the individuals' life style and its place in the socio cultural situation, aspects which are all believed to influence health.

Depending on its intensity, physical activity varies in terms of its long term effects on the organism. In the light of the current scientific evidences the physiological health effects of very light and light activities are estimated as minor and inconsistent, except for psychological and social benefits. The recent evidence indicates, however, that 'moderate' activity, at the level of, for example, brisk walking, if carried out continuously at least 30 min. daily, involves metabolic and physiological functions to such an extent that, with regular practice, important health benefits result in terms of weight control, blood pressure, glucose and lipid metabolism and reduced morbidity and mortality (Bouchard *et al.*, 1990–94; Fletcher *et al.*, 1995; Pate *et al.*, 1995). 'Heavy' and 'Very Heavy' activities when carried out at least 20 min. at a time, three or four times a week result in the same as or possibly in even greater health benefits than 'moderate' activity (Bouchard *et al.*, 1990–1994). Studies by Dishman and Sallis (1994) indicate that long-term activities with duration over 6 months help in successful maintenance of health (Emery, *et al.* 1992).

Regular physical activity reduces the risk of developing or dying from some of the leading causes of illness in the United States (U.S. Department of Health and Human Services, 1996). Regular physical activity improves health in the following ways. Reduces the risk of developing diabetes, high blood pressure, colon and breast cancer and promotes psychological well-being.

The investigator however feels that in their busy and hectic life schedules, many people cannot find time for physical exercise while the others, who do not give it sufficient importance, are not willing to find time for physical exercise. They would engage themselves in rigorous physical activities so that no extra physical exercises are needed.

Objective

A comparative analysis of physical activity level of diabetics and non-diabetics.

Hypothesis

There exists a significant difference in physical activity level of diabetics and non-diabetics, activity level of non-diabetics being higher.

Design

Ex-post facto research design.

Sample

The sample for the study consisted of two groups. Group I consisted of approximately 23 diabetic patients in the age range of 40 to 75 years taken from the clinics of physicians. Group II was a matched group of 23 non-diabetics who were matched with group I in terms of Age, Education, Marital Status, and Socio Economic Status. The following inclusion and exclusion criteria were followed for selection of diabetics in group I:

- Patients were diagnosed by doctor to have Type II diabetes and were under treatment for diabetes at least for last one year.
- The patients were 1st generation diabetic. The patients whose parents or grand parents had been diabetics were included in the sample.
- Age range of subjects between 40 to 75 years.
- Education at least class XII passed.
- Marital Status: Married.

Measures

1. Diabetes was diagnosed on the basis of doctors (Pathologist) report obtained during last six months. If the blood sugar level after fasting was beyond the normal value of 70–100 mg/dl, the person was called as a diabetic.
2. For measuring Activity level, Physical Activity level Scale prepared by the investigator herself was used. The responses were classified into four categories: (i) Physical inactivity (ii) Routine (light) Physical activity (iii) High Physical activity (iv) Rigorous Physical activity. A score of zero for physical inactivity, one for routine (light) activity, two for high physical activity, three for rigorous physical activity were awarded to each item of the scale. A total of all the scores in the scale was an indicator of physical activity of the individual.

Results

Table 1 indicates that a significant difference exists in activity level of diabetics and non-diabetics, activity level of non-diabetics being higher.

The t-value of rigorous physical activity is 2.594 with df = 44 which is significant at .01 level. It indicates that non-diabetics spend more time (M = 185.217, SD = 69.86) on rigorous physical activity (for example: Gardening, Physical Exercise, Yoga, Field work, Cycling, Walking, Swimming, Jogging and Sports and outdoor games) than the diabetic individuals (M = 123.91, SD = 89.22).

The table further indicates that the t-value of high physical activity is 2.002 with df = 44 which is significant at .05 level. It indicates that non-diabetics spend more time (M = 474.78, SD = 97.27) on high physical activity (for example: Marketing, Cooking, Manual Washing, Sewing, Dusting) than the diabetic individuals (M = 409.56, SD = 122.23).

Result Table 1: Physical Activity of Diabetics and Non-Diabetics

(N = 23 in each group)

Measures	*Non-Diabetic*		*Diabetic*		*t*
	Mean	*S.D*	*Mean*	*S.D.*	
Inactivity	558.26	153.96	663.91	185.44	2.102 (p < .05)
Light Physical Activity	161.73	61.17	187.82	60.82	1.450 (p > .05)
High Physical Activity	474.78	97.27	409.56	122.23	2.002 (p < .05)
Rigorous Physical Activity	185.217	69.86	123.91	89.22	2.594 (p < .01)

The table further indicates that the t-value of light physical activity is 1.45 with df = 44 which is not significant at .05 level. It indicates that there is no significant difference in light physical activity of diabetics (M = 187.82, SD = 60.82) and non-diabetics (M = 161.73, SD = 61.17).

The table further indicates that the t-value of inactivity is 2.102 with df = 44 which is significant at .05 level. It indicates that the significant difference in inactivity of diabetics (M = 663.91, SD = 185.44) and non-diabetics (M = 558.26, SD = 153.96).Thus physical activity of diabetics was found to be significantly low in comparison to non-diabetics. It is therefore proved that time duration of different levels of physical activity is an important cause of diabetes.

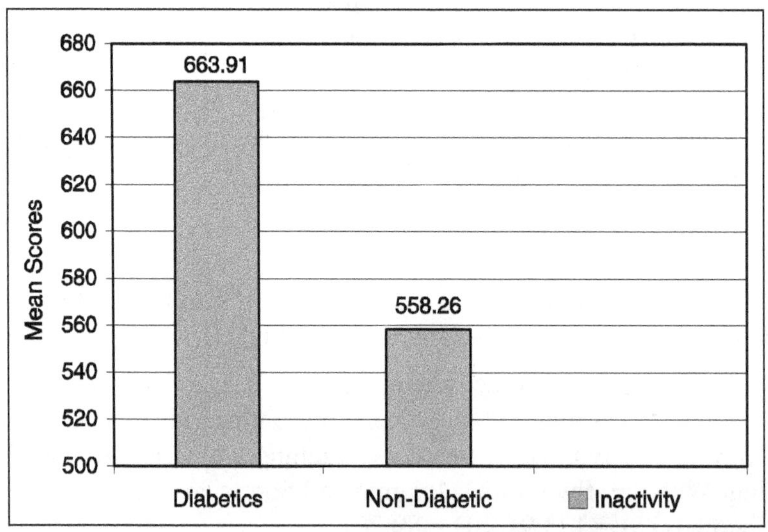

Graph 1: Inactivity of Diabetics and Non-Diabetics

Graph 1 indicated that diabetics remain inactive for grater time period, in comparison to non-diabetics. Similarly Graph 2 also indicated that diabetics spend most of their time in light physical activities, in comparison to non-diabetics.

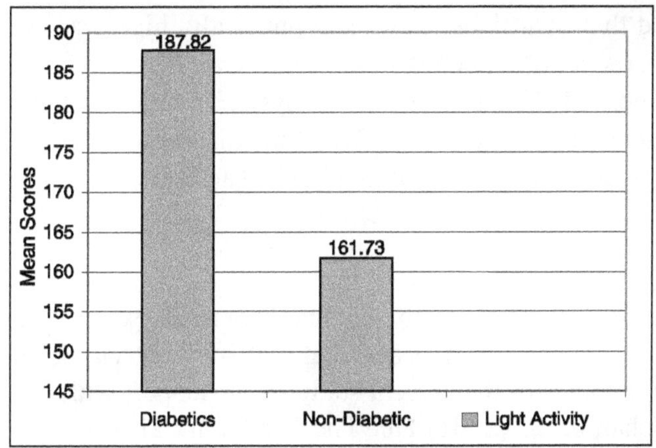

Graph 2: Light Physical Activity of Diabetics and Non-Diabetics

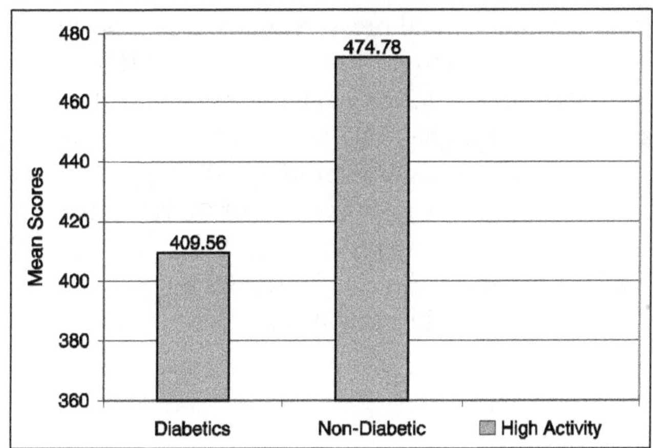

Graph 3: High Physical Activity of Diabetics and Non-Diabetics

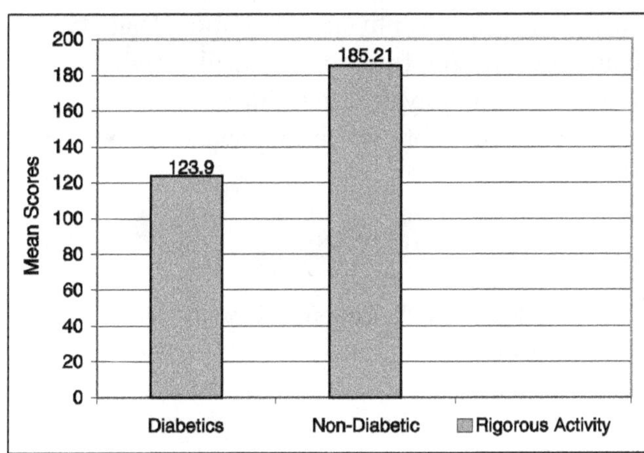

Graph 4: Rigorous Physical Activity of Diabetics and Non-Diabetics

Graph 3 indicated that non-diabetics remain physically highly active for greater time period, in comparison to diabetics. Similarly, Graph 4 also indicated that non-diabetics spend most of their time in high physical activities, and rigorous physical activities in comparison to diabetics. Therefore diabetics were advised to increase their rigorous physical activities and high physical activities.

DISCUSSION

The results of the present study led to conclude that there exist a significant difference in physical activity level of diabetics and non-diabetics, activity level of non-diabetics being higher. The findings of the present study are in support with that of Ramchandran *et al.* (2003), Mohan *et al.* (2001) *etc.* The results are also in agreement which the studies made by Paffenbarger, Hyde, Wing, *et al.* (1993) which indicate that physical activity has been shown to reduce the risk of developing or dying from heart disease, diabetes, colon cancer, and high blood pressure. On average, people who are physically active outlive those who are inactive. Ford, Liu *et al.* (1997) also found that it is important for individuals who are currently at a healthy weight to strive to maintain it since both modest and large weight gains are associated with significantly increased risk of disease. For example, a weight gain of 11 to 18 pounds increases a person's risk for developing type 2 diabetes to twice that of individuals who have not gained weight, while those who gain 44 pounds or more have four times the risk of type 2 diabetes. Tuomilehto, Lindstrom *et al.* (2001) found positive impact of regular physical activity mediated by weight control and other mechanism.

CONCLUSION

Thus the conclusion is that the major health benefit of regular physical activity is the prevention of type II diabetes. So diabetics are advised to spend minimum time on inactivity (sleep, relaxing) and light physical activities. Diabetics are also advised to develop a positive attitude towards rigorous physical activities and to spend more of their time on high and rigorous physical activities. Doing rigorous physical activity with productive output would be more interesting and at the same time more beneficial for their health.

REFERENCES

Bouchard, C., Shephard, R.J., Stephens, T., Sutton, J.R. and McPherson, B.D. (1990). "Exercise, Fitness and Health:" *A Consensus of Current Knowledge,* Human Kinetics, Champaign II.

Bouchard, C., Shephard, R.J. and Stephens, T. (1994). Physical Activity, Fitness and Health: *International Proceedings and Consensus Statement. Humans Kinetics,* Champaign II.

Butler R.N., Davis, R. and Lewis, C.B. (1998). "Physical Fitness: Benefits of Exercising for the Older Patient." *Geriatrics,* 53 (10) 46–62.

Carrol, P., Tiggemann, M. and Wade, T. (1999). "The Role of Body Dissatisfaction and Bingeing in the Self-esteem of Women with Type-II Diabetes." *Journal of Behavioral Medicine, 22,* 59–74.

Dishman, R.K. and Sallis, J.F. (1994). "Determinants and Interventions for Physical Activity and Exercise." In Bouchard, C., Shephared, R.J. and Stephens, T. (Eds). *Physical Activity Fitness and Health: International Proceedings and Consensus Statement.* Human Kinetics Champaign, II, 77–88.

Dishman, R.K., Sallis, J.F. and Orenstein, D.R. (1985). "The Determinants of Physical Activity and Exercise." *Public Health Reports*, 100, 158–171.

Emery, C.F., Hanck, E.R. and Blumenthal, J.A. (1992). "Exercise Adherence or Maintenance among Older Adults: 1 year Follow Up Study. " *Psychology and Aging*, 7, 466–470.

Fletcher, G.F., Balady, G., Froelicher, V.F., Hartley, L.H., Haskell, W.L. and Pollock, M.L. (1995). "Exercise Standards. A Statement for Healthcare Professionals from the American Heart Association." *Circulation*, 91, 580–615.

Ford, E.S., Williamson, D.F. and Liu, S. "Weight Change and Diabetes Incidence (1997): Findings from a National Cohort of US Adults." *Am J. Epidemiol,* 146(3), 214–22.

King, H., Aubert, R.E. and Herman, W.H. (1998). *Diabetes Care*, 21, 1414–1431.

Mohan, V., Deepa, M., Deepa, R., Shantirani, C.S., Farooq, S. and Ganesan, A. (2006). "Secular Trends in the Prevalence of Diabetes and Glucose Tolerance in Urban South India-the Chennai Urban Rural Epidemiology Study." *Diabetologiea,* 49, 1175–1178.

Mohan, V., Sandeep, S. Deepa, R., Shah, B. and Varghese, C. (2007). "Epidemiology of Type 2 Diabetes: Indian Scenario." *Indian Journal of Medical Research,* 125, 217–230.

Mohan, V., Shanthirani, S., Deepa, R., Premalatha, G., Sastry, N.G. and Saroja, R. (2001). *Diabetes Medicine,* 18, 280–287.

Mooradian, A.D., Perryman, K., Fitten, J., Kavonian, G.D. and Morley, J.E. (1988). "Cortical Function in Elderly No-insulin Dependent Dialectic Patients." *Archives of Internal Medicine,* 148, 2369–2372.

Old ridge, N.B. (1984). "Adherence to Adult Exercise Fitness Programs." In Matarazzo, J.O. (Ed.) *A Handbook of Health Enhancement and Disease Prevention,* New York: John Welay, 467–487.

Paffenbarger, R.S., Hyde, R.T. and Wing, A.L. (1993). "The Association of Changes in Physical-activity Level and Other Lifestyle Characteristics with Mortality among Men." *N. Engl. J. Med.,* 328(8), 538–45.

Pate, R.R., Pratt, M., Blair, S.N., Haskell, W.L., Maccra, C.A., Bouchard, C., Bouchner, D., Ettinger, W., Health G.W., King, A. C., Kriska, A., Leon, A.S., Macus, B.H., Morris, J., Paffenbarger, R.S., Patric, K., Pollock, M.L., Rippe, J.M., Sallies, J. and Wilmore, J.H. (1995). "Physical Activity and Public Health. A Recommendation from the Centers for Disease Control and Prevention and the American College of Sports Medicine." *Journal of American Medical Association,* 273, 402–407.

Ramchandran, A., Senhaltha, C. and Vijay, V. (2002). *Diabetes Research Clinical Practices,* 58, 55–60.

Ramchandran, A., Snehalatha, C., Kapur, A., Vijay, V., Mohan, V. and Das, A.K. (2001). "Diabetes Epidemiology Study Groups in India. High Prevalence of Diabetes and Impaired Glucose Tolerance in India: National Urban Diabetes Survey." *Diabetologia,* 44 1094–101.

Ramchandran, A., Snehalatha, C., Mary, S., Mukesh, B., Bhaskar A.D. and Vijay, V. (2006). "Indian Diabetes Prevention Programme. The I.D.P.P shows that Life Style Modification and Metformin Prevent Type-2 Diabetes in Asian Indian Subjects with Impaired Glucose Tolerancei." *Diabetologia,* 49, 289–297.

Spector, I.P., Leiblum, S.R., Carey, M.P. and Rosen, R.C. (1993). "Diabetes and Female Sexual Function: A Critical Review." *Annals of Behavioral Medicine,* 15, 257–264.

Talbot, F., Novwen, A., Gingras, J. Belanger, A. and Audet, J. (1999). "Relations of Diabetes Intrusiveness and Personal Control to Symptoms of Depression among Adults with Diabetes." *Health Psychology,* 18, 537–542.

Taylor, L.A. and Rachman, S.J. (1988). "The Effects of Blood Sugar Level Changes on Cognitive Function, Effective State, and Somatic Symptoms." *Journal of Behavioral Medicine,* 11, 279–292.

Taylor, S.E. (2006). "Heart Disease, Hypertension, Stroke, and Diabetes." *Health Psychology,* 6, 367–375.

The Diabetes Prevention Program Research Group (2002). "Reduction in the Incidence of Type 2 Diabetes with Lifestyle Intervention or Metformin." *N. Engl. J. Med.* 346, 393–402.

Tuomilehto, J., Lindstrom, J., Eriksson, J.G., Valle, T.T., Hamalainen, H., Ilanne-Parikka, P., Keinanen-Kiukaanniemi, S., Laakso, M., Louheranta, A., Rastas, M., Salminen, V. and Uusitupa, M. (2001). "Finnish Diabetes Prevention Study Group. Prevention of Type 2 Diabetes Mellitus by Changes in Lifestyle among Subjects with Impaired Glucose Tolerance." *N. Engl. J. Med.*, 344, 1343–1350.

U.S. Department of Health and Human Services (2002). *Leisure-time Physical Activity among Adults: United States, 1997–98.* U.S. Department of Health and Human Services, Centers for Disease Control and Prevention, National Center for Health Statistics.

U.S. Department of Health and Human Services (1996). *Physical Activity and Health: A Report of the Surgeon General. Atlanta, GA:* U.S. Department of Health and Human Services, Centers for Disease Control and Prevention, National Center for Chronic Disease Prevention and Health Promotion.

Vainio, H. and Bianchini, F. (2002). *Weight Control and Physical Activity*. IARC Handbooks of Cancer Prevention. IARC Press, 6.

Wankel, L.M. (1984). "Personal and Situational Factors Affecting Exercise Involvement: The Importance of Enjoyment." *Research Quarterly for Exercise and Sport,* 56, 275–282.

Ward, A. and Morgan, W.P. (1984). "Adherence Patterns of Healthy Men and Women Enrolled in an Adult Exercise Program." *Journal of Cardiac Rehabilitation,* 4, 143–152.

Weinhardt, L.S. and Carey, M.P. (1996). "Prevalence of Erectile Disorder among Men with Diabetes Mellitus: Comprehensive Review, Methodological Critique, and Suggestions for Future Research." *Journal of Consulting and Clinical Psychology,* 89, 77–84.

A Study of Stress, Problems and Recreational Activities of Adolescents Attending Coaching Classes for Admission in Professional Courses

Jaishree Sharma*[1] and Ravi Sidhu[2]

ABSTRACT

A large proportion of the adolescent population is diverging towards the coaching institutes for the preparation for admission in professional courses along with XI and XII classes. These adolescents are willing to sail on two boats simultaneously which seems to be a dangerous condition for their all round development. The present research investigated the problems and stress of such adolescent boys and girls and their involvement in recreational activities. A sample of 300 adolescents was drawn randomly from Coaching Institutes of Agra city. Self prepared Adolescent Stress Inventory (ASI), Problem Check-list for adolescent, and Recreational Activity Inventory were administered to get information from the subjects. The result of the present study revealed that adolescent girls experience higher level of stress and problems than did boys. Girls also show lower engagement in recreational and computer activities than boys. The problems were positively related with stress among both boys and girls.

INTRODUCTION

Work and recreation are the two important things for healthy life. Harmony between these two makes a person's life balanced. If one feels overloaded by work, lacks recreation, one may feel excited, anxious, sad, depressed, angry and may develop symptoms like sleeplessness, gastrointestinal upset, headache and muscular tension, all of which signal a disruption of psycho-biological balance. This disruption may be brief if one finds ways to meet the challenge and restores one's well-being. Resolving a change often becomes a positive growth experience. However if disruption in mind-body harmony is prolonged or severe, people experience stress (Edlin *et al.,* 2002). Prolonged, unresolved stresses can contribute to the development of several kinds of health disorders. In recent years the amount of research on pathological consequence of environmental stimuli perceived to be stressful has increased but research on problem of adolescents in the school age has been modest.

A large proportion of the adolescent population is diverging towards the coaching institutes for the preparation of professional courses. These coaching institutes are

---

*Corresponding author.

[1]Department of Home Science, Dayalbagh Educational Institute, Deemed University, Dayalbagh, Agra, UP, India. E-mail: [1]sharma.jaishri@gmail.com; [2]ragsuu@yahoo.co.in

often housed in a city different from their home town. In the present competitive world, adolescents are seen to adopt novel techniques to sharpen their skills and prove their mettle. Admission in educational programmes of their choice and desires gives them prestige, satisfaction and status. As a result they are motivated by the success stories of their seniors to adopt methods of studying which can guarantee success. The latest trend is that students join full time coaching classes after clearing their X class and neglect their schooling. The schools in which they are given admission assure them of fake attendance. For two years they are in the coaching institute and are preparing only for the competition exams. When time for board exams comes they suddenly divert their attention to schooling. Without much preparation they appear for + 2 boards. Parents, teachers and other well-wishers of these adolescents are willing to allow their wards to sail on two boats simultaneously. This indeed seems to be a dangerous condition for their all round development. The adolescents are likely to experience high level of stress and various types of problems since they are also uprooted from their home town which ultimately affects their health and well-being.

Developmentally adolescents are not initially too capable of handling much stress in their lives and it affects their feeling of well-being. Being an adolescent can be the most exhilarating time of one's life. New friends, new places, new challenges can all add up to a huge buzz. But all these things can also make the adolescent's life seem a total nightmare. There is an increasing amount of stress on adolescents these days to succeed and do extremely well; especially because their parents have invested a lot of money in their education and so they feel they have to do incredibly well. They are worried about their studies for both board and entrance examination and on the top of that the parents and teachers add to their worries by pressurizing them to perform equally well in both the examinations. This makes their conditions from bad to worse. Due to studies they are least involved in the extra curricular activities as a result they are deprived of the development of traits of personality other than intelligence. They are perhaps aware of their abilities in extra curricular activities but withdraw from participation to excel in educational pursuits which makes them emotionally strained. This reduces their ability to tolerate frustration, which in any case they will face in academics also. The sudden change to sedentary pattern of life affects their physique. This may not happen if these changes had to come one by one.

Students of these coaching institutes go into hibernation to prepare fully for entrance tests; they pay less attention to the recreational and social activities. The total environment is very demanding. The environmental expectations are translated to the adolescents by his parents and coaching institutes. He/she hardly gets any time for relaxation, making friends, recreation, extra curricular activities and stress relieving. The adolescent is faced with many challenges of independent life that he has to lead away from home. Added to this is the fact that there are no recreational and physical activities and their life is confined to table, chair and their books. There is no friend circle to enjoy with and truly speaking there is no one to help or support them. Their life begins from their room to coaching institute and again ends at their room. This dismal scenario increases the susceptibility of the adolescents to health problems.

Research shows that emotional reaction due to stress may aggravate pre-existing health problems, or produce new ones such as peptic ulcers, ulcerative colitis, migraine headache, asthmatic attacks, health disease, anxiety, apprehension, discomfort, bewilderment which may result in poor academic performance and poor physical health. This may ultimately become the cause of poor academic performance due to "hyper vigilance" and "premature closer" (Whiteman, 1985).

There are adolescents who seem to have a high tolerance level and appear to go on working under these circumstances. Yet in spite of high tolerance level they may reach their elastic limit and break down. One model that is useful in understanding stress among students is the person environmental model. According to one variation of this model, stressful events can be appraised by an individual as "challenging" or "threatening" (Lazaus, 1966), when students appraise their education as a challenge, stress can bring them a sense of competence and an increased capacity to learn. When education is seen as a threat, however stress can elicit feelings of helplessness and a foreboding sense of loss. Developmentally adolescents are not initially too capable of handling much stress in their lives and it begins to affect their health and well- being.

The effect of this latest academic scenario spelt in terms of stress and problems that they encountered when they attend a full time coaching institutes for higher academic ambition and give board exam without devoting adequate attention to it, is the major cause of concern of all academicians as it can have a major impact on the health. Hence the present investigation assesses the wisdom of this trend in terms of its affect on the adolescents.

OBJECTIVES

1. To study the differential stress among adolescent boys and girls attending coaching classes for admission in professional courses.
2. To study the differential problems of adolescent boys and girls attending coaching classes for admission in professional courses.
3. To study the engagement of adolescents in recreational activities.
4. To correlate stress and problems of adolescents.

METHODOLOGY

Sample

A sample of 300 adolescent boys and girls studying in XI and XII class between the age ranges of 16–19 years was selected randomly from coaching institutes of Agra city. These subjects were those who attended full time coaching institutes and did not attend school to prepare for board exams.

Tools

Self made questionnaires were used to assess.

Stress

The self made questionnaire for stress assessment was based on Bisht Battery of stress, which is a standardized tool prepared by Bisht (1971). Discussions and literature revealed that adolescents are exposed to self-inflicted stress, peer inflicted stress and parent-inflicted stress, which have been accepted as components of stress in the present study. The calculated reliability and validity of questionnaire to assess stress was 0.83 and 0.91 respectively.

1. *Involvement in recreational activity*—The engagement of adolescents in recreation or leisure was assessed through their involvement in music, cell phone games, daily exercises, participation in active games, movies, computer and newspaper reading. The calculated reliability and validity of recreational activity inventory was 0.75 and 0.87 respectively.
2. *Problems were assessed through a problem check-list*—The checklist attempts to identify different type of problems which may be academic problems, psychosomatic problems, problems with room mates and friends, financial problems, affective problems, food related problems and problems with the living conditions. The reliability of problem check-list was 0.77 and validity was 0.88 respectively.

RESULTS

Table 1: Mean, SD, and 't' Values of Adolescent Boys and Girls on Stress Scores

Components of Stress	*Boys (181)*		*Girls (119)*		*Statistical Value*	
	Mean	*SD*	*Mean*	*SD*	*'t'*	*p*
Self inflicted stress	26.34	2.54	26.56	2.38	0.773	> 0.05
Peer inflicted stress	24.28	3.33	25.50	2.85	3.292	< 0.01
Parent inflicted stress	25.50	3.74	26.66	3.02	2.825	< 0.01
Total stress	76.12	6.77	78.72	5.90	3.433	< 0.01

It is evident from the above table that adolescent girls experience more stress on all components of stress. Calculated 't' values show significant difference between two groups on peer inflicted stress, parent inflicted stress and total level. The scores indicate that both boys and girls are more or less equally ambitious as spelt by the self inflicted stress. The girls on the other hand experience significantly higher stress due to peers, parents as well as total stress.

Table 2: Mean, SD, and 't' Values of Adolescent Boys and Girls on Problem Scores

Problems	*Boys*		*Girls*		*Statistical Value*	
	Mean	*SD*	*Mean*	*SD*	*'t'*	*p*
Total Problem	32.48	11.56	37.41	11.03	3.680	< 0.01

Table 2 reveal, that girls have significantly higher number of problems than boys as is evident from the't' value 3.680 which is significant at 0.01 level of significance.

Table 3: Correlation of Problems with Stress of Adolescent Boys and Girls

Group	*Problems*	*Self Inflicted Stress*	*Peer Inflicted Stress*	*Parent Inflicted Stress*	*Total Stress*
Boys N = 181 Mean =	32.48	26.34	24.28	5.50	76.12
SD =	11.53	2054	3.33	3.74	6.77
r =	–	0.437	0.632	0.549	0.779
t-value =	–	6.500**	10.908**	8.785**	16.604**
Girls N = 119 Mean =	37.41	26.56	25.50	26.66	78.72
SD =	10.98	2.38	2.85	3.02	5.90
r =	–	0.261	0.350	0.253	0.404
t-value =	–	2.930**	4.041**	2.826**	4.777**

**Significant at 0.01 level.

It is clear from the above table that there is a positive and highly significant correlation of problems and stress among boys as is evident from the 't' values on self inflicted stress, peer inflicted stress, parent inflicted stress and total stress which are, 6.500, 10.908, 8.785, 16.604 respectively. The trend of positive and significant correlation is also seen among girls although t-values are not as high as obtained in the case of male sample.

Out of various recreational activities the subjects showed a preference for listening to music, playing game on mobile phone, and relaxing in park. However the time devoted to these activities was in the minimal time category. Other activities like exercise, active game and movies were rarely sought after by most respondents. Surprisingly most respondents felt that the entertainment equipments they possessed were adequate as against an almost same number who stated that they were not required at all. Newspaper reading was shown by most respondents (78.66%) but newspaper reading is not a purely entertainment activity.

Table 4: Engagement of Adolescent Boys and Girls in Recreational Activities

	Description	*Boys (181)*		*Girls (119)*		*Total (300)*	
		Number	*%*	*Number*	*%*	*Number*	*%*
A	*Listening Music*						
	a. 1–30 minutes	127	42.33	94	31.33	221	73.66
	b. 30 min.–1 hour	33	11	18	6	51	17
	c. More than 1 hour	21	7	7	2.33	28	9.33
B	*Playing game on mobile phone*						
	a. 1–30 minutes	150	50	106	35.33	256	85.33
	b. 30 min.–1 hour	24	8	12	4	36	12
	c. More than 1 hour	7	2.33	1	0.33	8	2.66
C	*Relaxing in park*						
	a. 1–30 minutes	152	50.66	101	33.66	253	84.33
	b. 30 min.–1 hour	24	8	13	4.33	37	12.33
	c. More than 1 hour	5	1.66	5	1.66	10	3.33
D	*Doing exercise*						
	a. Daily	46	15.33	28	9.33	74	24.66
	b. Depend on availability of time	90	30	49	16.33	139	46.33
	c. Never	45	15	42	14	87	29
E	*Participating in active games*						
	a. Daily	17	5.66	6	2	23	7.66
	b. Rarely	92	30.66	58	19.33	150	50
	c. Never	72	24	55	18.33	127	42.33
F	*Means of entertainment*						
	a. Adequate	70	23.33	61	20.33	131	43.66
	b. Inadequate	46	15.33	14	4.68	60	20
	c. Do not need	65	21.66	44	14.66	109	36.33
G	*No. of movies seen between last 2 test*						
	a. Zero	117	39	84	28	201	67
	b. 1–2	51	17	28	9.33	79	26.33
	c. More than 2	13	4.33	7	2.33	20	6.66
H	*News paper reading*						
	a. Yes	144	48	92	30.66	236	78.66
	b. No	37	12.33	27	9	64	21.33

Table 5: Different use of Computer for Entertainment by Adolescent Boys and Girls

	Involvement in Computer Activities	*Boys (181)*		*Girls (119)*		*Total (300)*	
		Number	*%*	*Number*	*%*	*Number*	*%*
A	Chatting	36	19.88	36	30.25	72	24
B	Playing game	68	57.45	37	31.09	105	35
C	Surfing	68	57.45	33	27.73	101	33.66
D	Listening music	84	46.40	39	32.77	123	41
E	Non users	57	31.49	40	33.61	97	32.33

The figures in Table 5 reveal a wide difference between boys and girls with respect to use of computer for entertainment. It shows that boys use computer more frequently for entertainment than the girls. Internet seems to be a great source of entertainment for the assessed adolescents but boys seem to enjoy surfing internet more (57.45%) rather than girls (27.73). Listening music is a major activity on computer in which the adolescents were involved and led the list with 41% of the total adolescent population in its favour.

Chatting is relatively a new source of entertainment and also a cheap means of communication with friends. Girls were much more involved in chatting (30.25%) rather than boys (19.88%). A total of 35% adolescents use computer for playing games. However if boys and girls are assessed separately than it becomes evident that a much higher percentage of boys (57.45%) play games on computer as compared to the girls (31.09%).

Out of 300 respondents more than 10% of the population identified as the nonusers of computer, thus 67.66% respondents use computer as a source of entertainment.

DISCUSSION

Stress is any situation that evokes negative thoughts and feelings in a person. The same situation is not evocative or stressful for all people and all people do not experience the same negative thoughts and feelings when stressed. Result of the present study reveal that girls have more academic stress than their counterparts. Perhaps the reason for this can be explained in the fact that girls appraise stressful events as more upsetting than boys (Grannis, 1992). Woodfield *et al.* (2005) has also confirmed that girls express higher level of anxiety and concerns about all aspects of their academic performance in comparison to boys. The result of the present study is consistent with that of a similar study conducted by Singh and Singh (2003) that shows that females exhibit higher degree of stress as compared to males. In a study conducted on girls on western sample it was found that parents and teachers were more conscious towards their academic achievements. Also, interference of elder makes them very stressful (Dubat *et al.,* 2007). Perhaps today Indian parents are very ambitious and concerned for the performance of not only their sons but also their daughters. Hence the results are consistent with studies conducted in west. Parents however still spend more on the education of male children as evidenced by the proportion of boys and girls in coaching institute which is tilted in favor of boys. Therefore perhaps these privileged girls seemed to face a higher risk of imaginary audience (Elkind, 1997), resulting in self consciousness, thereby increasing their susceptibility to stress. Anderson and Wallace (2007) confirmed that there were a significant gender difference in examination anxiety, level and the intensity and type of psychosomatic reaction to examination stress among secondary school students. Gender differences in reaction to stress may result from the socialization of males which teaches them that emotional expression is an admission of weakness and not muscularity (Davidson-Katz, 1991).

The results on problems faced are in agreement with those of Gierl and Rogers (1996) that female students tend to be more anxious and worry oriented which result in high level of problems among them. In Indian socio-cultural environment girls are reared up in an over protected environment, hence they are likely to find more problems from independent life than boys who are relatively more experienced in handling independence. Parents have higher expectations from sons in terms of education, employment and holding family responsibilities (Mythili *et al.,* 2004) as a result of high expectation parents are also likely to spend more willingly for their sons. Hence the boys are likely to be able to get better literature and academic provisions in comparison to girls. Society also offers more opportunity for education and employment to boys thus making them more reassured in comparison to girls. In a study by Sharma and Akhani (1996) it was found that females were more severely affected by health and physical fitness problems and home and family problems whereas males were not as severely affected in the same areas. The present study also investigated the health as a problem area and the result show a similar trend.

Studies also reveal that the changes and priorities of girls may be more complicated due to family and career choices affecting their lives (Chodorow, 1978; Gilligan, 1982 and Josselson, 1987) which may be the reason of higher problems among girls. Thus the present study seems to be in agreement with this perspective.

Although girls experience high level of stress and have more problems than boys yet correlation between problems and stress shows a stronger correlation in case of boys than girls. Perhaps the girls are using better management skills in handling stress, Misra *et al.* (2000) have infact found that girls have better ability to handle academic stress than boys. Also, a common experience or observation shows that girls are able to cathect their bottled up emotions by talking over, from which boys often refrain to prove their muscularity and maturity. Girls are also more sensitive and are often stressed out by minor problems; boys on the other hand remain unmoved by minor problems in an effort to conform to masculine expectation.

Participating in leisure and recreational activity can foster a range of positive experiences from simple relaxation, fun and enjoyment to personal development, fulfillment and improved health. Choices about types of activity and extent of involvement are not unilaterally made but are influenced by the demands and practicalities of everyday life.

The result reveal an over whelming majority of adolescents under study are interested in reading daily newspaper. Similar findings have been reported by Mahale (1987) who reasoned that as the child grows in to adolescence his horizons broadens. Now adolescents are interested in their community, national and in world affairs. The adolescents were found to read sections related to sports, movies, crime news and society news which perhaps thrills him. Newspaper is the only source which provide all the above. Hence the adolescents are very regular in reading newspaper. Result found that few adolescents are interested in leisure reading. The interest of adolescents in reading newspaper can be attributed to the fact that it takes less time to read news, the newspaper gives more scope for their knowledge to develop. Finally reading newspaper is cheaper and it keeps one informed about day to day happening hence newspaper reading was seen very frequently by them even when the leisure time is limited.

The poor involvement of adolescents in recreational activities is supported by Pranjic *et al.* (2007). The author stated that entertainment activities were rarely present in adolescent. Adolescents of the present study can be labeled as 'grind' because they are highly indulged towards their academic pursuits and least engaged in leisure activities. A study conducted by Kuh, Hu and Vesper (2000) stated that women are likely to be labeled as 'grind' where as men are much more likely to be recreators. Smith and Pino (2003) further explained that grind exhibit a high level of academic effort and recreators are involved with sports and exercise, students labeled as grind exhibited attitudes and behaviors very similar to those who have been identified as possessing an academic ethic (Rau and Durand, 2000). The importance of leisure can be explained through the study by Verma *et al.* (2002) who found that increase in leisure would raise the well-being of adolescent and this could be achieved without compromising academic work. However poor engagement in recreation in the present study can be explained through the study conducted by Kenny (1996) who reported that the hours spent in after school tutoring may prevent students from engaging in other developmental activities such as play, socialization with peers, sports and extra curricular activities, necessary for development of well adjusted and creative adults. Hickman *et al.* (2000) also reported that girls became less active during adolescence. Similar finding have been obtained in the present study.

Results reveal that more than half of the subjects used computer and internet for their entertainment. This result is consistent with that of Shubrahmanyam (2001) who found seventy five percent adolescents using internet and computer for recreation. Adolescents spend much time using computers for entertainment purposes, surfing the net and communicating through e-mail and chat rooms (Roberts *et al.,* 1999). Suler (1998) identified four basic categories of internet usage of adolescents namely website, e-mail, chat rooms and news groups. The first category is the web site, which provides documents or collections of documents that can be read for informational purposes. E-mail the second category is a rapid form of electronic letter communication. The third category is chat rooms. The fourth category newsgroups is like an electronic bulletin board all these forms of electronic media seemed equally popular with the subjects. In the present study researcher identified a number of uses of computer like chatting/e-mailing, playing game, surfing/researching information/ visiting website and listening music. Likewise Turow (1999) stated that using the computer to communicate is a popular activity among adolescents. Adolescents report that after academic work (home work, assignments *etc.*) e-mail and chat rooms are their most frequent computer activities.

Haffman, Kalsbeek and Novak (1996) conducted a survey to identify the use of internet by adolescents. Although their data suggested that people in the 16–24 age range, 22.1% were using the internet and World Wide Web at a high rate, while 15.5% did not use the internet or the web at all. It has been stated by Orleans and Walters (1996) that computer use increases among adolescents because probably they see their computer as a tool of personal expression and self involvement.

Although it is argued that playing games on computer is a sedentary activity, yet Lanningham *et al.* (2006) have shown that energy expenditure while playing computer games is 22% above resting value whereas while playing active games the energy expenditure is increased by 108%–172% above resting value.

The study reveals that boys were more involved in computer activity than girls. Study conducted by Furger (1998) supports these findings that boys consistently devoted more energy and time to the computer than girls. This may be due to the fact that girls prefer staying at home rather than enjoying outside as seen in previous section where girls prefer indoor over outdoor recreation activities. Due to low rates of personal computer ownership and broadband, internet cafes have become the only choice for adolescents to access the internet. A probable reason for poor female involvement in computer related activities could be due to the presence of undesirable elements in the internet cafes and also that the out side environment (cafes) is not perceived safe by female students.

Results reveal that females experience higher stress and lower participation in recreational activities than their male counterparts. Similar results have been obtained by Okasha *et al.* (1985) and Ragheb and McKinney (1993). Similarly Misra and Mckean (2000) found higher anxiety and lower leisure satisfaction and involvement among girls as compared to boys. Again the report of Mahoney, Schweder and Stattin (2002) also supports the results of the present study where it was reported that adolescents who participated in after school, activities had significantly lower level of depression and stress than those who did not participate in such activities. There is enough evidence to prove that daily rest (often consisting of simply relaxing in a chair, lying down or sleeping) and regular physical exercise of pleasant nature are helpful in overcoming the fatigue and tension associated with stressful situation which perhaps are less adequate in case of girls.

CONCLUSION

The study shows that the effect of engagement in sedentary table chair activities for long continuing duration has a negative effect on the mental health which is reflected by high level of stress. The study also throws light on the fact that adoption of this life style and non involvement in recreational activities can result in increase in their problems. Such adolescents have been found to face problems in mundane activities. No doubt academic pressure is at its peak but a balance between work and play, physical and mental work is still the call of the day. One cannot neglect health for a goal which is still an illusion.

REFERENCES

Anderson, J.K. and Wallace, L.M. (2007). "Gender Differences in the Psychosomatic Reactions to Students Subjected to Examination Stress." *Electronic Journal of Research in Educational Psychology,* 12, 5(2), 325–348.

Bisht, Abha Rani (1987). "Bisht Battery of Stress Scale", *National Psychological Corporation,* Agra.

Chodorow, Nancy (1978). *The Reproduction of Mothering: Psychoanalysis and the Sociology of Gender.* Berkeley, CA: University of California Press.

Davidson-Katz, K. (1999). *Gender Roles and Health.* In C.R. Snyder and D.R. Forsyth (eds.), Handbook of Social and Clinical Psychology: The Health Perspective, 179–196. New York: Pergamon.

Dubat, K., Punia, S. and Goyal, Rashmi. (2007). "A Study of Life Stress and Coping Styles among Adolescent Girls." *Journal of Social Sciences, 14(2)*, 191–194.

Edlin, G., Golanty, E. and Brown, K.M. (2002). *Health and Wellness* (7th ed.). Jones and Barlett Publishers.

Elkind, D. (1997). *Reinventing Childhood: Raising and Educating Children in a Changing World.* Rosemont, NS: Modern Learning Press.

Furger, R. (1998). *Does Jane Computer: Preserving our Daughters' Place in the Cyber Revolution.* New York: Warner Books.

Gierl, M.J. and Rogers, W.T. (1996). "A Confirmatory Factor Analysis of the Test Anxiety Inventory using Canadian High School Students." *Educational and Psychological Measurement,* 56(2), 315–32.

Gilligan, C. (1982). *In a Different Voice: Psychological Theory and Women's Development.* Cambridge, MA: Harvard University Press.

Grannis, J. (1992). "Students' Stress, Distress and Achievement in an Urban Intermediate School." *Journal of Early Adolescent,* 12, 4–27.

Hickman, M., Roberts, C. and deMatos, M.G. (2000). "Exercise and Leisure Time Activities." In C. Currie, K. Hurrelmann, W. Settertobulte, R. Smith and J. Todd (ed.) *Heath and Health Behavior among Young People.* WHO Policy Series: Healthy Policy for Children and Adolescents, 1, 73–82.

Hoffman, D.L., Kalsbeek, W.D. and Novak, T.P. (1996). "Internet and Web use in the United States: Baselines for Commercial Development." Retrieved September 28, 2000, from: http://commerce/vanderbilt.edu/baseline/Internet.demos.july9.1996.html.

Josselson, R. (1987). *Finding Herself: Pathways to Identity Development in Women.* San Francisco, CA: Jossey-Bass Publishers.

Kenny, D.T. and Faunce, G. (2004). "Effects of Academic Coaching on Elementary School Students." *The Journal of Educational Research,* 98,109–126.

Kuh, G.D., Hu, S. and Vespers, N. (2000). "They Shall Be Known by What They Do: An Activities-Based Typology of College Students." *Journal of College Student Development,* 41, 228–244.

Lanningham, F.L., Jensen, T.B., Foster, R.C., Redmond, A.B., Walker, B.A. and, Heinz D, *et al.* (2006). "Energy Expenditure of Sedentary Screen Time Compared with Active Screen Time for Children." *Pediatrics*, 118, 1831–1835.

Lazaus, R.S. (1966). *Psychological Stress and the Coping Process*. New York: McGraw-Hill.

Mahale, Meera (1987).*The Adolescents: Their Family Situations and Education*. India: Mittal Publications.

Mahoney, J.L., Schweder, A.E. and Stattin, H. (2002). "Structured After-School Activities as a Moderator of Depressed Mood for Adolescents with Detached Relations to Their Parents." *Journal of Community Psychology,* 30(1), 69–86.

Misra, Ranjita, McKean, M., West, S. and Russo, T. (2000). "Academic Stress of College Students: Comparison of Student and Faculty Perceptions." *College Student Journal.*

Misra, Ranjita. and McKean, M. (2000). "College Students' Academic Stress and its Relation to Their Anxiety, Time Management and Leisure Satisfaction." *American Journal of Health Science,* 16, 42–52.

Mythili, B. (2004). "Adjustment Problems of Adolescent Students." *Journal of Community Guidance and Research*, 21(1), 54–61.

Okasha, A., Kamel, M., Lataif, F., Khalil, A.H. and Bishry, Z. (1985). "Academic Difficulty among Male Egyptian University Students. II Association with Demographic and Psychological factors." *The British Journal of Psychiatry* 146, 144–150.

Orleans, M. and Walters, G. (1996). "Human-Computer Enmeshment: Identity Diffusion Through Mastery." *Social Science Computer Review*, 14(2), 144–156.

Pranjić, N., Brković, A. and Beganlić, A. (2007). "Discontent with Financial Situation, Self-rated Health, and Well-being of Adolescents in Bosnia and Herzegovina: Cross-sectional Study in Tuzla Canton." *Croatian Medical Journal,* 48(5), 691–700.

Ragheb, K. and Mekinney, J. (1993). "Campus Recreation and Perceived Academic Stress." *Journal of College Student Development,* 34, 5–10.

Rau, W. and Durand, A. (2000). "The Academic Ethic and College Grades: Does Hard Work Help Students to 'Make the Grade'?" *Sociology of Education,* 73, 19–38.

Roberts, D.F., Foehr, U.G. Rideout, V.J. and Brodie, M. (1999). "Kids and Media at the New Millennium": *A Comprehensive National Analysis of Children's Media Use*. Menlo park, CA: Kaiser Family Foundation Report.

Sharma, Neelam and Akhani, Panna (1996). "A Study of Selected Problems of College Going Youths and a Suggested Programme of Extra Curricular Activities." *Indian journal of Psychometry and Education,* 27(2), 73–76.

Singh, A.K. and Singh, Arpana (2003). "Impact of Sex and Birth Order upon Stressful Behavior." *Praachi Journal of Psycho Cultural Dimensions,* 19(2), 113–118.

Smith, W.L. and Pino, N.W. (2003). "College Students: The Academic Ethic, and Academic Achievement." *Unpublished paper*. Department of Sociology and Anthropology, Georgia Southern University.

Subrahmanyam, K., Greenfield, P., Kraut, R. and Gross, E. (2001). "The Impact of Computer use on Children's and Adolescents' Development." *Applied Developmental Psychology,* 2, 7–30.

Suler, J. (1998, June). *Adolescents in Cyberspace: The Good, the Bad, and the Ugly.* Retrieved September 28, 2000, from: http://www.rider.edu/users/suler/psycyber/ adoles.html.

Turow, J. (1999). *The Internet and The Family: The View from the Parents, The View from the Press* (report no. 27). Philadelphia: Annenberg Public Policy Centre of the University of Pennsylvania.

Verma, Suman, Sharma, Deepali and Larson, R.W. (2002). "School Stress in India: Effects on Time and Daily Emotions." *International Journal of Behavioral Development,* 26(6), 500–508.

Whitman, N.A. (1985). *Student Stress: Effect and Solution: ERIC Digest 85–1 Association for the Study of Higher Education (*Report no ED284514) Retrieved from the ERIC Database: http://www.ericdigests.org/pre-926/stress.htm

Woodfeild, R., Earl-Novell, S. and Salomon, L. (2005). "Gender and Mode of Assessment at University: Should We Assume Female Students Are Better Suited to Coursework and Male to Unseen Examination?" *Assessment and Evaluation in Higher Education,* 30, 35–50.

A Study of Maternal Stress and its Relationship with Neonatal Outcomes

Garima Srivastava[1] and Ravi Sidhu*[2]

ABSTRACT

Infant Mortality Rate (IMR) is regarded as an important and sensitive indicator of the health status of a community. India rates low on this indicator. The present study investigates maternal stress as a determinant of health status of neonates. The study was conducted on a sample of 100 mothers and their 100 neonates which could be SFD, pre-term and normal. All the mothers who delivered their child during the period of data collection (12 days) comprised of the sample. The sample consisted of uneducated women who belonged to low socio economic group. The tool used by department of Social Preventive Medicine for a welfare programme undertaken in Balrampur was used for collection of data. This tool was used to assess the stress (emotional, physical and pathological) of the mothers and the anthropometric measurements of the neonates were taken. Results show that there was no significant difference in the stress of women from different age group, family pattern and working and non-working status. Maternal stress was found to be highly significant with neonatal outcomes. Low maternal stress and normal neonatal status were highly significant X2 = 36.00. Mothers with high level of stress gave birth to the neonates who had poor anthropometric status. Out of the three stresses studied, the physical stress had the sharpest effect on anthropometric status of neonates which indicates that decrease in anthropometric measurements in neonate is an effect of maternal stress.

INTRODUCTION

The current state of neonatal health in India is indeed dismal to state the least. Three neonates are dying every minute in India and every 4th baby born is low birth weight! Out of 3.9 million neonatal deaths worldwide, India is accounting to 1.2 million or nearly 30% of global neonatal mortality! The present figure of 40 per 1,000 live births is too high. Furthermore, there is great diversity of NMR (Neonatal Mortality Rate) in different states and BIMARU states, of which Uttar Pradesh is one, together constitute over half of all newborn deaths in India. Most neonatal deaths are caused by preventable and/or treatable diseases. Infections, birth asphyxia, and prematurity are the leading causes of neonatal deaths in India (Thacker, 2007). Reduction in infant and child mortality is a major goal of the strategy to achieve health for all.

*Corresponding author.

[1, 2]Department of Home Science, Faculty of Arts, Dayalbagh Educational Institute, Deemed University, Dayalbagh, Agra, UP, India.

E-mail: [1]garima2984@gmail.com; [2]ragsuu@yahoo.co.in

During the last quarter of the century emphasis has been placed on reducing under-five childhood mortality largely through immunization, ORS and control of acute respiratory infections. Consequently, deaths among children over one month of age have no doubt declined in the last three decades. These changes, however, did not have a marked impact among neonates. Neonatal deaths in India now account for up to two-thirds of all infant deaths and half of under-five child mortality in developing countries. From many commonly accepted indices, it is evident that infant and maternal mortality rates are higher in many countries. Although exact figures remain elusive, an estimated 5,25,000 women continue to die from maternal causes (WHO, 2004). The neonatal mortality rates are higher in India as compared to the western countries. The neonatal period involves maximum risk in the life span of any human being and sequel of neonatal disorders usually means life long disability. The birth weight is a critical factor in the prognosis of a new born. Mean birth weight in India is 2500 grams. Among severely low birth weight, 10% of neonatal death occurs during first week of life.

The important hazard associated with pre-natal development is maternal stress which may be physical, pathological or emotional in nature. Maternal stress affects the developing child both before and after birth. Before birth severe and persistent stress may result in irregularities in the developing child and complications are greater because deliveries also become difficult. Hoffman (1990) established that ante-natal stress factors result in high risk of pregnancy. Georgas and Giakoumaki (1984) found the level of psychosocial stress experienced prior to delivery is positively associated with the occurrence of obstetric complications.

The question of whether stress increases the risk of pre-term delivery has interested epidemiologists for more than a quarter of a century. In one early investigation, Nuckolls *et al.* (2003) found that maternal stress during pregnancy was associated with poorer pregnancy outcomes. Stress during pregnancy and its association with adverse birth outcomes have been examined in a few studies, some of which found an association (Gorsuch and Key, 1974; Molfese 1987; Brooke, 1989) while others did not (Pagel, *et al.,* 1990; Peacock *et al.,* 1995; Wadhwa *et al.,* 1993; Norbeck and Anderson, 1989). One study found that pregnancy-related anxiety was associated with shorter gestations (Rini, 1999), and the present analysis supports this finding. When women with a history of adverse pregnancy outcome, the effect of stress was reduced but not eliminated, indicating that women who are anxious but do not have other medical conditions may be at increased risk of pre-term birth. Anxiety may be linked to some general malaise that is difficult to measure but may be indicative of problems with the pregnancy. Because some of the risk may be attributable to a physiologic response to anxiety, anxiety may influence gestational age at delivery (Norbeck and Anderson, 1989).

Fetal death is associated with Intrauterine Growth Retardation (IUGR) and conditions such as placental insufficiency that predispose the fetus to asphyxia. Neonatal deaths are associated with LBW and lethal congenital abnormalities. The affect of stress on neonatal outcomes can be easily measured through anthropometric measurements that includes mainly height, weight, head circumferences, chest circumferences and mid arm circumference. Thus this problem is a challenge to pediatricians and developmentalists especially for those in developing countries like India.

There is no doubt that women face greater number of risks to health. Especially pregnant women are a vulnerable group or a risk group. Stressful events can erode health. Stress can cause many complications of pre-gnancy and is the major affect of the poor neonatal outcome. It can result to SFD, LBW and preterm babies. The stress can be categorized as emotional stress (caused by worry, anxiety, fear, unwanted pregnancies, economic hardships, concern about the future of the unborn child, relations with other family members and difficulties of previous pregnancies), physical stress (attributed to extra work load, lifting heavy weight) and pathological stress (originated by Rh incompatibility, hypertension, anemia) which is aggravated by many environmental, social and even personal factors. The social and cultural context of pregnant women may add to or alleviate her level of distress. Ameliorating social environmental factors include intimate support, which has been associated with improved pregnancy outcomes in a number of studies (Rutter, 1990). Maternal stress and its association with neonatal outcomes have interested not only health psychologists and neonotologists but also developmentalists. The present study has focused on the problems related to this issue with special reference to low socio-economic status group. Thus the present study was conducted with the following objectives.

OBJECTIVES

- To study the differential maternal stress of the pregnant women from different backgrounds.
- To study the association of maternal stress and neonatal outcomes in high/low stressed mothers.
- To study the relationship between emotional, physical and pathological stress of the mothers and anthropometric measurements of the neonates.
- To study the pathological conditions of LBW, preterm and normal neonates.

RESEARCH METHODOLOGY

Selection of Sample

The sample of the study consisted of 100 mothers and their 100 neonates which could be SFD, preterm or normal. The sample has been selected from Balrampur hospital of Lucknow. The subjects of the sample were uneducated and belonged to low socio economic status. All the mothers who delivered children during the period of data collection were the mother population of the study. The neonates of these mothers were the neonates of the sample. The selection of sample was done purposively.

Tools

1. *A General Information Schedule:* It had two sections:
   Section 'a' obtains pathological information (obtained from the doctor).
   Section 'b' obtains information about anthropometric measurements.
2. *Stress Inventory:* This inventory had two sections which obtained information about physical and emotional stress. This test was administered as a schedule on the mothers.

Procedure

- Pathological information was obtained from the maternal history given by the doctor.
- Stress inventory was filled in the form of a schedule.
- Anthropometric measurements of the neonates were taken.
- The mothers were divided into high stress and low stress group by computing Q1 and Q3 for the stress scores.

RESULTS

Data obtained from the mothers and their neonates were analyzed and the obtained results are shown in the section below:

Table 1: Showing the Stress among Women of Different Age Group

Group No.	*Age Range*	*Mean*	*S.D*	*t-value*
1.	Up to 25 years	14.68	4.69	1.203 (Group 1 & 2)
2.	26–30 years	14.06	4.16	1.836 (Group 2 & 3)
3.	Above 30 years	14.68	5.35	1.284 (Group 1 & 3)

The results show that total stress of women in three groups is not significantly different as revealed by the t-values. The reasons may be that at least emotional stress arising from fears, anxieties and risks involved in pregnancy and child care were similar, since the data was homogeneous in nature with respect to socio economic status.

The results in Table 2 show that women of joint and nuclear families were equally stressed as evident from the obtained t-value 1.214 which shows insignificant difference. No doubt that there is a likelihood of joint family women being saddled with additional responsibilities of family but they also are assured of additional support which will be available for rearing the child immediately after birth and thereafter. On the other hand the women of nuclear families may be having fewer responsibilities at the present but the future anxieties, anticipated fears and non availability of constant family support in the time of need are likely to create stress. Thus women of both the families are equally stressed, though the causes of stress may be different.

Table 2: Showing the Stress of Women from Joint and Nuclear Families

S.No.	*Type of Family*	*Mean*	*S.D*	*t-value*
1.	Joint	14.40	3.86	1.214
2.	Nuclear	13.96	3.70	

Table 3: Showing Maternal Stress of Working and Non-working Women

S.No.	*Working Status*	*Mean*	*S.D*	*t-value*
1.	Working	14.28	3.50	0.404
2.	Non-working	14.10	3.93	

Table 3 indicates that there is no significant difference in the level of stress between working and non working women (t = 0.404). There is no doubt that working women have to cope up with the work during pregnancy but it is also true that non working mothers have to deal with stress arising from economic pressures and hardships. Also it is quite possible that the employees are compassionate with pregnant women and do not overstrain them with physical labor.

Table 4: Showing the Association of Maternal Stress and Neonatal Outcomes

Groups	*High Stress Group*				*Low Stress Group*			
Types of stress	*Physical*	*Pathological*	*Emotional*	*Total*	*Physical*	*Pathological*	*Emotional*	*Total*
Pre-term	3	5	2	10	2	5	2	9
SFD	4	9	3	16	2	4	3	9
Normal	2	4	2	8	5	10	3	18
Total	9	18	7	34	9	19	8	36

X2 = 27.019 X2 = 36.00

Table 4 reveals the distribution of the respondents of high/low stress according to neonatal outcomes. Significant association has been observed between neonatal outcomes (preterm, SFD or normal neonatal status) and stress of the respondents for both high and low stress groups (X2 = 27.019 and 36.00 for high stress and low stress group respondents). The obtained Chi- square values are highly significant indicating that there is a high association of normal neonatal status and low maternal stress and the reverse is true for high stressed mothers.

Table 5: Showing the Relationship between Emotional Stress of the Mothers and Anthropometric Measurements of SFD, Preterm and Normal Neonates

Anthropometric Measurements		*Preterm Infants*	*SFD Infants*	*Normal Infants*
Height	r	−0.304	−0.224	−0.161
	t	1.561(NS)	0.976(NS)	0.907(NS)
Weight	r	−0.275	0.253	0.049
	t	1.402(NS)	1.111(NS)	0.275(NS)
Head circumference	r	0.086	−0.217	0.147
	t	0.425(NS)	0.943(NS)	0.825(NS)
Chest circumference	r	−0.041	−0.419	0.096
	t	0.202(NS)	1.957(NS)	0.539(NS)
Mid-Arm circumference	r	−0.207	−0.744	0.029
	t	1.037(NS)	4.720(*)	0.161(NS)

*Significant and NS: Non-Significant

Table 5 shows that anthropometric measurements of neonates and emotional stress of mother shows a trend of negative relationship for both preterm and SFD babies. This means that with an increase in emotional stress there is a decrease in their anthropometric status. However this negative trend is significant for only mid arm circumference of SFD infants (t = 4.720). Normal neonates seemed to be unaffected by maternal emotional stress. Perhaps they have an advantage of healthier intrauterine life due to maternal age, diet and parity.

Table 6 shows a negative relationship between the physical stress and the anthropometric measurements of the SFD and the preterm infants. This means that with the increase in physical stress of the mothers the anthropometric measurements are decreasing. But the t-values are significant only for head circumference (3.253), chest circumference (3.623) and the mid arm circumference (2.740) of the preterm neonates. Whereas in SFD babies, weight (2.644) and mid arm (2.267) values are significant. Again the normal infants are least affected by maternal physical stress.

Table 7 shows that there is a negative relationship between the pathological stress of the mothers and the anthropometric measurements of SFD and preterm neonates. Only one positive relation is found in height of the SFD babies *i.e.,* 0.102., which however is insignificant. Again SFD babies were at highest risk of maternal pathological stress as the obtained three t-values, that is head circumference (2.132), chest circumference (2.918) and mid arm circumference (4.071) are significant.

Table 6: Showing the Relationship between Physical Stress of the Mothers and Anthropometric Measurements of SFD, Preterm and Normal Neonates

Anthropometric Measurements		*Preterm Infants*	*SFD /Infants*	*Normal Infants*
Height	r	−0.319	0.242	−0.088
	t	1.649(NS)	1.056(NS)	0.496(NS)
Weight	r	−0.103	0.529	−0.214
	t	0.505(NS)	2.644(*)	1.217(NS)
Head circumference	r	−0.553	−0.146	0.168
	t	3.253(*)	0.627(NS)	0.951(NS)
Chest circumference	r	−0.595	−0.281	−0.010
	t	3.623(*)	1.241(NS)	0.058(NS)
Mid-Arm circumference	r	−0.488	−0.471	0.119
	t	2.740(*)	2.267(*)	0.668(NS)

*Significant and NS: Non-Significant

Table 7: Showing the Relationship between Pathological Stress of the Mothers and Anthropometric Measurements of SFD, Preterm and Normal Neonates

Anthropometric Measurements		*Preterm Infants*	*SFD Infants*	*Normal Infants*
Height	r	−0.247	−0.381	0.115
	t	1.249(NS)	1.748(NS)	0.644(NS)
Weight	r	−0.067	0.102	0.195
	t	0.328(NS)	0.433(NS)	1.109(NS)
Head circumference	r	−0.154	−0.449	0.151
	t	0.764(NS)	2.132(*)	0.849(NS)
Chest circumference	r	−0.244	−0.567	0.105
	t	1.231(NS)	2.918(*)	0.588(NS)
Mid-Arm circumference	r	−0.302	−0.692	0.028
	t	1.551(NS)	4.071(*)	1.156(NS)

*Significant and NS: Non-Significant.

Table 8 shows that there is a negative relationship between the total stress of the mothers and all parameters of anthropometric measurements of the SFD and pre-term neonates. The values for height (2.244), head circumference (2.296), chest circumference (3.022) and mid arm circumference (2.982) in pre-term babies and in SFD babies the values for weight (2.233), chest circumference (2.164) and mid arm circumference (4.370) were found to be significant. Rest all the values are non- significant.

Table 8: Showing the Relationship between Total Stress of the Mothers and Anthropometric Measurements of SFD, Preterm and Normal Neonates

Anthropometric Measurements		*Preterm Infants*	*SFD Infants*	*Normal Infants*
Height	r	–0.416	0.007	–0.114
	t	2.244(*)	0.030(NS)	0.637(NS)
Weight	r	–0.202	0.466	–0.144
	t	1.008(NS)	2.233(*)	0.812(NS)
Head circumference	r	–0.424	–0.271	0.232
	t	2.296(*)	1.194(NS)	1.326(NS)
Chest circumference	r	–0.525	–0.454	0.042
	t	3.022(*)	2.164(*)	0.233(NS)
Mid-Arm circumference	r	–0.520	–0.718	0.124
	t	2.982(*)	4.370(*)	0.698(NS)

*Significant at 5% and NS: Non-Significant.

Table 9: Showing the Pathological Conditions of the Neonates at the Time of Birth

Pathological Conditions	*LBW (n = 41)*		*Pre-term (n = 26)*		*Normal (n = 33)*	
	No.	*%*	*No.*	*%*	*No.*	*%*
Respiratory Distress Syndrome	11	26.84	10	38.48	7	21.21
Jaundice	4	9.70	2	7.69	7	21.21
Anemia	4	9.70	2	7.69	3	9.09
Odema	3	7.31	2	7.69	0	0
Infections	10	24.30	8	30.7	7	21.21
Asphyxia	9	21.90	2	7.69	9	27.27

Table 9 shows the pathological conditions of the neonates at the time of birth. It is evident from the table that LBW, preterm as well as normal neonates were having bad pathological conditions at the time of birth. Most neonates were having same type of infections in the form of fever.

Again respiratory distress syndrome which is normally seen in unhealthy children was also very prevalent even in normal born neonates. The reason for pathological problems can be related to high maternal stress, their low socio economic status and poor maternal care.

DISCUSSION

A majority of newborn problems are specific to pre-natal period, and are the results of maternal stress, poor maternal health and inadequate care during pregnancy, inappropriate management and poor hygiene during the delivery, lack of newborn care and discriminatory care (Thacker, 2007). Similar results are also obtained in the present study with reference to stress which has been found to be significantly related to pregnancy outcome. Again a study done by Forde (1992) also supports the findings and suggests that women experiencing high level of stress were 80% more likely to deliver preterm babies than those who have low level of stress. Similarly findings of Cooper *et al.* (1996) also reported that women who score high on stress are also higher on the risk of IUGR. The results of the study are consistent with Dunken (1998) where it was reported that maternal anxiety and stress are linked to low birth weight of babies.

Stress is a negative emotional experience accompanied by predictable biochemical, physiological, cognitive and behavioral changes that are directed either towards altering the stressful event or accounting to its effect (Baum, 1990). Chronic stress during pregnancy has been related to a variety of adverse health related outcomes including the likelihood of giving birth prematurely (Wadhwa and Sandman, 1999). Simmons (1990) studied the psycho-social aspects of pregnant women. Results reveal that these mothers were under great stress to meet the multiple demands resulting in high stress and fatigue. There are evidences that gender related roles may create stress that could adversely affect pregnancy outcomes. For example, chronic strain in household role was found to be associated with both preterm delivery and low birth weight (Pritcahrd, 1995). The present study shows that total stress was significantly related to most anthropometric measurements in case of SFD and preterm babies whereas in case of normal infants no relationship was significant. This shows that greater the stress of the mother, greater is the risk of not having normal delivery. The present study specifically shows the major affect of physical stress on the neonatal outcomes. This finding is consistent with the study done by Caplan *et al.* (1993), which states that workload is a chief factor that produces a high level of physical stress. Women who are required to work too long and too hard at too many tasks, practice poor health habits. Such women sustain more health risks than do women not suffering from overload. It was stated that problems are particularly acute for pregnant women and effects the neonatal outcomes. Nayeye (1982) has also highlighted the impact of physical stress on neonatal status. A negative correlation is found between emotional stress and anthropometric measurements of SFD and preterm infants; however mid arm circumference was significantly related to emotional stress of the SFD babies. The result is consistent with a similar study done by Istvan (1998) that shows that emotional stress, birth weight and gestational age have a negative relationship. Pathological stress also affects the neonatal outcomes. This is also supported by James and Miller (1996) that women having medical problems are likely to experience a low birth weight and preterm delivery. Reduction in infant and child mortality is a major goal of the strategy to achieve health for all. No doubt the role of maternal stress during pregnancy needs a more serious handling approach.

CONCLUSION

The current status of neonatal health services in the country is quite slapdash and disorganized. The results of the study indicate that the maternal stress in any form has negative consequences on the health status (as assessed by anthropometric measurements) of neonates. If a comparison of the individual stress is done, physical stress has the maximum ill effect since most correlation values were significant. Also, if the mother is leading an otherwise healthy life, the risk of maternal stress is minimized, hence the normal neonates were least effected. Healthy mothers are vital to national development and so are the healthy neonates as they are the future of the country. Neonatal deaths can not be substantially reduced without efforts to reduce maternal mortality and improving maternal health. Maternal health means ensuring that all women receive the care they need to be safe and healthy throughout pregnancy and childbirth. Safe motherhood encompasses social and cultural factors, as well as addresses health systems and health policy. A woman dies from complications in childbirth every minute—about 529,000 each year—the vast majority of them in developing countries. Improving maternal health is one of the eight Millennium Development Goals, and great efforts have been put forth to achieve that goal. On the basis of findings it is concluded that maternal stress has a negative influence on the neonatal health outcomes. Therefore every effort must be made to keep the mother under relaxed condition. Life cannot be controlled but having a good social support network which can include family; friends and relatives can help relieve the stress of pregnant women. A number of stress reduction techniques can be used successfully to reduce stress like meditation, guided mental imagery and yoga (for pregnant women). Need to prioritize interventions based on the NMRs of different states can also not be ignored.

REFERENCES

Baum, S.A. (1990). "Maternal Stress and Preterm Delivery." *Prenatal and Neonatal Medicine,* 3, 39–42.

Brooke, O.G., Anderson, H.R. and Bland, J.M., *et al.* (1989). "Effects on Birth Weight of Smoking, Alcohol, Caffeine, Socioeconomic Factors and Psychosocial Stress." *BMJ*, 298, 795–801.

Caplan, R.D. and Jones, K.W. (1993). "Effects of Work Load, Role Ambiguity and Typey—A Type Personality on Anxiety, Depression and Heart Rate." *Journal of Applied Psychology*, 60, 713–719.

Cooper, R.L., Goldenberg, R.L., Das, A., Elder, N., Swain, M. and Norman, G., *et al.* (1996). "The Preterm Prediction Study." *American Journal of Obstetrics and Gynecology,* 175, 1286–92.

Dunken-Schettar, C. (1998). 'Maternal Stress and Preterm Delivery." *Prenatal and Neonatal Medicine,* 3, 39–42.

Forde, R. (1992). 'Pregnant Women's Ailments and Psychosocial Conditions." *Faculty Practitioner*, 9(3), 270–73.

Georgas, J. and Giakoumaki, E. (1984). "Psychosocial Stress and its Relation to Obstetrical Complications", *Psychotherapy Psychometric,* 41(4), 200–06.

Gorsuch, R.L. and Key, M.K. (1974). "Abnormalities of Pregnancy as a Function of Anxiety and Life Stress." *Psychosom. Med.,* 36, 352–62.

Istvan, E.D. (1998). "Stress, Support and Pregnancy Outcomes: A Reassessment Based on Recent Research." *Pediatric and Perinatal Epidemiology*, 10, 380–405.

James, E.J. and Miller, C.A. (2006). "Critical Review of Dietary Caffeine and Blood Pressure. A Relationship that Should be taken More Seriously." *Psychometric Medicine*, 66, 63–71.

Krieger, N., Rowley D.L. and Herman, A.A., *et al.* (1993). "Racism, Sexism, and Social Class: Implications for Studies of Health, Disease, and Well-Being." *Am. J. Prev. Med.*, 9, 82–122.

McLean, D.E., Hatfield-Timajchy, K. and Wingo, P.A., *et al.* (1993). "Psychosocial Measurement: Implications for the Study of Preterm Delivery in Black Women." *Am. J. Prev. Med.*, 9, 39–81.

Molfese, V.J., Bricker, M.C. and Manion, L.G., *et al.* (1987). "Anxiety, Depression and Stress in Pregnancy: A Multivariate Model of Intra-Partum Risks and Pregnancy Outcome." *J. Psychosom. Obstet. Gynecol.*, 7, 77–92.

Nayeye, R.L. (1982). "Effect of Maternal Under-Nutrition and Heavy Physical Work during Pregnancy on Birth Weight." *Br. Journal of Obstetrics Gynecology,* 87, 222–226.

Norbeck, J.S. and Anderson, N.J. (1989). "Life Stress, Social Support, and Anxiety in Mid- and Late-Pregnancy among Low Income Women." *Res. Nurs. Health*, 12, 281–287.

Nuckolls, K.B, Kaplan, B.H and Cassel, J. (2003). "Psychological Assets, Life Crisis and the Prognosis of Pregnancy." *American Journal of Epidemiology*, 95, 431–441.

Pagel, M.D., Smilkstein, G. and Regen, H., *et al.* (1990). "Psychosocial Influences on New Born Outcomes: A Controlled Prospective Study." *Soc. Science Med.*, 30, 597–604.

Peacock, J.L., Bland, J.M. and Anderson, H.R. (1995). "Preterm Delivery: Effects of Socioeconomic Factors, Psychological Stress, Smoking, Alcohol, and Caffeine." *BMJ*, 3, 11: 531–5.

Pritcahrd, C.W. (1995). "Preterm Birth, Low Birth Weight and Stressfulness of the Household Role for the Pregnant Women." *Social Science and Medicine,* 7, 346–351.

Rini, C.K., Dunkel-Schetter, C. and Wadhwa, P.D., *et al.* (1999). "Psychological Adaptation and Birth Outcomes: The Role of Personal Resources, Stress, and Socio-Cultural Context in Pregnancy." *Health Psychology*, 18, 333–45.

Rutter, D.R. (1990). "Inequalities in Pregnancy Outcomes: Review of Psychosocial and Behavioral Mediators." *Social Science and Medicine,* 30, 553–568.

Sammons, L.N. (1990). "Psychosocial Aspects of Second Pregnancy NAACOGS Clinical Issues." *Prenatal Women's Health Nurse,* 1(3), 317–24.

Stancil, T.R., Hertz-Picciotto, I. and Schramm, M., *et al.* (2000). "Stress and Pregnancy among African-American Women." *Paediatric Perinatal Epidemiol*, 14, 127–35.

Thacker, N. (2007). "Improving Status of Neonatal Health in India." *Indian Pediatrics,* 44, 891–892.

Wadhwa, P.D.and Sandman, C.A. (1999). "Stress, Infection and Preterm Birth: A Bio-behavioral Perspective." *Pediatric and Perinatal Epidemiology,* 15, 17–29.

World Health Organization (WHO) (2004). *Maternal Mortality in 2000: Estimates Developed by WHO, UNICEF and UNFPA.*

Role of Parents and Family in the Development of Self-Esteem of Children—A Behavior Modification Approach

Surila Agarwala*[1] and Satya Singh[2]

ABSTRACT

The study was undertaken with the purpose to compare the self-esteem among orphan and non-orphan children and to study the effectiveness of behavior intervention in enhancing self-esteem of children. The study was conducted in two parts. Part 'A' deals with the comparison of self-esteem of orphan and non-orphan children. Part 'B' deals with the study of effectiveness of behavior intervention in enhancing self-esteem of orphan and non-orphan children. In part 'A', matched group design was used for the study. The sample of the study consisted of two groups of children: Group I comprised 50 orphan children (25 girls and 25 boys) and Group II comprised 50 non-orphan children (25 girls and 25 boys). Results showed that orphan children have lower self-esteem than non-orphan children. In part 'B', pre and post design was used for the study. The sample of this part of the study consisted of two groups of children: Group I comprised 10 orphan children and Group II comprised 10 non-orphan children, having low self-esteem. Results of self-esteem measures of part 'A' of the study were utilized for the selection of the sample. Results showed effectiveness of behavior intervention in enhancing self-esteem of both orphan and non-orphan children.

INTRODUCTION

Self-esteem is a major key to success in life. The development of a positive self-concept or healthy self-esteem is extremely important to the happiness and success of children and adults. Self-esteem is how we feel about ourselves, and our behavior reflects those feelings. Self-esteem is a set of attitudes and beliefs that a person brings within him or herself, when facing the world. The term Self-esteem refers to the evaluation a person makes and customarily maintains with regard to him or herself.

Self-esteem is a ratio or relationship between our achievements and our aspirations (James, 1890). Self-esteem is an evaluative measure of one's self image (Coopersmith, 1967). The National Association for Self-Esteem defined Self-esteem as, "The experience of being capable of meeting life's challenges and being worthy of happiness."

---

*Corresponding author.

[1,2] Department of Psychology, Faculty of Social Sciences, Dayalbagh Educational Institute (Deemed University) Dayalbagh, Agra, UP, India.

E-mail: [1]surilaagarwala@gmail.com; [2]zeitgeist_2110@yahoo.com

Self-esteem includes a person's subjective appraisal of himself or herself as intrinsically positive or negative to some degree (Sedikides and Gregg, 2003).

Self-esteem expresses an attitude of approval or disapproval and indicates the extent to which a person believes him-or-herself capable, significant, successful and worthy. In short, a person's self-esteem is a judgment of worthiness that is expressed by the attitude he or she holds toward the self. It is a subjective experience conveyed to others by verbal reports and overt expressive behavior.

The term self-esteem includes cognitive, affective and behavioral elements. It is cognitive as one consciously thinks about oneself as one considers the discrepancy between one's ideal self, the person wishes to be, and the perceived self or the realistic appraisal of how one sees oneself. The affective elements refer to the feelings or emotions that one has when considering that discrepancy. The behavioral aspects of self-esteem are manifested in such behaviors as assertiveness, resilience, being decisive and respectful of others.

Children are not born with concerns of being good or bad, smart or stupid, lovable or unlovable. They develop these ideas. They form self-images—pictures of themselves—based largely on the way they are treated by the significant people, the parents, teachers and peers, in their lives. The self-image is the content of a person's perceptions and opinions about him-or-herself. The positive or negative attitudes and values by which a person views the self-image and the evaluations or judgments he or she makes about it form the person's self-esteem.

Self-esteem originates early in life and its structure becomes increasingly elaborative over the childhood years. The foundation of self-esteem is laid early in life when infants develop attachment with the adults who are responsible for them. When adults readily respond to their cries and smiles, babies learn to feel loved and valued. As young children learn to trust their parents and others who care for them to satisfy their basic needs they gradually feel wanted, valued and loved.

Our self-esteem is very dependent on factors within our environment. It is formed as a result of our years of experiences (especially the early ones). It could be said that one's eyes and ears record the message they receive from others, especially those most important to them. One unconsciously accepts all words and emotions as facts no matter how legitimate or based in reality. One's self-esteem is being continuously constructed and reconstructed by what is encountered in the mirror of others verbal and non-verbal messages.

The development of self-esteem is influenced by various factors. Family and social factors play a significant role in the development of self-esteem in children. Among the various social groups the family occupies the first and the most significant influence for the development of the child. It does not provide only the hereditary transmission of basic potentials for his development but also provides environmental conditions, personal relationships and a cultural pattern, favorable or unfavorable, positive or negative as reflected from its structure and the pattern of mutual relationship and emotional state among its members.

Parents, more than anyone else influences their child's self-esteem. Children who did not receive adequate parental love, acceptance and approval tend to develop a pattern of insatiable needs (Horney, 1945). Love, warmth and acceptance by parents have been determined to be extremely important in terms of developing a high degree of self-esteem (Coopersmith, 1967). Children develop high self-esteem simply because they have supportive parents. Children who experience a warm and affectionate relationship with their parents, who are accepted by their parents and who are aware of their parents' attitudes towards them, are most accepting of themselves (Sears, 1970). Early and continued parental acceptance contributes to a child's self-acceptance, which in turn enables him to be accepting of others. A positive self-concept in terms of self-esteem and self-acceptance is the foundation for healthy personality development. One's self-esteem is the quality and amount of parental attention and acceptance one received as a child (Loeb *et al.*, 1980; Gorden *et al.*, 1981). Parental attachment had mostly direct effects on self-esteem (Laible *et al.*, 2004). Parental support and monitoring would be associated with higher self-esteem and less risky behavior during adolescence (Parker *et al.*, 2005). A child who does not feel safe or is being abused at home will suffer immensely from low self-esteem (Lan, 2005).

Conflict between a parent and an adolescent may be indicative of problems of family cohesion and may predict poor self-esteem (Brien *et al.*, 1997; Bagley *et al.*, 2001). A child who is exposed to parents who fight and argue repeatedly may become depressed and withdrawn (Lan, 2005). Parental time given towards their children has significant influence on self-esteem, mastery and educational aspiration of children (Passmore, 2005).

Healthy self-esteem is a child's armor against the challenges of the world. Children who feel good about them seem to have an easier time handling conflicts and resisting negative pressures. They tend to smile more readily and enjoy life. A child or teen with high self-esteem will be able to act independently, assume responsibility, take pride in his accomplishments, tolerate frustration, attempt new tasks and challenges, handle positive and negative emotions, and offer assistance to others. A child who has healthy self-esteem tends to enjoy interacting with others. He or she is comfortable in social settings and enjoys group activities as well as independent pursuits. When challenges arise, he or she is able to work toward finding solutions. He or she voices discontent without belittling her or others. He or she knows his or her strength and weaknesses, and accepts them. A sense of optimism prevails. A person with high self-esteem is fundamentally satisfied with the type of person he is, yet he may acknowledge his faults while hoping to overcome them (Rosenberg, 2001).

The most important key of success in life is a favorable self-image. Children with high self-esteem feel better about their abilities to perform and who expect to do well actually perform better in school (Bodwin and Bruck, 1962; Bledsoe, 1964; Thomas and Patterson, 1964). Feelings of confidence and self-respect are as important in school performance as they are in other areas of life (Quimby, 1967). Self-esteem is significantly related to creativity, academic achievement, resistance to group pressures, willingness to express unpopular opinions, perceptual constancy (Coopersmith, 1967), selection of difficult tasks (Goodstadt and Kipens, 1971), perceived popularity (Simon, 1972), general and test anxiety (Many, 1973), effective communication between parents and youth (Matterson, 1974), family adjustment (Matterson, 1974) and perceived reciprocal liking (Simon and Bernstein, 1975). High levels of self-esteem are said to lead to a host of positive attributes such as well-adjusted children (Buri, Kirchner and Walsch, 1987), happy marriages (Thornstan, 1992), and a healthy sex life (Hally and Pollack, 1993). Persons having high esteem maintain their distinctness as individual and constant images of their capabilities (Meaux, 1996; Darlene, 1997). Children with higher self-esteem showed higher intrinsic motivation and better academic performance (Redden, 2000). Self-esteem can affect many aspects of children's lives, such as improving school performance and efforts toward achieving goals (Guest and Biasini, 2001).

Life satisfaction is thought to be the subjective part of quality of life *i.e.,* the feelings of the persons concerned about their functioning and circumstances. The feelings are influenced by self-esteem, the positive or negative attitude toward oneself, as well as life satisfaction and the effect of loneliness on self-esteem. The higher the self-esteem of an individual, the higher the life satisfaction and lower the feelings of loneliness experienced (Izonichak and Kleftaras, 2002).

People with high self-esteem report more positive attitudes, feelings, and life satisfaction and less anxiety, hopelessness and depressive symptoms (Crocker, 2002). People high in self-esteem claim to be more likeable and attractive, to have better relationships, and to make better impressions on others than people with low self-esteem (Vohs *et al.*, 2003). High self-esteem makes people more willing to speak up in groups and to criticize the group's approach. Leadership does not stem directly from self-esteem, but self-esteem may have direct effects. Relative to people with low self-esteem, those with high self-esteem show stronger in-group favoritism, which may increase prejudice and discrimination. Children with a healthy sense of self-esteem feel that the important adults in their lives accept them, care about them, and would go out of their way to ensure that they are safe and well (Schoenberg *et al.*, 2005).

On the other hand, a child with low self-esteem will avoid trying new things, feel unloved and unwanted, blame others for his own shortcomings, feel or pretend to feel emotionally indifferent, be unable to tolerate a normal level of frustration, put down his own talents and abilities, be easily influenced. A child who has low self-esteem may not want to try new things. He or she may frequently speak negatively about himself or herself. A child may exhibit a low tolerance for frustration, giving up easily or waiting for somebody else to take over. Children with low self-esteem tend to be overly critical of and easily disappointed in them. Children with low self-esteem see temporary setbacks as permanent, intolerable conditions. Low esteem children tend to be more reactive and pessimistic (Rosenberg and Owens, 2001).

Children with poor self-esteem are inclined to stop trying and just give up (Shaw and Alves, 1963; Brookover, 1965; Quimby, 1967). Children with poor self-esteem, do poorly in school, they blame the school or the teacher for their poor performance (Leafley, 1974). Low levels of self-esteem are not only a central cause of various psychological problems, but are also an important contributing factor to a multitude of social problems (Smelser, 1989). Low levels of self-esteem have been linked to such widely varying issues and problems as teenage pregnancy (Crockenberg and Soby, 1989), homicide (Lowenstein, 1989), Suicide (Choquet, Kovess and Poutiganat, 1993) and fires tarting (Stewart, 1993). The frequency and intensity of the affects of loneliness correlated inversely with self-esteem (Ginter *et al.*, 1994).

Individual with low self-esteem exhibit contingency expectations involving their interpersonal acceptance and rejection (Baldwin *et al.*, 2004). Lower self-esteem in childhood can lead to the development of a variety of emotional disturbance and an increased risk of suicide (Thompson, 2004). Children with low self-esteem feel that the important adults and peers in their lives do not accept them, do not care about them very much, and would not go out of their way to ensure their safety and well-being (Schoenberg *et al.*, 2005). Low self-esteem can actually trigger higher levels of stress, anxiety, sleeplessness and many other healths—depriving symptoms (Tobias, 2006). A person with low self-esteem experiencing feelings of worthlessness and not belonging, can unfortunately lead to thoughts of suicide.

Hence there is a need to enhance the self-esteem of children because low self-esteem can lead to many psychological problems. There are many possible interventions that can be initiated for children or adults with low self-esteem. Reinforcement, extension punishment, stimulus control, respondent conditioning *etc.* are some basic principles to modify the behavior. Goal of behavior modification is to decrease the occurrence of undesirable behaviors and increase the desirable behaviors that are not occurring frequently enough. There are many ways or procedure that psychologist usually consider for the behavior change such as self-management, respondent conditioning to decrease fear and anxiety, and to change cognitive behavior. There are three ways in which self-esteem can be raised—The first way, using self–deception and self-enhancement. The second way, is from within, through self-contact and autonomy.

The third way, is to boost people's self-esteem by being accepting and approving of them (Vonk *et al.*, 2006).

Parents, more than anyone else can promote their child self-esteem. If parents want to raise a responsible child, they needed to be attentive to the building of self-esteem at a very early age. It is important for parents to identify child's irrational beliefs about self, whether they are about perfection, attractiveness, ability, or anything else (Sheldon *et al.*, 2000). Eagle (2002) warns parents that if they did not work on building their child's self-esteem, the child was at risk of becoming an "insecure, unhappy teenager." Thompson (2004) favors the development of self-confidence and adds that there are many indirect ways to help a child to increase his/her self-esteem. He suggested to the parent of a child, "You can provide an environment in which the children feel secure, and you can try to teach them self-confidence and instill in them a love of learning by rewarding them when they succeed."

Considerable evidence indicates that self-esteem can be increased, if parents, teachers, or others create an atmosphere characterized by acceptance and freedom from anxiety, which tends to promote and encourage curiosity and exploratory behaviors. Responsive classroom environment is one of them. The central idea behind it is that schools can give children an awareness of their power and help them recognize that they can make a difference in their lives. Even a minimal, short-term interaction with a caring adult can have a positive impact on young Children (Anderman *et al.,* 2001; Daniels *el al.,* 2001).

Cognitive behavior that elicits unpleasant conditions, such as anger, anxiety, can be decreased with cognitive behavior modification procedures. Praise statements or critical statements from others can serve as reinforcers or punishers for behavior change. (Borowski and Muthukrishna, 1995; Larkin and Thyer, 1999). School system may consider to have additional classroom technologies for the purpose (Page, 2000).

Enhancement of self-esteem among children having low self-esteem is a great liability on the part of parents, teachers, psychologists, social workers *etc.* The enhancement was undertaken with the objectives—(a) To compare the self-esteem of orphan and non-orphan children (b) To study the effectiveness of behavior intervention in enhancing self-esteem of orphan and non-orphan children.

METHOD

The study was conducted in two parts. In part 'A', role of parents and family in the development of self-esteem of children was studied. To study the importance or role of parents and family in the development of children's self esteem, self-esteem of orphan and non-orphan children was compared and in part 'B', the effectiveness of behavior intervention in enhancing self-esteem of children was studied.

Part–A

Hypothesis

Orphan children have lower self-esteem than non-orphan children.

Sample

Sample consisted of two groups. Group I comprised of 50 orphan children (25 boys and 25 girls) and Group II comprised of 50 non-orphan children (25 boys and 25 girls). The age range of these children is 8–15 years. Orphan children have been selected from the orphanage of Agra and Vrindavan. Non-orphan children have been selected from those schools where orphan children are also enrolled.

Design

In the study, matched group design (matching by pairs—age, gender and educational level) was used.

Variables

Independent Variable - Orphan and Non-orphan Conditions
Dependent Variable - Self-Esteem
Controlled Variables - Age, gender, educational level

Measure

Self-esteem Inventory (SEI) developed by Coopersmith (1975) was used to measure self-esteem of orphan and non-orphan children. Its school form was used in the present research. Retest reliability for the SEI was reported by Coopersmith to be 0.88 and by Bedeian *et al.* (1977) as 0.80 for males and 0.82 for females. Kokens (1974, 1978) reported and confirmed the SEI's construct validity. In the present study Hindi translation of school form of the measure (done by the researcher) was used. The English and Hindi versions showed a correlation of 0.96 ($n = 100$).

Procedure

The SEI was administered on the children selected in the sample. The subjects were given the test booklets and requested to complete the entries of name, age, sex, school name, class, date *etc.* given on the first page. Then the instructions were read out loudly which were printed on the first page of the booklet.

The completed questionnaires were collected after being completed and the subjects were thanked for their co-operation.

Part–B

Hypothesis

Behavior intervention is effective in enhancing self-esteem of children.

Sample

10 orphan and 10 non-orphan children having low self-esteem were included in the sample. Results of self-esteem measures of part 'A' of the study were utilized for selection of the sample.

Design

Pre and post design was used.

Procedure

Self-esteem of orphan and non-orphan children was measured in part 'A' of the study, which served as baseline or pre-measure. Behavior intervention for 2 months was given to children included in the sample for the purpose of enhancing their self-esteem. The intervention included the following steps:

Initially Parents/guardians of each child were told that they should give extra attention and care to their child, encourage the child by helping and praising and behave in a friendly manner with the child so that the child can freely express himself/herself.

Other family members of each child were also told that they should give extra attention and care to their child, and encourage the child.

All the teachers teaching the children were given a list of these children. Teachers were requested to give special/extra attention to those children in the class, encourage them, give them maximum opportunities for participation in the class room activities and give them proper and immediate feedback for their performance/activities.

The researcher also met each child at least twice a week and talked to the child about his/her performances and achievement, praised and encouraged the child for still better results.

The above intervention was continued for two months. After intervention, the data were again collected on the measure.

ANALYSIS OF DATA AND RESULTS

Part–A

In part 'A' of the study, self-esteem of orphan and non-orphan children was compared. To compare the self-esteem of orphan and non-orphan children, Wilcoxon-Mann-Whitney test was used. Results are presented in result Table 1.

Result Table 1: Showing Value of z_U and Critical Value of z_U at 0.01 Level of Significance

Groups	*N*	z_U	*Level of Significance*	*Critical Value*
Orphan	50	–6.44	0.01	2.58
Non-orphan	50			

It can be observed from Result Table 1 that the value of z_U is –6.44. The observed value of –6.44 exceeds the critical value of 2.58 at $\alpha = 0.01$. Thus, the obtained value of z_U is significant at 0.01 level of significance. Therefore, we accept the hypothesis that orphan children have lower self-esteem than non-orphan children.

Part–B

In part 'B' of the study, Wilcoxon *T* Test was applied to test the significance of difference between pre and post measures of self-esteem of orphan and non-orphan children. Results are presented in Result Table 2, as well as Figures 1 and 2.

Result Table 2: Showing Value of 'T' for Both Groups

Groups	*N*	*Sum of Ranks with Positive Signs*	*Sum of Ranks with Negative Signs*	*T*
Orphan	10	55	0	0
Non-orphan	10	55	0	0

It can be observed from Results Table 2 that $T = 0$. According to Appendix Table, with $N = 10$ subjects, *T* must be less than or equal to 5 (on one tail test at $\alpha = 0.01$) in order to accept the hypothesis. *T* observed (0) for both groups is less than the table value of *T*, so we conclude that behavior intervention is effective in enhancing self-esteem of orphan as well as non-orphan children.

It is indicated in Figures 1 and 2 that results are not only statistically significant but they are significant clinically also. The statistical significance represents that behavior intervention is effective in the enhancement of self-esteem, while the clinical significance is helpful in accepting the hypothesis as well, as it is representative of the fact that behavior intervention is effective not only in few particular individual cases but in case of all who have low self-esteem.

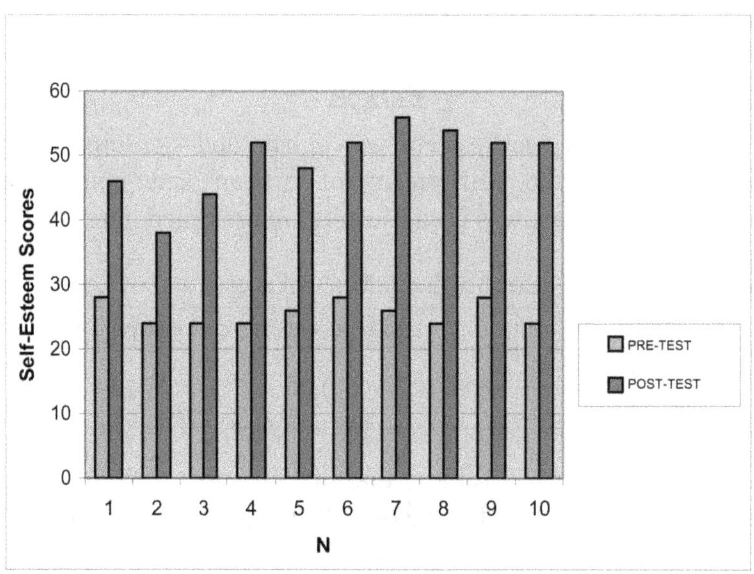

Figure 1: Showing Pre and Post Test Scores of Orphan Children

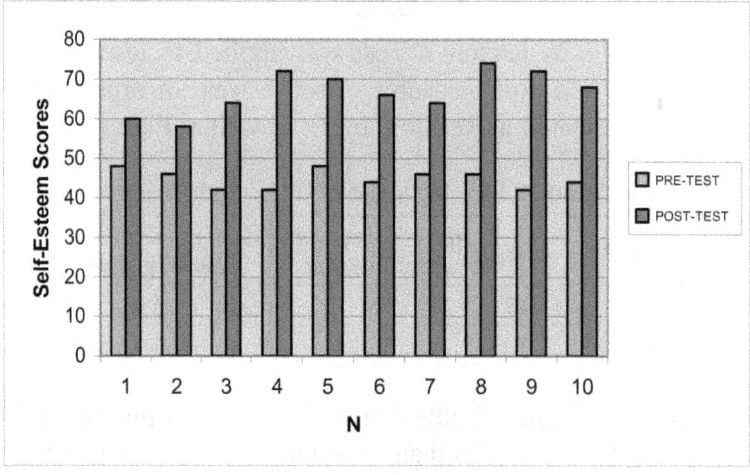

Figure 2: Showing Pre and Post Test Scores of Non-Orphan Children

DISCUSSION

Part–A

Results of part 'A' of the study showed that orphan children have lower self-esteem than non-orphan children. The children who have both their parents and are living with them in a family atmosphere of love, care and security have higher self-esteem than the orphan children, living in an orphanage. Parents play an important role in building and development of child's self-esteem. An orphan child remains devoid of parental love, care and protection, which affects the development of child's self-esteem

Children, who receive parental love, care, protection and acceptance, tend to be outgoing, active and adjustive. They tend to have positive, friendly and co-operative attitude with their peer groups. Children who remain devoid of parental love, care, protection and acceptance tend to have a variety of adjustment problems at home, in school and with their peer groups.

Love, warmth and acceptance by parents have been determined to be extremely important in terms of developing a high degree of self-esteem. Children who did not receive parental love and acceptance tend to develop low levels of self-esteem (Kernis *et al.*, 2000). Children of caregivers, who are warm and responsive, consequently develop relatively positive self-views (Arend *et al.*, 2000). Being accepted by parents is a major contingency for everyone. Parental rejection or disapproval produces sharp declines in children's self-esteem; these effects occurred regardless of their initial self-esteem level and regardless of whether they themselves acknowledged that their self-esteem depended on others (Leary *et al.,* 2003). Self-esteem is strongly related to the levels of parenting dimensions (responsiveness and demanding ness) (Slicker *et al.*, 2004).

The quality and amount of parental love, attention and acceptance is the critical factor as an antecedent to one's self-esteem. Therefore orphan children who remain devoid to parental love, attention and acceptance tend to develop low levels of self-esteem.

Part–B

The result of part 'B' of the study revealed that there is significant increase in the self-esteem of orphan and non-orphan children after intervention. These results indicated that, behavior intervention is effective in enhancing self-esteem of children. Figure 1 and 2 also represents that behavior intervention is effective in the enhancement of self-esteem. If we compare Figures 1 and 2, it will be evident that although behavior intervention has positive effect on the enhancement of self-esteem in both orphan and non-orphan children yet the self-esteem of orphan children has increased to a greater degree as compared to non-orphan children. The reason could be that orphans are devoid of parental love, care and acceptance to a greater extent. Therefore, when some love, care, approval and acceptance were given, their self-esteem enhanced more than the self-esteem of non-orphans.

Self-esteem has been positively linked to a wide range of behaviors, including mastery and achievement, subjective well-being and health. Low self-esteem has been identified as a risk factor for aggression, delinquency, depression, poor school performance and so forth. Having low self-esteem has been found to be associated with a tendency to withdraw and isolate one's self from others (Gibson, 1981; Peck and Kaplan, 1995; Rosenberg and Owens, 2001). Low self-esteem individuals tend to be more reactive and pessimistic (Rosenberg and Owens 2001). An essential element of the low self-esteem is shame. It is a highly negative emotional state. In shame the entire person seems to feel unworthy.

Hence there is a need to enhance self-esteem of children. Enhancement of self-esteem among children is of great importance from individual as well as social point of view. The important way is to boost people's self-esteem by being accepting and approving of them. If parents, family members, teachers or others create an atmosphere that is characterized by acceptance and freedom from anxiety, which tends to promote and encourage curiosity and exploratory behavior, children would learn to honor their strength and maintain their high self-esteem. Building self-esteem in children requires collaboration between parents, family members, school personnel and the child (Elliot and Dweck, 1988; Wells *et al.*, 2002).

One way to experience high self-esteem would be to rethink what is important. When people follow their actual strengths rather than some standard given to them by society, their parents or their peers, they begin to develop high self-esteem. When their skills are being appreciated by other people, it can result in a rapid improvement in self-esteem.

To increase individual's self-esteem, it is necessary to change their self-concept (Griffin *et al.*, 2001). They need to perceive themselves as possessing the resources to get the important things they want from life. Much of what people want reflects the values of society, parents and peers. If they have skills consistent with those values, they are more likely to experience high self-esteem. Should their strengths be elsewhere, they might need to change their values, so that they can derive self-esteem from the skill that they have.

This study suggests that parents, family members and teachers can provide individualized support for children's progress and create an atmosphere that sends a clear message that children can learn, and improve their performance and behavior.

CONCLUSION

Result of part 'A' of the study leads to the conclusion that orphan children have lower self-esteem than non-orphan children. The quality and amount of parental and familial love, attention and acceptance is the critical factor as an antecedent to one's self-esteem. Therefore orphan children who remain devoid of parental and familial love, care and protection tend to develop low levels of self-esteem. Result of part 'B' of the study leads to the conclusion that behavior intervention is effective in enhancing self-esteem of orphan as well as non-orphan children. It is possible to change their 'pessimistic' view and turn into 'optimistic', with the help of some intervention strategies.

REFERENCES

Anderman, E.M., Eccles, J.S., Roeser, R. and Blumenfeld, P. (2001). "Learning to Value Mathematics and Reading. Relations to Mastery and Performance-oriented Instructional Practices." *Contemporary Educational Psychology*, 26, 76–95.

Arend, M. and Gove, F. (2000). "Continuity of Individual Adaptation from Infancy to Kindergarten: A Predictive Study of Ego-resiliency and Curiosity in Preschoolers." *Child Development,* 50, 950–959.

Bagley, C., Bertrand, L. and Mallick, K. (2001). "Discrepant Parent Adolescent Views on Family Functioning." *Journal of Comparative Family Studies, 32*(3), 393–403.

Bedeian, A.G., Geagud, R.J. and Zmud, R.W. (1977). "Test-retest Reliability and Internal Consistency of the Short Form of Coopersmith's Self-Esteem Inventory." *Psychological Reports,* 41, 1041–1042.

Bledsoe, J.C. (1964). "Self-concepts of Children and their Intelligence, Achievement, Interests and Anxiety." *Journal of Individual Psychology,* 20, 55–58.

Bodwin, R. and Bruck, M. (1962). "The Relationship between Self-concept and the Presence and Absence of Scholastic under Achievement." *Journal of Clinical Psychology,* 18, 181–182.

Borkowski, J.G. and Muthukrishna, N. (1995). "Learning Environments and Skills Generalization: How Context Facilitate Regulatory Processes and Efficacy Beliefs." In Weiner, F. and Schneider, W. (Eds.), *Memory Performance and Competence: Issues in Growth and Development*, Hillsdale, N.J.: Erilbaum, 283–300.

Brien, M., Bahadur, M.A. and Cee, C. (1997). "The Influence of a Big Brothers Programme on the Adjustment of Boys in Single-parent Families." *Journal of Psychology,* 13(2), 143–156.

Brookover, W.B. (1965). *Self-concept of Ability and School Achievement II: Improving Academic Achievement Through Student's Self-concept Enhancement.* U.S. Office of Education, Co-Operative Research Project No. 2831. East Lansing, MI: Office of Research and Publications, Michigan State University.

Buri, J., Kirchner, P. and Walsh, J. (1987). "Familial Correlates of Self-esteem in Young American Adults." *Journal of Social Psychology,* 127, 583–588.

Choquet, M., Kovess, V. and Poutignat, N. (1993). "Suicidal Thoughts among Adolescents: An Intercultural Approach." *Adolescence,* 28, 649–659.

Coopersmith, S. (1967). *The Antecedents of Self-esteem*. Palo, Alto, CA: Consulting Psychologists Press, Inc., 3–10.

Coopersmith, S. (1975). *Developing Motivation in Young Children.* Palo Alto, CA: Consulting Psychologists, Press, Inc.

Crockenberg, S. and Soby, B. (1989). "Self-esteem and Teenage Pregnancy." In A. Mecca, N. Smelser and J. Vasconcellos (Eds.), *The Social Importance of Self-Esteem.* Berkeley: University of California Press, 125–164.

Crocker, J. (2002). "Self-esteem that's Based on External Sources has Mental Health Consequences." *Journal of Social Issues, 58*(3), 16.

Daniels, D.H., Kalkman, D.L. and McCombs, B.L. (2001). "Yong Children's Perspectives on Learning and Teacher Practices in Different Classroom Contexts: Implications for Motivation." *Early Education and Development,* 12, 253–273.

Eagle, C. (2002). *All That She Can Be.* New York: Simon and Schuster.

Elliot, E.S. and Dweck, C.S. (1988). "Goals: An Approach to Motivation and Achievement." *Journal of Personality and Social Psychology,* 54, 5–12.

Ginter, E.J., Dwinell, E. and Patricia, L. (1994). "The Importance of Perceived Duration Loneliness and its Relationship with Self-esteem and Academic Performance." *Journal of College Student Development,* 35(6), 456–460.

Goodstadt, B. and Kipens, D. (1971). *Report on Achievement Instruction Materials.* Philadelphia: Research for Better Schools.

Gordon, D., Nowicki, S. and Wichern, F. (1981). "Observed Maternal and Child Behaviors in Dependency Producing Task a Function of Children's Locus of Control Orientation", *Merrill Palmer Quarterly,* 27, 43–51.

Griffin, D.W., Bellavia, G. and Rose, P. (2001). "The Mismeasure of Love: How Self-doubt Contaminates Relationship Beliefs." *Personality and Social Psychology Bulletin,* 27(4), 423–436.

Guest, K.C. and Biasini, F.J. (2001). "Middle Childhood, Poverty and Adjustment: Does Social Support have an Impact?" *Psychology in the Schools,* 38(6), 549–560.

Horney, K. (1945). *Our Inner Conflicts.* A Constructive Theory on Neuroses, New York: Norton.

Izonichak, I. and Kleftaras, G. (2002). "Paraplegia from Spiral and Injury: Self-esteem, Loneliness and Life Satisfaction." *Psychological Abstracts,* 89, 10.

James, W. (1890). *The Principles of Psychology, 1,* New York: Holt.

Kernis, M.H., Brown, A.C. and Brody, G.H. (2000). "Fragile Self-esteem in Children and its Associations with Perceived Patterns of Parent-child Communication." *Journal of Personality,* 68(2), 225–252.

Kokenes, B. (1974). "Grade Level Differences in Factors of Self-esteem." *Developmental Psychology,* 10, 954–958.

Kokenes, B. (1978). "A Factor Analytic Study of the Coopersmith's Self-Esteem Inventory." *Adolescence,* 13, 149–155.

Lan, C.H. (2005). "Relationship among Socioeconomic Status, Parenting, Academic Achievement and Self-esteem in Early and Middle Adolescence: A Longitudinal Study." *Psychological Abstracts International,* 65(12–A), 4519.

Larkin, R. and Thyer, B.A. (1999). "Evaluating Cognitive Behavioral Group Counseling to Improve Elementary School Student's Self-esteem, Self-control and Classroom Behavior." *Behavioral Interventions,* 14(3), 147–161.

Leafley, H.P. (1974). "Social and Familial Correlates of Self-esteem among American Indian Children." *Child Development,* 45, 829–833.

Leary, M.R., Gallagher, B., Fors, E. and Mills, A. (2003). "The Invalidity of Disclaimers about the Effects of Social Feedback on Self-esteem." *Personality and Social Psychology Bulletin,* 29, 623–636.

Loeb, R.C., Horst, L. and Horton, P.J. (1980). "Family Interaction Patterns Associated with Self-esteem in Pre-adolescent Girls and Boys." *Merrill Palmer Quarterly,* 26, 203–217.

Many, M. (1973). "The Relationship between Anxiety and Self-esteem in Grades 4 through 8 (Doctoral Dissertation)", In S. Coopersmith's SEI, Palo Alto. CA 94303.

Matterson, R. (1974). "Adolescent Self-esteem, Family Communication and Satisfaction." *Journal of Psychology,* 86, 35–47.

Meaux, M. (1996). "A Comparative Investigation of Self-esteem, Achievement Motivation, Learning Style and Parental Relationship Across Black While Gifted Talented Adolescent Group (Doctoral Dissertation, University of Chicago, 1995)." *Dissertation Abstracts International,* 56, 4706 A.

Page, M.S. (2000). "A Comparison of Student Achievement Self-esteem and Classroom Interactions in Technology Enriched and Traditional Elementary Classroom with Low Socio-economic Students (Doctoral Dissertation, Louisiana Technical University, 1999)." *Dissertation Abstracts International,* 60, 3975A.

Parker, J.S. and Benson, M.J. (2005). "Parent-adolescent Relations and Adolescent Functioning: Self-esteem, Substance Abuse and Delinquency." *Family Therapy,* 32(3), 131–142.

Passmore, N.L., Gerard, J., Sandra, F. and Evans, B. (2005). "Parental Bonding and Identity Style as Correlates of Self-esteem among Adult Adoptees and Non-adoptees." *Family Relations: Interdisciplinary Journal of Applied Family Studies,* 54(4), 523–534.

Quimby, V. (1967). "Difference in the Self-ideal Relationship of an Achieved Group and an Underachieved Group." *California Journal of Educational Research,* 18, 23–31.

Rascoe, B.J. (2002). "Effect of Competing Power Dynamics of Science Teachers and Gifted Black Male's Interactions in the Science Learning Environment." (Doctoral Dissertation, University of Georgia, 2001). *Dissertation Abstracts International,* 62, 3025377 D.A.

Redden, S.A. (2000). "Self-esteem and Intrinsic Motivational Effects of Using a Constructivist and Behaviorist Approach to a Computer Usage in Fifth Grade Hispanic Classrooms." (Doctoral Dissertation, NOVA, South Eastern University, 2000). *Dissertation Abstracts International,* 62, 464A.

Rosenberg, M. and Owens, T.J. (2001). "Low Self-esteem People: A Collective Portrait." In T.J. Owens, S. Stryker and N. Goodman (Eds.), *Extending Self-esteem Theory and Research: Sociological and Psychological Currents* (pp. 400–436). New York: Cambridge University Press.

Sears, R.R. (1970). "Relation of Early Socialization Experiences to Self-concept and Gender Role in Middle Childhood." In C.J. Ronald and Gene, R. Medinnus's *Behavior and Development,* New York, 267–289.

Sedikides, C. and Gregg, A.P. (2003). "Portraits of the Self." In M.A. Hogg and J. Cooper (Eds.), *Sage Handbook of Social Psychology*. London: Sage Publications, 110–138.

Shaw, M. and Alves, G. (1963). "The Self-concept of Bright Academic Underachievers II." *Personal Guidance Journal,* 42, 401–403.

Simon, R.G. and Bernstein, F. (1975). "Sex, Sex Roles and Self-image." *Journal of Youth and Adolescence,* 4, 229–258.

Thomas, P. and Patterson, S.E. (1964). "Self-concepts of Children and their Intelligence, Achievement, Interests and Anxiety." *Journal of Individual Psychology,* 20, 59–60.

Thompson, A.H., Roger, H. and Battle, K. (2004). "The Relative Age Effect and the Development of Self-esteem." *Educational Research,* 46(3), 313–320.

Tobias, E., Lichtenstein, P. and Granlund, M. (2006). "Long Term Relationship between Symptoms of ADHD and Self-esteem in a Prospective Longitudinal Study of Twins." *Acta Paediatrica,* 95(6).

Vohs, K.D., Baumeister, R.F., Campbell, J.D. and Krueger, J.I. (2003). "Does High Self-esteem Cause Better Performance, Interpersonal Success, Happiness, or Healthier Lifestyles?" *Psychological Science in the Public Interest,* 4(1), 1–44.

Vonk, R., Jolij, J. and Boog, I. (2006). *Effects of Unconditional Positive Regard and Self-Reflection on Self-esteem.* Manuscript in Preparation.

Wells, D., Miller, M. and Clanton, R. (2002). "Using a Psycho-educational Approach to Increase the Self-esteem of Adolescents at High Risk for Dropping Out." *Psychological Abstracts*, 89, 31678.

Depression and Self-Esteem: A Behavior Modification Approach

Surila Agarwala*[1] and Shraddha Sharma[2]

ABSTRACT

The study was undertaken with the purpose to compare the self-esteem among subjects having high depression and those having low depression and to study the effect of behavior intervention in reducing depression. The study was conducted in two parts. Part 'A' deals with the comparison of self-esteem among individuals having high depression and low depression. Part 'B' deals with the study of effectiveness of behavior intervention in reducing depression and to study the effect of reduced depression on level of self-esteem. In Part 'A' matched group design was used. The sample of Part 'A' consisted of two groups. Group I comprised 5 subjects having high depression and Group II consisted of 5 subjects having low depression. Results show that the individuals having high depression have lower level of self-esteem than those having low level of depression. In Part 'B' pre and post design was used. Results of depression measure of Part 'A' were utilized in Part 'B' for the selection of the sample. Sample consisted of 5 subjects having high depression. Results of Part 'A' were utilized as baseline measure for Part 'B'. Results revealed the effectiveness of behavior intervention in reducing depression and reduction in depression leads to enhancement of self-esteem.

INTRODUCTION

Health Psychology is the field within Psychology, devoted to understand psychological influences on how people stay healthy, why they become ill, and how they respond when they get ill. Health Psychology consists of such issues and promotes interventions to help people stay well or get over illness. It applies psychological principles and research for the improvement of health, treatment and prevention of illness. We are more likely to think of health as the absence of disease rather than as the absence of a debilitating battlefield injury. A Person, who is free from disease but still leads a depressed, stressful life, wouldn't be called healthy. Good health is not limited only to physical well being; mental health is also included in it. In 1946 charter, the WHO defined health as "a state of complete physical, mental, and social well-being and not merely the absence of disease or infirmity. Health is a positive multi-dimensional state that involves three domains: Physical health, Psychological health, and Social health."

---

* Corresponding author.

[1, 2] Department of Psychology, Faculty of Social Sciences, Dayalbagh Educational Institute, Deemed University, Dayalbagh, Agra, UP, India.

E-mail: [1]surilaagarwala@gmail.com; [2]shraddhasharma09@gmail.com

Psychological health is being able to think clearly, have good self-esteem and to enjoy a general feeling of well being. It includes creativity, problem solving skills and emotional stability. It is also characterized by self-acceptance, openness to new ideas and general hardiness of personality. Each domain of health is influenced by the other two domain, *e.g.,* an emotionally stable person who has good problem solving skills (Psychological health) will probably have good healthy social relationships (Social health) than a depressed person who is not able to care for personal and social relationships. Conversely person with poor physical health faces challenges, to his/her self-esteem (Psychological health) and to relationships with her/his family and friends (Social health).

Depression is one of the most common psychological problems and is called the common cold of mental health. Depression presents a person with depressed mood, loss of interest or pleasure; feeling of guilt or low self-esteem, disturbed sleep or appetite, low energy, and poor concentration. These problems can become chronic or recurrent and lead to substantial impairment in an individual's ability to take care of his/her everyday responsibilities. The term "Depression" itself refers to a heterogeneous set of phenomena, ranging from a normal mood, which is common and probably affects most of us at some point in our lives. Everyone of us faces various ups and downs. Most people may become mildly depressed in response to these ups and down in their lives, but only a few react with a severe affective state (Gotlib and Hammen, 1998). Everyone feels down, blue, bummed, hopeless, or pessimistic from time to time. Almost everyone feels depressed, at least in its mild forms. When loss and pain occur we go into mourning and react to loss with some of the symptoms of depression. We become sad and discouraged, apathetic and passive, the future looks bleak, and some of the zest goes out of living. Normal depression differs in degree from clinical disorder. The line between a "normal" depressive disturbance and a clinically significant depressive disorder is blurry. There are three dimensions of depression.

Frequency—How often one feels down or depressed? Everyday? Three times a week? Once in a month? All the time?

Severity—How bad is it? Does one feel suicidal? Totally hopeless and stuck in as dark hole? Or just kind of lousy and negative?

Duration—How long does it last? Until one is with own partner? Until one goes to home for the weekend? Just a couple of hours? Does it drag on for days, weeks, or even months? Has one felt somewhat depressed throughout the whole life?

Depression has been determined by the World Health Organization (WHO) as one of the most disabling disorders in the world. It affects roughly 25% women and 10% men at some point in their life time. It has been estimated that at least 12% of the adult population have at least one episode of "depression" serious enough that individual should seek professional help (Schuyler and Ketz, 1998). A review of studies from a number of countries estimated that between 17% and 22% of youth under 18 years of age experience emotional and behavioral problems (Soloman *et al.*, 2003). Large random population surveys commonly report that 25 to 30% of adolescents describe themselves as currently feelings at least somewhat depressed (National Institute of Mental Health, Delhi, 2004). It is estimated that one of every 20 adolescents suffers from clinical depression (Tredeau, Michelle, 2006). It is thus estimated more than 340 million people worldwide suffer from depression at any particular time. A high recurrence rate may be associated with genetic vulnerability, early symptoms onset, poor diagnosis and treatment, and inadequate emphasis on prevention. The overwhelming burden of depression may also be compounded by co-morbidity with medical disorders such as diabetes, stroke and cardiovascular disease and other psychiatric disorders such as anxiety disorders, substance abuse and alcoholism. Untreated depression often leads to personal, marital, familial, and career difficulties, and is associated with a high rate of suicide, approaching 15% of patients with major depression. Although the exact cause of depression is unknown but the thinking is that depression is associated with mental illness, and is often associated with current or early life stress. This combination of genetic and environmental factor causes specific changes in brain chemicals such as Serotonin, Nor-epinephrine or Dopamine that may explain some of depressive symptoms. It is also feared that the more frequent the episode, the high the likelihood that some form of brain damage in the form of brain tissue degeneration will occur.

Depression is a combination of biological, genetic and psychological factors. At the biological level, depression results from abnormal levels of certain neurotransmitters in the brain. This can be caused by changing levels of hormones. Depression is not just a state of mind; it is related to chemical imbalance in the brain that carries signals in brain and nerves. These chemicals are called neurotransmitters. In fact all psychological problems have some physical manifestations, and all physical illnesses have psychological components. Depression during adolescence has been associated with a number of factors including a failure, insecure attachment, friction, hostility, lack of affection (Gottib and Hammen, 1999; McCauley, Greenberg, Burike and Mitchell, 2002), and family atmosphere (Batt, 2001; Sinha, R.C. (2004). The important role of parental depression and their interaction patterns have been noted in the occurrence of depression (Sanford, 1996; Allen *et al.* 1997; Chen and Robin, 1998; Hammen and Brennan, 2003).

The good news about depression is that safe and effective treatment is available for most forms of the disease. There are various treatment options such as counseling, psychotherapy; trauma focused therapy, combination of antidepressant and other therapies, electro convulsive therapy *etc.* Treatment depends on the cause and severity of depression and, to some extent, on personal preference. In mild and moderate depression, psychotherapy is often the most appropriate treatment. In combined treatment, medication can relieve physical symptoms quickly, while psychotherapy enables the patient to learn more effective ways of handling his problems. Counselling and psychotherapy can be particularly helpful in treating depression. In Cognitive behavior Therapy, a form of psychotherapy, clients learns to replace dysfunctional self-speech (Such as I knew I'd never be able to cope with this job) with adaptive alternatives (The job's not going well, but I am capable of working out a plan to overcome the problems). Cognitive-behavioral treatment for depression includes attempts to improve interpersonal problem-solving skills. The objectives of Cognitive behavior Therapy typically are to identify irrational or maladaptive thoughts, assumptions and beliefs that are related to debilitating negative emotions and to identify how they are dysfunctional, inaccurate, or simply not helpful. The aim is to reject the distorted cognitions and to replace them with more realistic and self-helping alternatives. A person's core beliefs (often formed in childhood) contribute to thoughts that pop up in everyday life in response to situations. Cognitive Practitioners hold that clinical depression is typically associated with negatively biased thinking and irrational thoughts. Cognitive Behavior Therapy (CBT) helps subject in distinguishing between problems that can be and, can not be resolved and develop better coping skills. Cognitive therapy has been proved as effective without the negative side effects. Cognitive behavior therapy was actually reported superior on 9 of 10 outcome measures (self reported) at the end of treatment (Antonuccio, 1995). The U.S. Food and Drug Administration (2001) studied the effectiveness of CBT and found that there are 56% improvements in depressive symptoms, when CBT was provided to subjects.

Depression and self-esteem may be viewed as vicious cycle. The inability to relate positively in social situation may lead to low self-esteem that leads to depression. The depression then leads to further inability to relate with others or be fully accepted in social groups, which then adds to the feelings of low self-esteem. The term 'self-esteem' refers to the evaluation a person makes and maintains with regard to him or herself. Self-esteem expresses an attitude of approval or disapproval and indicates the extent to which a person believes himself or herself capable, significant, successful and worthy. Self-esteem has become a widely used concept. James (1890) first talked about self-esteem in; he described it as a ratio or relationship between our achievements and our aspiration. According to Coopersmith (1967), "Self-esteem is an evaluative measure of one's self image." Branden (1997) defined self-esteem as "The disposition to experience oneself as being competent to cope with the basic challenges of life and of being worthy of happiness." The National Association for self-esteem (1997) modified this to define self-esteem as "The experience of being capable of meeting life's challenges and being worthy of happiness." According to Reasnor (2000), member of National Association for self-esteem, the term self-esteem includes cognitive, affective and behavioral elements. It is cognitive as one consciously thinks about oneself and considers the discrepancy between one's ideal self, the person wishes to be, and the perceived self or the realistic appraisal of how one sees oneself. The affective elements refer to the feelings or emotions that one has while considering that discrepancy. The behavioral aspect refers to the state when self-esteem is manifested in such behaviors as assertiveness, resilience, being decisive and respectful of others. According to Sedikdes and Greg (2003) "Self-esteem includes a person's subjective appraisal of himself or herself as intrinsically positive or negative to some degree.

Self-esteem has been found to be affected by many factors such as parental ambition and expectations (Gordon *et al.,* 2001). Maternal depression also affects level of self-esteem (Laura *et al.,* 1999). Gender difference is also found to be related with level of self-esteem (Block, 1991; Kling *et al.*, 2003). Friends and peers also play a significant role in the development of self-esteem. A high quality friendship is associated with high self-esteem (Pomerantz and Saxon, 2001; Bloger, 2004). Socio-economic status is also one of the important factors that affect self-esteem of the individual (Kim and Alison, 2000; Marsh *et al.* 2004). Perceived physical appearance, personal identity, academic performance and academic quality were also found to be related with development of self-esteem (Meaux, 2005).

High self-esteem is said to be a host of positive attitudes such as good academic performance (Agarwala, and Raj, 2003), well adjusted children (Kirchner, and Walsh, 1999), good health, general wellness behavior (Abood and Conway, 2004), optimism about the future and with positive belief about one's skills and abilities (Brown, 1999; Campbell, 2000). In contrast low level of self-esteem has been linked to behavioral problems and poor school performance (Agarwala, and Raj, 2003), anxiety, fear, suicides and maladjustment (Brown and Mcgill, 2002). It is found that low self-esteem leads to psychological problems *e.g.,* depression, loneliness, alienation (Leary, 2004). Low level of self-esteem is strongly associated with friendship problems and social treatment (Crocker and Lutithnen, 2003). Low level of self-esteem is strongly correlated with negative mental models of self in relationships (Griffin and Bartholomew, 1999) and is associated with feeling that one is not valued by or valuable to others (Murry, Holmes, Griffin, Bellovia and Rose, 2005). For some people, low level of self-esteem is not only a central cause of various psychological problems, but is also an important contributing factor to a multitude of social problems. Echoing this view, Neil Smelser (1999) stated "Many, if not most, of the major problems plaguing society have roots in the low self-esteem of many of the people who make up society."

The present study was undertaken with the purpose to study depression and self-esteem among undergraduate students. According to Feldman and Elliot (2003), the peak age of depression and low self-esteem coincides with the transition from school to college. When student enters into college life, it is particularly important phase of life because individuals are faced with challenging problems and struggle for their educational and professional career as well as personal life settlement. The present study is designed to examine effect of behavior modification in reducing depression. It also explores the effects of reduced depression on the level of self-esteem of subjects. Students of today are the professionals of tomorrow. If we wish for a healthy and prosperous society, it is necessary that individuals should be physically as well as mentally healthy. Depression is the 4th leading contributor to the global burden of disease (DALYs) in 2000 and diagnosed as one of the leading causes of mental illness. By the year 2020, depression is projected to reach 2$_{nd}$ place in the ranking of DALYs (Disability Adjusted Life Years) calculated for all ages, both sexes. Today, depression is already the 2$_{nd}$ cause of DALYs in the age category 15–44 years for both sexes combined.

Objectives

- To compare the self-esteem of the subjects having high depression and the subjects having low depression.
- To study the effectiveness of behavior intervention in reducing depression.
- To study the effect of reduced depression on level of self-esteem.

Hypotheses

- Subjects having high depression have lower level of self-esteem as compared to the subjects having low level of depression.
- Behavior intervention is effective in reducing depression.
- Reduced level of depression leads to enhancement of self-esteem.

Method

The study was conducted into two parts. In part 'A' self-esteem of the subjects having high level of depression and low level of depression was compared and in part 'B' the effectiveness of behavior intervention in reducing level of depression and the effects of reduced depression on self-esteem of the subjects were studied.

Sample

The sample for part 'A' of the study consisted of two groups of subjects. Group 'I' comprised 5 subjects undergoing high depression and Group 'II' comprised 5 subjects having low depression. While selecting the subjects care was taken to match them on selected variables like age, sex, and education. The sample for part 'B' of the study comprised 5 subjects having high depression. Results of depression measure in part 'A' were utilized for the selection of the sample in part 'B'.

Tools

Following tools were used in the present study:

1. Depression of subjects was measured with the help of highly standardized Beck Depression Inventory developed by Beck (1996). Its second edition (BDI-II) is a 21 items self-reported instrument for measuring the severity of depression. The reliability coefficient of this inventory by test-retest method was found to be .93.
2. Self-esteem Inventory developed by Coopersmith (1975, was used to assess the level of self-esteem of the individual having high level of depression and those having low level of depression. Its adult form used in the present research. Test-retest reliability for the Self-Esteem Inventory was reported by Coopersmith to be .88 and by Bedeian *et al.* (1977) .88 for males and .82 for females. In the present study Hindi translation of adult form of the measure (done by researcher) was used. The English and Hindi versions showed a correlation of .96 (n = 20).

Procedure

In part 'A' of the study investigator met each subject personally. Rapport was established with the subjects. All the respondents were asked to fill up the Beck Depression inventory by themselves. They were assured that their responses would be kept confidential. The scoring of the inventories was done with the help of the manual. The subjects who were found highly depressed on the basis of scores obtained by them and those who were found, having low depression were divided into two different groups; Group I and Group II respectively. Then the self-esteem of the subjects having high depression and subjects having low depression was measured with the help of Self-esteem inventory developed by Coopersmith (1996). In part 'B' of the study subjects having high depression were selected. Initial measures of depression of subject served as baseline measures. Behavior Intervention for 2 months was given to subjects for the purpose of reducing depression. Behavior intervention included Cognitive Restructuring through Counseling and Jacobson's Progressive Muscle Relaxation. Cognitive Restructuring helped the subjects in modifying their internal sentences like what they say to themselves. The subjects also became aware of how their internal sentences caused their emotional problems. Jacobson's Progressive Muscle Relaxation Therapy involved tensing and releasing various voluntary muscles groups throughout the body in an orderly sequence.

The intervention was given for 40–45 minutes daily for a fortnight, then twice a week for next fortnight, after that once a week for a fortnight and finally once in a fortnight. Subjects were asked to do relaxation at home at least for once in a day. Thus the intervention continued for two months. Then the post measure of depression and self-esteem were conducted. The measurement conditions maintained during pre-measure were in effect during post measure also.

ANALYSIS OF DATA AND RESULTS

The data collected were tabulated group wise and subjected to statistical analysis with the help of Wilcoxon Mann Whitney 'U' test in part 'A' of the study.

Table 1: 'U' Value for the Self-esteem of the Subjects having High Depression and the Subjects having Low Depression at 0.01 Level of Significance

Groups	*N*	*'U'*	*Level of Significance*	*Result*
Subjects having high depression	5			
Subjects having low depression	5	1	0.01	Significant

The result in Result Table 1 indicates that obtained 'U' value has been found significant at .01 level, which proves one of the underlying hypothesis that the subjects having high level of depression have lower level of self-esteem than the subjects having low level of depression.

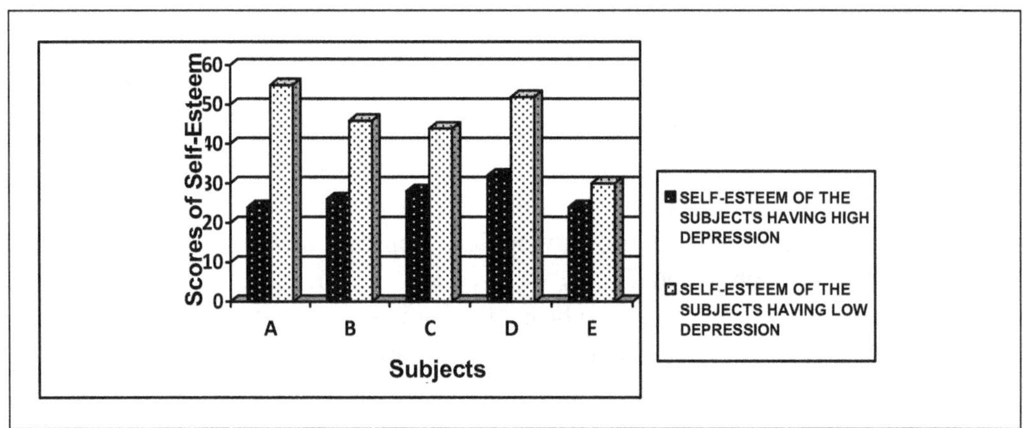

Figure 1: Comparison among Self-esteem Scores of Subjects having High Depression and Those Having Low Depression

Figure 1 represents the difference between self-esteem of the subjects having high depression and the subjects having low depression. Graphical presentation shows that majority of the subjects having high depression have lower level of depression except the one because individual differences can not be avoided.

In 'Part B' of the present study it was hypothesized that behavior modification reduces the level of depression. A-test was applied to test the significance of difference between pre-intervention and post-intervention scores of depression. Result is presented with the help of Result Table 2.

Result Table 2: Showing Value of 'A-test' for Pre-Intervention and Post-Intervention Scores of Depression

Group	*N*	*'A'*	*Level of Significance*	*Results*
Subjects Received Behavior Intervention for Reducing Depression	5	.2	.01	Significant

Results, presented in Result Table 2 show that obtained 'A' value is .2 and is significant at a given level if it is equal to or less than the value given in the table. The value given in the table at .01 level is .238. Thus, the obtained value .2 is less than the critical value .238 and it proves that there is significant difference between the pre-intervention scores and post intervention scores of depression.

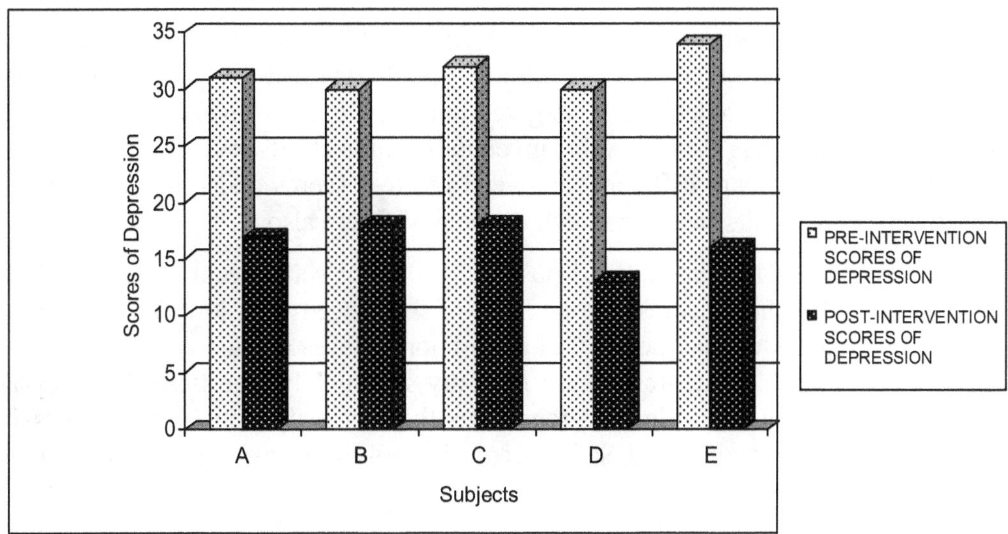

Figure 2: Showing Pre-Intervention and Post-Intervention Scores of Depression

In Figure 2 pre intervention and post intervention scores of depression are compared to show the effect of behavior intervention on depression and it can be observed that as the effect of behavior intervention, post intervention scores of depression are lower than the pre intervention scores in case of each subject. Results are significant statistically as well as clinically. It is the representative of the fact that behavior intervention is effective not only on one particular individual but on all those who have high depression. It can be observed that effectiveness of behavior intervention varies in relation to each subject. Results show that most of the subjects having high depression have reduced the level of depression from severe to mild and in one case depression has been reduced from severe level to minimal level. Effectiveness of behavior intervention varies due to the individual differences. It is the fact that minimal level of depression is common to all. In adolescents the minimal and mild level of depression is usually found because it is the phase of life when they turn from school to colleges, face social changes, and especially they suppose to be conscious for success in their career (Eccles, *et al.*, 1993).

Another hypothesis in part 'B' of the study was that the reduced level of depression leads to enhancement of self-esteem. Again A-test was applied to test the significance of difference between pre and post measures of self-esteem. Results are presented in Result Table 3.

Result Table 3: Showing Value of 'A-test' for Pre and Post Measure of Self-esteem

Group	*N*	*'A'*	*Level of Significance*	*Result*
Subjects Received Behavior Intervention For Reducing Depression	5	.2	.01	Significant

Results presented in Result Table 3 reveal that obtained 'A' value is .20 and it has been mentioned above that is significant at a given level if it is equal to or less than the value given in the table. The value given in the table at .01 level is .238. Thus, the obtained value .2 is less than the value given in the table at .o1 level so it is significant. Thus there is significant difference between pre test scores and post test scores of self-esteem. The results are shown with the help of figure also.

Figure 3 represents the pre test and post test scores of self-esteem. It is shown that when subjects had high depression the level of self-esteem was low. When behavior intervention was given and the level of depression reduces (Figure 2) the self-esteem enhances (Figure 3). Thus, results are not only statistically significant but they are clinically significant also. Figure 3 represents the fact that 'reduction in depression level leads to enhancement of self-esteem' it applies on all subjects not on one particular individual.

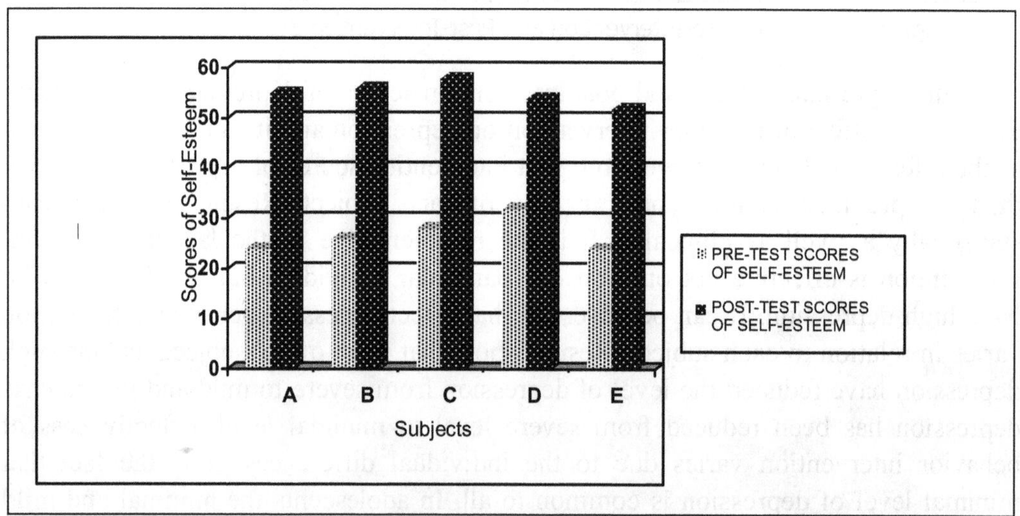

Figure 3: Showing Pre-Test Scores and Post-Test Scores of Self-esteem

CONCLUSIONS

- Subjects having high depression have lower level of self-esteem than those having low level of depression.
- Behavior Intervention is effective in reducing level of depression among young adults.
- Reduction in level of depression to enhancement of self-esteem among young adults.

DISCUSSION

The findings of the present research are in conformity with previous research reports. It is found that the subjects having high depression have lower level of self-esteem as compared to those having low level of depression. The one who has high depression often feels sad, pessimistic, blue, down, and hopeless. As the result of depression the condition of social withdrawal, feeling of insecurity, fear of failure arises and one's self-esteem level goes down. The present finding is consistent with the findings of various researches (Clark, 1995: Compas and Lema, 1997). A study was conducted on private sector employees and found that those who have high depression share low level of self-esteem (Klings *et al.*, 2003).

Another finding reveals that behavior intervention is effective in reducing depression. Many researchers have proved that Cognitive Behavior Therapy is effective in reducing depression. Cognitive Behavior Therapy (CBT) helps people in distinguishing between problems that can be and, can not be resolved and develop better coping skills. Cognitive therapy proved as effective without the negative side effects. Cognitive behavior therapy was reported superior on 9 of 10 outcome measures (self reported) at the end of treatment (Antonuccio, 1995). A study was done with the aim to study the effectiveness of Cognitive behavioral therapy for depression and Enhancing self-esteem and self-control. Cognitive behavior treatment for depression included attempts to improve social functioning, reduce cognitive biases, and improve interpersonal problem-solving skills. However, many depressed clients reported problems caused by low self-esteem. The research described the cognitive behavioral approach for the improvement in self-esteem in depressed clients. Psychosocial exploration was used to gather detailed information about client's view of self, and help both therapist and client understand the various component of self-esteem. Then, adaptive change was structured around four general issues: (1) Expanding the client's perspective to include a more balanced view of both positive and negative events (2) Increasing the frequency of self-reinforcement by praising areas of success (3) Modifying the client's coping strategies so as to maximize the likelihood of successful performance, and (4) Revising the client's goal and standards that underlie the self-evaluation process. Using a combination of these approaches, the therapists helped the clients in improving their self-esteem and reduce the likelihood of depression (Overholser, 2004). The U.S. Food and Drug Administration (2001) studied the effectiveness of CBT and found that there are 56% improvements in depressive symptoms, when CBT was provided to subjects. The enhancement of self-esteem among adolescents is of great importance from individual as well as social point of view. If we wish to effectively target adolescent's depression, there is need to target self-esteem. The approach to improving self-esteem should be different from traditional view of individualized pep talks. Self-esteem can only be improved when environment, in the person lives, improves: improvement in terms of inter-personal skills and social acceptance. If parents, teachers and others create an atmosphere that is characterized by acceptance and freedom from anxiety, which tends to promote and encourage curiosity and exploratory behavior, adolescents would learn to honor their strength and maintain their self-esteem.

REFERENCES

Abood, D.A. and Conway, T.C. (2004). "Health Values and Self-esteem as Predictors of Wellness Behavior." *Health Values*, 16, 21–27.

Agrawala, Surila and Raj, Pritam (2003). *Relation of Self-esteem with Behavioral Problems and School Performance of Children: A Behavior Modification Approach.* Unpublished Ph.D's Thesis. Dayalbagh University, Agra, India.

Antonuccio (1995). "Treatment for Chronic Depression: Cognitive Behavioral Analysis System of Psychotherapy Integration." *Journal of clinical Psychology.*13, 241–263.

Batt, K. (2001). "Familial Correlates of Depression in Young American Adults." *Journal of Clinical Psychology*, 32, 374–386.

Bellovia, Janice and Rose, Dors. (2005). "Self-esteem (Dominance Feeling) in Women." *Journal of Social Psychology*, 151, 259–263.

Bolger, Rose (2004). *Society and Adolescent Self-image.* Princeton: Princeton University Press.

Brown, J.D. and Mcgill (2000). "Suicidal Thoughts among Adolescents: An Intercutural Approach." *Journal of Youth Development*, 28, 649–657.

Brown, J.D. (1999). "Evaluations of Self and Others; Self-enhancement and Biases in Social Judgment." *Social Cognition*, 4, 353–376.

Campbell, J.D. (2000). "Similarity and Uniqueness: The Effects of Attribute Type, Relevance, and Individual Differences in Self-esteem and Depression." *Journal of Personality and Social Psychology*, 50, 281–294.

Chen and Rubin (1998). "Comparisons of Children of Depressed and Non-depressed Parents: A Social-environmental Perspective." *Journal of Abnormal Child Psychology*, 11, 463–485.

Chen and Rubin (1998). "Comparisons of Children of Depressed and Non-depressed Parents: A Social-environmental Perspective." *Journal of Abnormal Child Psychology*, 11, 463–485.

Clark, G. (1995). "Depression in Older Adults and the Elderly." *Journal of Mental Health*, 21, 469–482.

Compass, S. and Lema, R. (1997). "Affective and Cognitive Characteristics of Depression in Adults." *Journal of Personality and Social Psychology*, 49, 194–202.

Coopersmith, S. (1981). *The Antecedents of Self-esteem.* Palo Alto, CA: Consulting Psychologists Press.

Crocker, J. (2003). "The "What" and "Why" of Goals Pursuits: Human Needs and Self-Determination of Behavior." *Journal of Social Issues*, 58, 596–613.

Eccles, J., Midgley, C., Wigfield, A., Buchanan, C., Reuman, D., Flanagan, C. and Maciver, D. (1993). *Development during Adolescence. American Psychologist*, 48, 90–101.

Feldman, S. and Elliot, G. (1990). "Adolescence: Path to a Productive Life or a Diminished Future?" *Carnegie Quarterly*, 35, 1–13.

Gordon, John (2001). "Familial Correlates of Self-esteem in Young American Adults." *Journal of Social Psychology*, 27, 583–588.

Gottib and Hammen (1999). "Adolescence: Path to a Productive Life or a Diminished Future?" *Journal of School Health*, 65, 390–394.

Greenberg, J., Soloman, S., Psyzczynski, T., Rosenblatt, A., Burling, J., Lyon: D. and Simon, C. (1999). "Assessing the Terror Management Analysis of Self-esteem: Converging Evidence of an Anxiety-buffering Function." *Journal of Personality and Social Psychology*, 67, 913–922.

Griffin, D. and Bartholomew, K. (1999). "Models of Self-other: Fundamental Dimensions Underlying Measures of Adult Attachment." *Journal of Personality and Social Psychology*, 67, 430–445.

Hammen and Brenan (2003). "General and Specific Depression in Late Adolescent Students: Race X Gender X Sex Effect." *British Journal of Clinical Psychology*, 20, 555–566.

Kim, William and Allison Gary (2000). "Social Interaction and the Self-concept." *Journal of Education and Psychology*, 30, 201–207.

Kirchner, J.G. and Walsh, Brein (1999). "Self-Concept of Ability and School Achievement." *Sociology of Education*, 42, 271–278.

Kling, Bushan (2003). "Sex Differences in Covert Aggression and Self-conceptions among Adolescents." *Journal of Health and Personality*, 25, 267–284.

Laura, E.L. (1999). "Parenting Styles and Mental Health of Palestinian-Arab Adolescents in Israeli." *Transcultural Psychiatry*, 41, 503–513.

Leary, M.R. (2004). *Understanding Social Anxiety: Social Personality and Clinical Perspective.* Beverly Hills, CA: Sage.

Levy, R. and Aumgardener, E.L. (2003). "Self-Esteem and Adjustment in Early Adolescence: A Social Contextual Perspective." *Journal of Youth and Adolescence*, 38, 263–269.

Marsh, K.E. (2004). "Factors in Social Environment as Related to Emotional Security-Insecurity Syndrome." *Psychological Studies*, 20, 55–58.

McCauley, Greenberg, Burke and Mitchell (2002). "Development during Adolescence." *American Psychologist*, 48, 90–101.

Meaux, T.E. (2005). "Attribution for Negative Life Events and Depression. The Role of Perceived Control." *Journal of Psychotherapy Integration*, 16, 241–263.

Murry, Holmes, Griffin, Bellavin, G. and Rose, P. (2005). "Peers Group and Social Factors as Predictors of Self-esteem." *Journal of Social Issues*, 27, 423–436.

Overholser, James C. (2004). "Cognitive-behavioral Treatment of Depression, Part V: Enhancing Self-esteem and Self-control." *Journal of Contemporary Psychotherapy*, 34, 1573–3564.

Pomerantz, C. Saxon (2001). Relational and Overt Form of Victimization: A Multidimensional Approach." *Journal of Consulting and Clinical Psychology*, 73, 337–347.

Schyler, S. and Ketz, P. (1998). "Level and Instability of Day-to-day Psychological Well-being and Risk for Depression." *Journal of Personality and Social Psychology,* 60, 129–138.

Sinha, R.C. (2004). "Perceived Causes of Depression in Family." *Journal of Clinical Psychology*, 29, 289–306.

Soloman, S. (2003). "Why do We Need What We Need? A Terror Management Perspective on the Roots of Human Social Motivation." *Psychological Inquiry*, 8, 1–20.

Strub, O. Richard (2002). *Health Psychology*. New York: Worth Publishers.

Tredeau, M and Michelle, S. (2006). "Attribution for Negative Life Events and Depression", *Journal of Personality and Social Psychology,* 66, 316–322.

World Health Organisation (WHO) (2000). *The World Health Report 2000; Health System: Improving Performance*. Geneva, Switzerland: United Nation.

Latest Trends in Internet Addiction Disorder: Concepts, Symptoms, Theories, Triggers and Coping Strategies

Saran Kumari Sharma*

ABSTRACT

The paper entitled "Latest trends in Internet Addiction Disorder (IAD): concepts, symptoms, theories, triggers and coping strategies" is a descriptive, informative and explanatory paper. Main focus of the paper is on behavioral problems and symptoms which arise due to extensive use of internet, coping strategies of reduction of this latest clinical disorder with some pleasure deriving skills which are practical and within the reach of everyone are also discussed. Reading of latest research findings which are included in this paper will facilitate the individual in leading a happy, healthy, peaceful and energetic life. In the end author has given some humble suggestions for making the atmosphere of schools, colleges and community congenial and relaxing in the interest of progressive global community.

INTRODUCTION

In the first decade of 21st century we have done a very rapid and fast technological changes and advancements. But these advancements are not giving relaxation to our children, youngsters and adults which is the basic requirement of this stressed era in which we are living. Modern means of communication are shrinking distances between people and has flattered the world into a compact and easily accessible global community. It means we are saving time and dependency on other persons but side by side these are giving some behavioral problems like withdrawal, depression, worry and anxiety which are very near to psychiatric disorders. Out of the many other psychiatric/mental disorders, internet addiction disorder is the most common disorder of recent times. Youngsters are openly admitting to being addicted to the internet and it is already becoming an addiction.

This mental disease needs immediate attention of educationists, policy makers, psychiatrist, psychologists, social workers and religious leaders who are concerned with the well-being of individuals' global peace and health. This paper is an attempt to give right direction to students, teachers, patients, and general public for reducing this dangerous disease for the betterment of mankind.

*Department of Correspondence Studies, Panjab University, Chandigarh, Punjab, India.

MEANING AND CONCEPT

Meaning of Internet

The Internet is a worldwide, publicly accessible series of interconnected computer networks that transmit data by packet switching using the standard Internet Protocol (IP). It is a "network of networks" that consists of millions of smaller domestic, academic, business, and government networks, which together carry various information and services, such as electronic mail, online chat, file transfer, and the interlinked web pages and other resources of the World Wide Web.

Meaning of Addiction

The term addiction does not appear in the most recent version of the DSM-IV (American Psychiatric Association, 1995). Of all the diagnoses referenced in the DSM-IV, substance dependence may come the closet to capturing the essence of what has traditionally being labeled addiction, and provides a workable definition of addiction. The seven criteria considered under this diagnosis are withdrawal, tolerance, pre-occupation with the substance, heavier or more frequent use of the substance then intended, centralized activities to procure more of the substance, loss of interest in other social, occupational and recreational activities and disregard for the physical or psychological consequences caused by the use of the substance.

While many believe the term addiction should only be applied to cases involving chemical substances (Walker, 1998; Rachlin, 1990), similar diagnostic criteria have been applied to a number of problem behaviors such as pathological gambling (Griffiths, 1990), eating disorders (Lacey, 1993; Lesieur and Blume, 1993), generic technological addictions (Griffiths, 1995), and video game addiction (Soper, 1983; Keepers, 1990; Griffiths, 1991 and 1992). Escaping through watching televisions, eating chocolate or surfing the internet are what some people termed as soft addiction (Ganahi, 2003). However, when such activities result in negative physical, mental, interpersonal, professional or social consequence, they move out of the realm of the soft addictions.

Meaning of Internet Addiction

According to Bratter and Forest (1985), like all other addiction, Internet addiction is a psycho physiological disorder involving tolerance (the same amount of usage elicits less response; increased amounts necessary to evoke the same amount of pleasure), withdrawal symptoms (especially tremors, anxiety and moodiness), affective disturbances (depression, irritability), and interruption of social relationships (a decline or loss, either in quality or quantity).

The term internet addiction disorder was coined by Dr. Evan Goldverg in 1995. The term Internet addiction is defined as spending so much time online that internet use adversely affects marriages, family and social life, academics, work and psychological and physical well-being. Due to the nature of internet addiction disorder (failed impulse control without involving an intoxicant), internet addiction disorder is said to be closest to pathological gambling as defined by the diagnostic and statistical manual of Mental disorders–IV, published by the American Psychiatry Association (APA), 1995.

To be diagnosed as having internet addiction disorder, a person must meet certain criteria as prescribed by the APA, 1995. Three or more of these criteria must be present at any time during a 12 month period.

1. *Tolerance:* These refer to the need for increasing amounts of time on the internet to achieved satisfaction or significant diminishing effects with continued use of the same amount of time on internet.
2. Two or more withdrawal symptoms developing within days to one month after reduction of internet use or cessation of internet use, and these must cause distress or impair social, personal or occupational functioning. These include psychomotor agitation, *i.e.,* trembling and tremors; anxiety obsessive thinking about what is happening on the internet; voluntary or involuntary type movements of the fingers.
3. Use of the Internet is engaged in to relieve or avoid withdrawal symptoms.
4. The Internet is often accessed more often, or for longer periods of time than was intended. A significant amount of time is spent in activities related to internet use *e.g.,* Internet books, trying out new World Wide Web browsers, researching Internet vendors, *etc.*
5. Important social, occupational, or recreational activities are given up or reduced because of Internet use.
6. The individual risks the loss of a significant relationships, job, educational or career opportunities because of excessive use of the internet.

In a recent research, Egger and Rauterberg (1996) identified some other characteristics *viz.* feeling of restlessness or irritability when attempting to cut down or stop internet use. The second is that the internet is used as a way of escaping problems or relieving feelings of helplessness, guilt, anxiety or depression. The third characteristic is that the user lies to family members or friends to conceal the extent of involvement with the internet. And finally, the user returns repeatedly excesses fees.

Young (1996) developed brief eight-item criteria to provide a screening instrument for addictive internet use. Patients were considered addicted when answering yes to five (or more) of the questions. Young (1996) stated that the cut off score of five was consistent with the number of criteria used for pathological gambling and was seen as an adequate number of criteria to differentiate normal from pathological addictive internet use. Further, Young (1996) pointed out that internet dependent spent an average of 38 hours per week surfing the internet.

SYMPTOMS OF INTERNET ADDICTION

Young (2000), the founder of the Center for Online Addiction, has identified eight key symptoms. According to her, if five or more apply, one needs to consider it as an addiction.

1. *Preoccupation*—one thinks constantly about previous online activity or keeps looking forward to the next online session. Some people crave time on the internet the way a smoker craves a cigarette.
2. *Increased use*—one needs to spend increasing amounts of time online to achieve satisfaction.
3. *Inability to stop*—one can't cut back on one's internet use, even after several attempts. Some people can't stop visiting chat rooms while at the office, even though they know their bosses are monitoring the sites they visit.
4. *Withdrawal symptoms*—one feels restless, moody, depressed or irritable when one attempts to stop or cut down internet use.
5. *Lost sense of time*—everyone lets time slip by occasionally while on the internet. This should be considered a problem only if it happens consistently and the person also experience some of the other symptoms on this list.
6. *Risky behaviors*—these include jeopardizing a significant relationship, job or educational or career opportunity because of internet.
7. *Telling lies*—This includes lying to family members, a therapist, or others to conceal the extent of one's involvement with the internet. Someone who's seeing a therapist for depression might not tell the therapist about her internet use.
8. *Escape to the Internet*—one uses the internet as a way to avoid thinking about problems, or to allay depression or feelings of helplessness.

The symptoms of internet addiction can be classified under two broad categories as given:

Psychological Symptoms

1. Having a sense of well-being or euphoria while at the computer.
2. Inability to stop the activity.
3. Craving for more and more time on the internet.
4. Feeling empty, depressed, and irritable when not at the computer.
5. Using on line services every day without skipping.

6. Losing track of time after making a connection.
7. Going out less and less.
8. Spending less and less time on meals at home or at work, and eating in front of the monitor.
9. Denying spending too much time on the Net.
10. Others complaining of your spending too much time in front of monitor.
11. Checking on your mailbox too many times a day.
12. Logging onto the Net while already busy at work.
13. Sneaking online when spouse or family members are not at home, with a sense of relief.

Physical Symptoms

1. Dry eyes.
2. Migraine headache.
3. Backache.
4. Eating irregularities, such as skipping meals.
5. Failure to attend to personal hygiene.
6. Sleep disturbances, change in sleep pattern.
7. Gastroentitis.

REVIEW OF RELATED LITERATURE

Individuals who are dissatisfied or upset by a particular area or multiple areas of their lives have an increased chance of abusing internet, to avoid an unhappy situation such as marital or job satisfaction, medical illness, unemployment, or academic instability.

Several withdrawal symptoms are related to internet addiction including nervousness, agitation, and aggression, as well as an addiction syndrome that includes the presence of withdrawal symptoms, increasing tolerance, and loss of control. A high rate of comorbid mental disorders has also been reported, especially depressive symptoms and social impairment.

Philips and Reddie (2007) reported that technological predispositions, decisional styles, and self-esteem may potentially influence the extent to which people use e-mail at work. Higher levels of email use in the workplace could be predicted by avoidant decisional styles such as procrastination and buck passing.

Metheson (2006) reported that parental overprotection is a risk factor for number of psychological problems in overprotected subjects. Such regulatory excess has been linked in studies to drug addiction (Andersson and Eisemann, 2003), disruptive behavior disorders (Rey and Plapp, 1990; Joyce *et al*., Mak 1996), depression (parker *et al*., 1987), likelihood of being bullied (Rigby *et al.,* 1999), antisocial personality disorder (Reti *et al.,* 2002), school phobia (Torma and Halstic, 1975), agoraphobia (DeRuiter, 1994). Obsessive-compulsive disorder (DeRuiter 1994), anxiety disorder (Clayer *et al.*, 1984), dependent personality disorder and failures of autonomy (Howe and Madgett, 1975; Ruchkin, 1998), over inhibited personality (Wergeland, 1979), and dissociation (Offen *et al.,* 2003).

Sun *et al.* (2005) reported that less parental monitoring and more unsupervised time were positively related to e-mail use, chat room use.

Matheson (2006) reported parental overprotection involving disaffected subjects' moral character negatively, in the sense that it tends to vitiate the conditions required for the subject to develop moral virtues.

Young (1996) found that 58% of students reported a decline in study habits, a significant drop in grades, missed classes or being placed on probation due to excessive internet use. A survey initiated by counselors at university of Texas at Austin found that 14% of the students met the criteria for internet addiction (Scherer, 1997). This led the counseling center to initiate an internet addiction Support Group when they noticed academic impairment and poor integration in extracurricular activities due to excessive internet use on campus. Brady (1996) stated that 43% of the normally successful students failed due to extensive patterns of late night log-ons to the university computer systems.

A recent online survey at two campus—conducted at the university of Texas (Scherer, 1997) and Bryant College (Morahan—Martin, 1997) have further documented that pathological internet use is problematic for academic performance and relationship functioning.

Scherer (1997) found that excessive internet use becomes problematic when it results in impaired functioning such as compromised grades or failure to fulfill responsibilities. Internet Relay Chat (IRC) and instant messaging are widely used by college students to meet and get to know one another. 33% of the students prefer communicating online rather than meeting face to face.

Gender Differences in Internet Usage

In a study on Multiusers, Cherney (1994) found that men tend to use more physically violent imagery, and that women are overall more affectionate towards other characters. Scherer (1997) and Greenfield (1999) reported a preponderance of male internet addicts.

The online social behavior is an extension of traditional social behavior, as females tend to be higher on intimacy than males. They also communicate over the internet with family and friends more frequently than men. (Hussong, 1997; Pew, 2000).

Cooper (2000) found that men and women addicts seem to prefer sites that fit behavioral stereotypes of their own gender. Women were more likely to spend time flirting or having Cybersex with others in sexually oriented chat rooms, while men were drawn to porn web sites. Men prefer visual stimuli and more focused sexual experiences, while women are more interested in relationships and interactions.

Stevenson and Scealy (2002) reported that males were more likely to use the internet for downloading entertainment. Shy males were more likely to use the internet for recreation/leisure activities. Ko *et al.* (2005) found that subjects who played online games were predominantly male. Gender differences were also found in the severity of online gaming addiction and motives for playing. Older age, lower self esteem, and low satisfaction with daily life were associated with more severe addiction among males, but not among females.

Theories of Internet Addiction

Ferris (2003) listed the following theories to explain Internet Addiction:

Biomedical Theories

These explanations focus on the role of hereditary and congenital factors, chemical imbalances in the brain and neurotransmitters. According to this perspective, these factors cause some people to be more susceptible to addiction (Sue, 1994). There is definitive research that shows that some drugs act to fill in the gaps of the neurons in the brain, fooling the brain into sending out faulty information. This, it is thought, is one reason for the high one gets from engaging in activities such as running, drug use and gambling. This might apply to internet addiction also, since many opportunities on the internet generate fun and excitement.

Psychodynamic Theories

Psychodynamic theorists and personality theorists account for addiction through early childhood traumas, correlation with other personality traits or other disorders, and inherited psychological dispositions (Sue, 1994). A dispositional model or diathesis—stress model of addiction might help in understanding internet addiction disorder. Certain people, due to a variety of factors may be predisposed (diathesis) to developing an addiction to something, be it alcohol, heroin, gambling, sex, shopping, or on-line computer services. They could go through their entire lives never developing any kind of addiction. On the other hand, if stress or a combination of stressors, affect the person at a critical time, the person may be more inclined to develop an addiction. If the person begins drinking alcohol even occasionally, but continues to increase consumption, he may develop a dependency on alcohol. The same premise holds for internet addiction. The right combination of time, person and event, may lead to addiction.

Behavioral Theories

These explanations are based on B.F. Skinner's studies on operant conditioning. The person performs a behavior. This applies to addictions, specifically internet addiction in the following way: Being hooked to drugs, alcohol, sex, gambling, the internet, and shopping offer many rewards. They offer love, excitement, physical, emotional, and material comfort, and the means to escape from reality. These can all be rewards. If an individual wants these rewards and learns that the internet will allow him to escape, or receive love, or have fun, he will probably turn to the internet the next time he feels these needs. This becomes reinforcing, and the cycle continues.

Socio-cultural Theories

According to Sue (1994), addictions may vary according to gender, age, socioeconomic status, ethnicity, religion and country. Some addictions are more common among persons of different categories *e.g.,* alcoholism is most common in the middle socioeconomic classes. Not enough data is available yet about those persons addicted to the internet to determine if a particular class is most predominant though some researchers. Sun *et al.* (2005) report that higher socioeconomic status and Asian ethnicity were associated with higher internet use.

TRIGGERS OF INTERNET ADDICTION

According to the center for Internet Addiction Recovery, internet addiction affects people of varying ages, cultural backgrounds occupations and educational levels. The following problems are likely triggers of internet addictions.

Substance Abuse—Over half of internet addicts suffer from other addictions, mainly to drugs, alcohol, smoking and sex.

Mental Illness—Trends shows that internet addicts suffer from emotional problems such as depression and anxiety related disorders and often uses the fantasy world of the internet to psychologically escape unpleasant feelings or stressful situations.

Relationship Troubles—In almost 75% of cases, internet addicts use applications such as chat rooms, instant messaging or online gaming as a safe way of establishing new relationships and more confidently relating to others.

COPING STRATEGIES

Internet addiction disorder can be treated by many simple techniques which are not only simple but also give pleasure and relaxation to the patient suffering with internet addiction.

Table 1 gives the list of simple pleasure deriving techniques out of which internet addict can use any technique according to environment and his/her needs, interest and aptitudes:

Table 1: List of Simple Pleasure Deriving Techniques

Yoga Meditation and Dhyan	Theater
Clapping	Positive thought
Laughing	Creative writing, craft work, cooking
Shopping	Sitting and spending time with nature
Occupational	Weekend break with family and friends
Aroma	Eating nutritive and balanced diet
Long Drive	Collection of good quotations
Brisk Walking	Playing with pets
Relaxation through party	Gardening
Get together of like minded persons	Reading books and journals
Music—Vocal, Instrumental and dance	Playing games
Massage	Watching television
Acupressure	Be a good listener

Table 2 gives an insight for coping strategies of internet addiction disorder. These strategies are very useful for recovering from the disorder. Skills given above can be used for reducing stress level, worry and tension.

Physical strategies can prevent the build of physical tension and provide immediate tools to control situational stress and situational stress reactions.

Intellectual strategies are also beneficial in interrupting the stress cycle by altering the perception of a specific event as stressful. Social strategies tend to increase the individual skill in dealing with potentially stressful situation and receiving support from others.

The list of emotional and spiritual strategies for managing stress is much shorter and is based primarily on clinical observation. These techniques may be helpful at any stage of the stress cycle.

Environmental strategies help individual assess and alter the stress producing aspects of their surroundings as well as change habitual behavior that tend to disrupt and complicate their environment.

Table 2: Coping Strategies of Internet Addicts

Physical strategies	Intellectual/Mental strategies
Progressive relaxation	Cognitive restructuring
Biofeedback	Systematic desensitization
Visualization	Thought - stopping
Sensory Awareness	Reframing
Deep breathing	Values clarification
Hot tubs (Jacuzzi, sauna)	
Massage	
Yoga	
Exercise	
Diet	
Social strategies	Emotional strategies
Interpersonal skill training	Catharses/emotional discharge
Assertiveness	Self-awareness
Support Groups	Withdrawal
Networking	
Spiritual strategies	Environmental strategies
Meditation	Time Management
Prayer	Problem Solving
Faith/Hope	Goal setting
	Lifestyle assessment
	Decision Making

HUMBLE SUGGESTIONS

1. As internet addiction disorder is more prevalent in youngsters, counseling sessions in schools and colleges should be given to diagnose internet addicts and students in general by expert administrators, academicians, sociologists, psychologists, psychiatrists, social workers and religious leaders.
2. Internet users should be advised to use internet giving breaks in the form of some recreational activities of their choice-like listening music, playing any indoor or outdoor game, socializing with friends, taking nature therapy or taking any therapeutic technique which gives them peace of mind and relaxation.
3. Introvert patients of this disorder should be counseled for breaking their isolation habit by parting and spending much time with their intimate friends, parents and family members.
4. Strict rules should be observed in cyber cafes, schools and colleges for limited use of internet.

5. Sites which are making our adolescents and youth characterless should be discouraged by authorities.
6. Sites which inculcate good heritage and moral values should be encouraged.
7. Exhibitions and posters display exclusively should be arranged for the awareness about IAD in a beautiful and attractive style.
8. Seminars, workshop and conferences should be exclusively arranged on the disease in which patients of this disease, family of patients and other supportive groups, organizations and institutes must be involved with psychologists, psychiatrists and social workers.
9. Multi-disciplinary approach *i.e.,* social sciences, pure sciences, languages, commerce and education faculties should be given responsibilities for viewing social, family and other problems of this disease and simple and practical ways must be suggested to solve these problems with co-coordinated approach.

CONCLUSION

To sum up, the present paper of 'Latest trends in Internet Addiction Disorder: Concepts, Symptoms, Theories, Triggers and Coping Strategies', is a theoretical and self explanatory paper on internet addicts which is spreading it's wings at an alarming rate in present day scenario. Theoretical explanations and review of related literature which are useful for eliminating this dangerous disease are given. Emphasis is given on coping strategies and skills for fighting with this behavioral disorder in the interest of individual herself/himself, family, society, community and universe as a whole.

REFERENCES

Anderson, P. and Eisemann, M. (2003). "Parental Rearing and Individual Vulnerability to Drug Addiction: A Controlled Study in a Swedish Sample." *Nordic Journal of Psychiatry,* 57, 147–156.

Bhagat, G. (2007). *A Study of Psychological Correlates of Internet Addiction (Ph.D. Synopsis) Supervisor.* Meena Sehgal. P.U. Chandigarh.

Brady, K. (1996). "Dropouts Rise a Net Result of Computers." *The Buffalo Evening News*, 1.

Bratter and Forest (1985). Internet Addiction Disorder: Causes, Symptoms, and Consequences. Available at: www.ndri.com/article/nternet_addiction_disorder causes symptoms and consequences.

Brenner, V. (1997). "The Results of an On-line Survey for the First Thirty Days." *Paper Presented at the 105th Annual Meeting of the American Psychological Association,* August Chicago, IL.

Cherney, L. (1994). "Gender Differences in the Text-Based Virtual Reality Available:" www.lucien.berkeley.edu/MOO/Gender/MOO.ps.

Clayer, J., Ross, M. and Campbell, R. (1984). "Disclosure as Social Exchange: Anticipated Length of Relationships, Sex Roles and Disclosure Intimacy." *Western Journal of Speech Communication,* 49, 43–56.

Cooper, A. (2000). "Sexual Addiction and Compulsion." *The Journal of Treatment and Prevention.*

DeRuiter, C. (1994). "Anxious Attachment in Agoraphabia and Obsessive—Compulsive Disorder: A Literature Review and Treatment Implications." *Parenting and Psychopathology.* New York:Wiley, 281–307.

Egger, O. and Rauterberg, M. (1996). "Internet Behavior and Addiction." *Semester Thesis;* Swiss Federal Institute of Technology, Zurich. www.ifap.bepr.ethz.ch/~egger/ibq/res.htm.

Ferris, J.R. (2003). "Internet Addiction Disorder: Cause, Symptoms, and Consequences." [Web Page] www.rider.edu/~ruler/psycyber/cybaddict.html.

Ganahl, J. (2003). "The Softer Side of Addiction." *San Francisco Chronicle.*

Griffiths, M. (1990). "Psychological Characteristics of Compulsive Internet Use: A Preliminary Analysis." *Cyber Psychology and Behavior*, 2, 403–412.

Griffiths, M. (1991). "Amusement Machine Playing in Childhood Adolescence: A Comparative Analysis of Video Game and Fruit Machines." *Journal of Adolescence*, 14, 53–73.

Griffiths, *M. (1992). Pinball Wizard: The Case of Pinball Machine Addict.* Psychological Reports, 71, 161–162.

Griffiths, M. (1995). "Technological Addictions." *Clinical Psychology Forum*, 71, 14–19.

Howe, M.G. and Madgett, M.E. (1975). "Mental Health Problems Associated with the Only Child." *Canadian Psychiatric Association Journal*, 20, 189–194.

Hussong, A.M. (1997). "Gender Differences in Adolescent Friendships and Adjustment." *Dissertation Abstracts International*, 57 (7–B), 4710.

Keppers, D. (2000). "Most Employees Disciplined for Internet Abuse." New Bytes News Network.

Ko, C.H., yen, J.Y., C.C., S.H., Wu, K and Yen, C.F. (2006). "Tridimensional Personality of Adolescents with Internet Addiction and Substance use experience." *Canadian Journal of Psychiatry*, 51 (14).

Kraut, R., Patterson, M., Lundmark, V., Keisler, S., Mukopadhyay, T. and Scherlis, W. (1998). "International Paradox: A Social Technology that Reduces Social Involvement and Psychological Well Being?" *American Psychologist*, 53(9), 1017–1031.

Lacey, H.J. (1993). "Self Damaging and Addictive Behavior in Bulimia Nervosa: A Catchment Area Study." *British Journal of Psychiatry*, 163, 190–194.

Lesieur, H.R. and Blume, S.B. (1993). "Pathological Gambling, Eating Disorder and the Psychoactive Substance Use Disorders." *Journal of Addictive Diseases*, 12(3), 89–120.

Matheson, D. (2006). "Overprotection, Surveillance and the Development of Virtue." Available at: www.idtrial.org/files/Matheson%20–%20 Overprotection.pdf.

Mitchell, P. (1993). "Gambling as a Rational Addiction." *Journal of Gambling Studies*, 9(2), 121–151.

Morahn-Martin, J. and Schumacher, P. (1997). "Incidence and Correlates of Pathological Internet Use in College Students." *Paper Presented at the 105th Annual Meeting of the American Psychological Association,* Chicago, IL.

Murphey, B. (1996). "Computer Addiction Entangle Students, The APA Monitor."

Offen, L,. Thomas, G., Waller, G. (2003). "Dissociation as a Mediator of the Relationship between Recalled Parenting and the Clinical Correlates of Auditory Hallucinations." *British Journal of Clinical Psychology*, 42, 321–341.

Parker, G., Kiloh, L. and Hayward, L. (1987). "Parental Representations of Neurotic and Endogenous Depressive." *Journal of Affective Disorders,* 13, 75–82.

Pew Internet and American life Project (2000). "Tracking Online Life: How Women Use the Internet to Cultivate Relationships with Family and Friends." [on-line] Available at www.perointernet.org/reports/pdfs/PIP Time Spent_Online.pdf.

Phillips, J.G. and Reddie, L. (2007). "Decisional Style and Self-Reported E-mail Use in the Workplace." *Computers in Humar Behavior.* 23(5), 2414–2428.

Rachin, H. (1990). "Why do People Gamble and Keep Gambling Despite Heavy Loses?" *Psychological Science,* 1, 294–297.

Reti, I.M., Samuels, J.F., Eaton, W.W., Bienvenue III, O.J., Costa Jr., P.T., Nestadt, G. (2002). "Adult Anti-social Personality Traits are Associated with Experiences of Low Parental Care and Maternal Overprotection." *Acta Psychiatrica Scandinavica,* 106, 126–133.

Rey, J. and Plapp, J. (1990). "Quality of Perceived Parenting in Oppositional and Conduct Disordered Adolescents." *Journal of the American Academy of Child and Adolescent Psychiatry,* 29, 382–385.

Rigby, K., Slee, P. and Cunningham, R. (1990). "Effects of Parenting on the Peer Relations of Australian Adolescents." *The Journal of Social Psychology,* 139, 387–388.

Scherer, K. (1997). "College life Online: Healthy and Unhealthy Internet Use": *Journal of College Student Development,* 38(6), 655–665.

Sharma, S.K. (2000). "Job Stress and its Management." *Recent Researches in Education and Psychology,* III–IV, 116–117.

Soper, B.W. (1983). "Junk-time Junkies: An Emerging Addiction among Students." *School Counsellor,* 31, 40–43.

Stevenson, R. and Scealy, M. (2002). "Shyness and Anxiety as Predictors of Internet Usage." *Cyber Psychology and Behavior,* 5(6), 507–515.

Sue, D., Sue, D. and S. (1994). "Understanding Abnormal Behavior." Boston: Houghton Mifflin.

Sun, P., Unger, J.B., Palmer, P.H., Gallaher, P., Chou, C.P., Baezconde—Garbanti, L., Sussman, S. and Johnson, C.A. (2005). "Internet Accessibility and Usage among Urban Adolescents in Southern California: Implications for Web-Based Health Research." *Cyber Psychology and Behavior,* 8(5), 441–453.

Torma, S. and Haisti, A. (1975). "Factors Contributing to School Phobia and Truancy." *Psychiatric Fennica,* 209–220.

Walker, M.B. (1989). "Some Problems with the Concept of "Gambling Addiction". Should Theories of Addiction be generalized to include Excessive Gambling?" *Journal of Gambling Behavior,* 5, 179–200.

A Cross Cultural Comparison of Emotional States and Moods among Indian and Kenyan Students

Gur Pyari Prakash*

ABSTRACT

The present study attempts to evaluate the different emotional moods amongst Indians and Kenyan college going students. The sample consisted of 20 Indian and 20 Kenyan college going students of age group 18 to 25 years. The results point out difference in some of the areas *viz.* anxiety, depression and guilt amongst Indian and Kenyan students.

INTRODUCTION

In the present scientific age people are facing anxiety, stress, depression and many other such problems. These mental problems are result of the environment in which the person lives in. These anxiety, stress, depression, regression, fatigue, guilt, extroversion and arousal are said to be cultural phenomenon. It is obvious that people living in western culture with fast pace of life would have more stress and anxiety compared to those living in slower pace of life. Cattell and Scheiner (1961), using an abbreviated version of anxiety scale questionnaire, found that Indian college students were more anxious than American college students.

Gupta (1973) conducted a study comparing the anxiety of American and Indian college students. In his findings indicated reverse of Cattell's results. He found higher anxiety in American students than in Indian students. Gupta (1990) administered the IPAT anxiety scale questionnaire to 113 American and 136 Indian students. ANOVA yielded a culture × sex interaction on a total anxiety scale indicated that the American males were less anxious than Indian males, but American females were more anxious than Indian females.

As the Kenyan students migrate to India for a limited period to complete their studies, they might be facing a lot of problems in communication with the Indians. Therefore, this study is conducted to find out the difference in the level of some emotional moods amongst the Indian and Kenyan students.

It is hypothesized that there is no significant difference in the anxiety, stress, depression, regression, extroversion arousal, fatigue, and guilt level of Indian and Kenyan college going students.

*Department of Psychology, Bundelkhand University, Jhansi, UP, India.
E-mail: gurpyari.prakash@gmail.com

METHODOLOGY

Design

The present endeavour was to study emotional states and moods among Indian and Kenyan students. Out of 40 students, 20 Indians and 20 Kenyans were selected. The subjects were administered eight stage questionnaires by Cattell *et al.*

Sample

The study was conducted at Jhansi, comprising 40 college going Kenyan and Indian students, age ranging from 18 to 25 years. The sample was selected through random sampling procedure, *i.e.,* 20 students each (10 Kenyan and 10 Indian) from the two colleges of Jhansi as shown in Table 1. All the forty students belonged to the Middle income group.

Table 1: Sample Characteristics

	Bundelkhand Degree College (Arts)	*Bipin Bihari Degree College (Science)*
Kenyan	10	10
Indian	10	10

Measure

The Eight State Questionnaire (8SQ) was designed specifically for measuring eight important emotional sates and moods (Cattell, 1972; Barton, Cattell and Corner, 1972). The theoretical importance of measuring emotional states lies in the fact that any prediction of how a person will act or how he will perform depends as much on his present state as on his usual. The descriptions of the states measured by 8SQ are as follows:

Anxiety

An intense emotional condition with apprehensiveness of some dreadful happening.

Stress

Feeling a lot of pressure, unable to take time off and relax, constantly on the go experiencing great strain and lots of demands.

Depression

Unhappy, disagreeable, pessimistic in poor spirits, disappointed.

Regression

Confused, unorganised, unable to concentrate, experiencing difficulty in coping.

Fatigue

Exhausted sluggish and below par in performance.

Guilt

Regretful, concern about own misdeeds, dissatisfied with self.

Extroversion

Sociable, outgoing, adventure-some, talkative, enthusiastic.

Arousal

Alert, keyed-up, excited, stimulated, keen and sharp senses.

Both forms of the 8SQ contain 96 items; 12 of which measure each state. The 8SQ test used in this study is original and not adopted. The test may be administered individually or in a group. The test was constructed to be used with adults and adolescents of approximately 16 years of age group or above. A deliberate choice of language has been observed to make the test of equally appropriate for various English speaking groups.

An inspection of values found in the test reveals that the concept reliability for each of the psychological states ranged from excellent (.89) to moderate (.74).

An inspection of the values found in the test reveals that the concept validity for each of the psychological states ranged from excellent (.96) to moderate (.40).

RESULT ANALYSIS

As the object of the study was to compare the emotional states and moods of the Indian and Kenyan students, the 8SQ was administered on them. In order to find out the significance of difference between the two groups in eight emotional states, 't' values were calculated. As shown in Table 2(a) and 2(b) the sten scores of both the groups were categorised mostly in average except in three areas placing Indians in slightly deviant category and these areas are Anxiety, Depression and Guilt.

Table 2(a): Means, Sten Scores and Description of Sten Scores of Indian Students according to Eight State Questionnaire

Indians			
Area	*Mean*	*Sten Score*	*Description*
Anxiety	16.8	7	Slightly Deviant
Stress	16.5	6	Average
Depression	17.3	7	Slightly Deviant
Regression	15.55	6.5	Average
Fatigue	15.5	5.5	Average
Guilt	17.55	7	Slightly Deviant
Extroversion	18.95	5	Average
Arousal	19.75	5	Average

Table 2(b): Means, Sten Scores and Description of Sten Scores of Kenyan Students according to Eight State Questionnaire

Kenyans			
Area	*Mean*	*Sten Score*	*Description*
Anxiety	12.55	7	Average
Stress	15.05	6	Average
Depression	11.9	5	Average
Regression	12.25	6	Average
Fatigue	13.05	5	Average
Guilt	13.1	5	Average
Extroversion	22.85	6	Average
Arousal	23.05	6	Average

According to the results shown in Table 3, the 't' test values of Indians and Kenyans show significant differences in the areas of anxiety ($D = 4.25$, $t = 2.66$, $P < .05$); Depression ($D = 5.4$, $t = 3.33$, $P < .01$); Guilt ($D = 4.45$, $t = 2.32$, $P < .05$) and extroversion ($D = 3.95$, $t = 2.12$, $P < .05$).

Table 3: 't' Scores and Significance Level of Indians and Kenyans in Eight Areas (As per 8SQ)

8SQ Areas	*Indians (M1)*	*Kenyans (M2)*	*Difference*	*'t' score*	*Significant Level*
Anxiety	16.8	12.55	4.25	2.66	0.05
Stress	16.5	15.05	1.45	1.09	Not significant
Depression	17.3	11.9	5.4	3.33	0.01
Regression	15.55	12.25	3.3	1.74	Not significant
Fatigue	15.5	13.05	2.45	1.42	Not significant
Guilt	17.55	13.1	4.45	2.32	0.05
Extroversion	18.95	22.85	3.95	2.12	0.05
Arousal	19.75	23.05	3.3	1.85	Not significant

DISCUSSION AND CONCLUSION

Analysis of the results reveals the fact that there is significant difference between the Indians and Kenyans in the area of anxiety, depression, guilt and extroversion. The mean score of Indian group in anxiety is 16.8 and their sten score is 7, which shows that Indian students are slightly inclined towards anxiety. This implies that they are more worried, easily rattled, tense and emotional upset and short tempered as compared to Kenyans whose sten score is 6 which places them in average category. The mean score of Indians and Kenyans in the area of Depression are 17.3 and 11.9 respectively, their 't' value 3.33 shows significant difference at .01 level. Again the sten score 7 displays slightly deviant characteristics of Indians in depression as compared to Kenyans who again scored 5 sten score. Conclusively, Indians are unhappier, pessimistic and disappointed as compared to the Kenyans. Indian students again proved themselves to be slightly inclined towards the area of 'guilt' by scoring 17.55 mean score with sten score 7. Kenyans were found to be average in the area of guilt with their mean score 13.1 and sten score 5. 't' value is 2.32 shows significant difference between the two groups at .05 level. Indians are more regretful, concerned about their own misdeeds, dissatisfied with self in comparison to Kenyans. The fourth area in which significant difference was observed was extroversion; 't' value '2.12' shows that the difference is significant at .05 level.

According to the mean score, Kenyans (mean = 22.85) are more social outgoing, adventure-some, talkative and enthusiastic as compared to Indians (mean = 18.95).

Stress, regression, fatigue and arousal are four areas in which no significant difference was found between the two groups.

It may be concluded that Indian students though living and studying in their own motherland are more anxious, unhappy, in poor spirits, dissatisfied as compared to those Kenyans students who are studying in a foreign land (India), living among foreigners (Indians) with language problem and many other problems. In spite of all those adversities they are happy, sociable, outgoing and enthusiastic. Our hypothesis is partially rejected as out of eight areas significance difference is observed in four areas, while in rest of the four areas, no significant difference was found.

REFERENCES

Barton, K., Cattell, R.B. and Conner, D.V. (1972). "The Identification of 'State' Factors through p-Technique Factor Analysis." *Journal of Clinical Psychology,* 28, 459–463.

Cattell, R.B. and Scheiner, I.H. (1961). *The Meaning and Measurement of Neuroticism and Anxiety*. New York: Ronald Press Company, 273–281.

Gupta, Naim C. (1973). "A Cross Cultural Investigation of Test Anxiety, General Anxiety and Self Concept amongst American and Indian College Students." *Reports of Research Conducted at Ball State University*, Muncie, Indiana.

Gupta, Naim C. (1990). "Comparison of Anxiety among American and Indian College Students." *Journal of Indian Academy of Applied Psychology,* 16(1).

A Study of Differential Health Status of the Aged from Different Demographic Backgrounds

Seema Kashyap[1] and Ravi Sidhu*[2]

ABSTRACT

Health is a primary concern especially in old age, because the weak social support system does little to improve their lot. In a country like India knowledge and attitude towards health is poor. Poverty, ignorance and marginalization of aged compounds the health problem manifold. Epidemiological survey of elderly report increasing prevalence of hypertension, diabetes, joint pain, peptic ulcer, paralysis etc. in them. The present study was conducted on randomly selected 300 aged living in Agra city. CMI (Cornell Medical Index) developed and standardized by Pershad and Verma (1973) was used to assess the health status . The results show that senescent enjoyed better health than senile aged (t = 18.711), male have better health than female aged (t = 4.437), economically independent aged have better health than economically dependent aged (t = 14.773), aged with spouse have better health than their counterparts (t = 12.836), and lastly aged of nuclear family have a better health than joint family aged (t = 4.973).

INTRODUCTION

The pace of population aging varies widely among countries. Generally, developing countries are aging faster than more developed ones. "Global aging is occurring at a rate never seen before and we will need to pay close attention to how countries respond to the challenges and opportunities of growing older," Nancy Gordon (2001), the Census Bureau's associate director for demographic programs.

Old age is a period of physical decline; the physical condition depends partly upon hereditary constitution, temperament, the manner of living, environmental factors vicissitude of living, diet, infectious intoxication, gluttony, rest, work, stress, endocrine and other environmental conditions. To most people getting older means losing beauty, strength and vigor. Physical changes while occurring throughout adulthood rarely have much effect on a person's everyday life in the early and middle adult years. It is only in later life that the cumulative changes tend to catch up with the individual and begin to interfere with daily patterns and habits.

Health is a primary area of concern in old age. India, where knowledge of health and attitude towards health is poor, health gets tied up to poverty, ignorance and to some

*Corresponding aurthor.

[1,2] Department of Home Science, Faculty of Arts, Dayalbagh Educational Institute, Deemed University, Dayalbagh, Agra, UP, India.

E-mail: [1]docoment84@gmail.com; [2]ragsuu@yahoo.co.in

extent with the marginalization of the elderly. The epidemiological surveys on Indian elderly reported that hypertension, diabetes, joint pain, ulcer, limb paralysis, gastro intestinal cancers are highly prevalent diseases of the elderly. These are but a few examples that indicate poor health status of the aged in our country.

Health and hygienic practices at individual level and advances in medicine have saved the lives of many but have also increased the number of disabled and infirm elderly. Thus problem of elder care has become more problematic with a greater proportion of the elderly being infirm or partly disabled, developing new predicament in the Indian family.

The physical problems and deterioration in biological capabilities of the old age are coupled with a number of psychological problems and complications. In fact, to certain extent they reinforce each other, because most of the diseases and problems are psychosomatic in nature. Bose (1982) has reported that older men and women suffer from rolelessness, powerlessness and depression. With aging there is decline in many functions that lead to feeling of inadequacy and insecurity.

Due to the passage of time and gradual progress in all fields especially medicine, life expectancy has drastically increased; however it still varies at places around the world. This increase in the life expectancy has resulted in phenomenal increase in 'Old Age' population. Longer lives are not necessarily healthier lives. So health for aged is an important area of concern, this fact deeply motivated the investigator to select health as the subject of the study of this growing section of society.

Objective

To assess the health condition of the aged.

Method

The present study was conducted on randomly selected 300 aged between 65 yrs. to 85 yrs. in Agra city.

Tools

CMI (The Cornell Medical Index) health questionnaire developed and standardized by Wig, Pershad and Verma (1973) was used to assess the health status, the tool is standardized and its reliability and validity has been worked out. Higher scores are indicative of higher health distress and therefore poor health.

RESULTS AND DISCUSSION

The collected data were analyzed and the results are presented in the following sections.

Table 1: Showing Mean, S.D. and 't' Values on Health Components among the Senescent and Senile Group

Components of Health	*Senescent*		*Senile*		*Statistical Values*	
	Mean	*S.D.*	*Mean*	*S.D.*		
n =	176		124		t	p
Physical	71.24	8.39	86.02	8.14	15.211	< 0.01
Emotional	27.65	3.79	36.18	3.60	19.596	< 0.01
Total	98.89	11.50	122.20	9.24	18.711	< 0.01

Table 1 above shows mean, S.D. and t-value of obtained health score from aged of two groups one of 65 yrs. to 70 yrs. (senescent) and other of 71 yrs. to 85 yrs. (senile). All the indicators show that the chronological decline in physical, emotional and total health of the aged is higher among the senile subjects than the senescent subjects.

The decline in physical health is due to the advancement of age. It is a well-known phenomenon that the physical health of the aged people shows great decline in later years of life as compared to early aged stage. Along with some chronic physical health problems usually senile aged also experience organ or multi organs dysfunction, disorder or failure. Ramamurti and Jamuna (1993) have also stated that old age is associated with ill health, physical and sensory impairments, heightened sensitivity and increased susceptibility to disease.

Such chronological and radical decline in physical health leads to inadequacy, depression, anxiety, sensitivity, anger and tension that finally lead to a decline in emotional health. The decline in the physical and emotional health results in decline of total health. It is evident from the above results that decline in physical, mental and total health is higher in senile population as compared to senescent population.

Table 2: Showing the Mean, S.D. and 't' Values on Health Components among Aged Male and Female Population

Components of Health	*Male*		*Female*		*Statistical Values*	
	Mean	*S.D.*	*Mean*	*S.D.*		
N =	143		157		t	p
Physical	74.12	8.61	80.30	12.11	5.050	< 0.01
Emotional	30.34	5.13	31.93	5.91	2.477	< 0.05
Total	104.46	13.29	112.23	16.66	4.437	< 0.01

Table 2 indicates the mean, S.D. and t-value of physical, emotional and total health of male and female among the aged population under study. Females show higher health scores as compared to males. The significant t-values of physical, emotional and total health are 5.050, 2.477 and 4.437 respectively; they clearly show that physical, emotional and total health of male population is significantly better and improved as compared to the female population.

The above table shows poor physical, emotional and total health status of females than the males. In India the gender bias at early as well as later life is a common problem, where women may downplay their morbidities, attempt home remedies and seek traditional medical treatment before reaching the modern health care system. It seems that women have not only poor access to the health care system but are inclined to use it less. Poor health and gender discrimination always has adverse emotional effects. Several health problems afflict elderly women such as changes in the skeletal, cardiovascular, nervous, skin, genito-urinary and gastro-intestinal systems caused by declines in ovarian hormonal levels triggered by menopause. Due to the absence of ovarian steroids, chronic diseases such as osteoporosis, coronary heart disease and cerebro-vascular develop (Tinker *et al.,* 1994).

Table 3: Showing Mean, S.D. and 't' Values of Health Scores of Economically Independent and Dependent Aged

Components of Health	*Economically Independent*		*Economically Dependent*		*Statistical Values*	
	Mean	*S.D.*	*Mean*	*S.D.*		
N =	162		138		t	p
Physical	71.43	8.40	84.30	9.60	12.384	< 0.01
Emotional	27.73	3.69	35.22	4.70	15.451	< 0.01
Total	99.16	11.35	119.52	12.51	14.773	< 0.01

Table 3 indicates the mean, S.D. and t-value of economically independent and economically dependent aged subjects. These values indicate that the mean score of economically dependent aged were significantly higher as compared to the economically independent aged in all three components of health.

The great social changes such as migration of working force, urbanization, individualism, lack of funds, increase in general cost of living, breaking of joint family system as well as decreased cohesiveness of family and social bonds with change in the values and norms have made the position of aged in general and economically dependent aged specially more vulnerable, they are being often abused of their existence even. Such social changes have resulted in decline of the status enjoyed by the aged traditionally (Ramamurti and Jamuna, 1993). Financial and economic dependence of aged has put them farther from medical aids and their basic health care needs. This loss of status has made the aged feel helpless, isolated, ignored, stressful, economically dependent and out thrown (Kumar, 1995). On the other hand economically independent aged feel motivated and live with pride and honour such happiness and satisfaction keep them more physically and emotionally healthy as compared to the dependent aged.

Table 4 indicates the mean, S.D. and t-value of health scores of aged with and without spouse. The aged without spouse have lower health status showing higher mean score on all three components of health. The calculated significant t-values of physical, emotional and total health are 10.192, 15.358 and 12.836 respectively. During this period of life time spouse is a real companion.

Table 4: Showing Mean, S.D. and 't' Values on Components of Health of Aged with and Without Spouse

Components of Health	*Without Spouse*		*With Spouse*		*Statistical Values*	
	Mean	*S.D.*	*Mean*	*S.D.*		
n =	142		158		t	p
Physical	83.25	9.66	72.05	9.36	10.192	< 0.01
Emotional	35.10	4.72	27.65	3.66	15.358	< 0.01
Total	118.35	12.98	99.70	12.18	12.836	< 0.01

In the present times where offspring are busy with their studies, employment or with modern recreation means and both the members of the young couples mostly employed, the aged gets less attention from inside their family. The public health care system is mostly preoccupied with population control or care of mother and child, so both the spouse proves buddy for each other. It is also seen that the elderly as they grow older and older lose their contemporaries such as friends, relatives, colleagues, neighbours and people with whom they had grown up and shared ethos and their experiences of life; at such juncture of life losing of spouse usually have compounded setback effect on them. Living without spouse adversely affects the emotional and physical health of aged.

Table 5: Showing the Mean, S.D. and 't' Values on Components of Health of Aged Living in Joint and Nuclear Families

Components of Health	*Nuclear Family*		*Joint Family*		*Statistical Values*	
	Mean	*S.D.*	*Mean*	*S.D.*		
n=	202		98		t	p
Physical	75.36	10.15	81.46	11.62	4.652	< 0.01
Emotional	30.16	4.98	33.27	6.22	4.666	< 0.01
Total	105.52	14.32	114.72	16.40	4.973	< 0.01

Table 5 presents the mean, S.D. and t-value of health scores of aged living in joint and nuclear families. The table shows that the aged living in joint families have poor health as compared to the aged living in nuclear families. Scores of t-value of physical, emotional and total health are significant between both the groups.

Apparently these findings sound unusual that aged people living in nuclear families are healthier as compared to aged living in joint families. It seems that the aged population covered by the investigator was more oriented towards nuclear family system. The aged living all by themselves in a nuclear family system are bound to be younger, mobile and economically more stable as compared to their counter parts. Nuclear family phenomenon is widely acknowledged in present times. Bursting of joint families into nuclear families seems inevitable due to the massive social changes and formation of certain pressures in joint family systems. The joint family system seems to take care of the aged but perhaps it does little to provide quality care that contributes to improving health status. On the other hand, nuclear family has probably been able to look after, motivate and ensure aged for quality health care. It can be concluded that aged people have started accepting this social change and phenomenon of nuclear family system and they are showing the signs of adopting and adjusting with it rather blindly refuting and protesting against it.

CONCLUSION

On the basis of the obtained results it is concluded that health of the aged chronologically declines, health of the aged female population is poorer as compared to aged male population, aged having spouse are healthier than the aged without spouse, independent aged shows better health than the dependent aged and aged living in nuclear families are healthier than the aged living in joint families. Illness and diseases in aged are mostly chronic and of long term as health problems start from young age they are usually overlooked. Health status of an aged is an outcome of many, variables, however it has deep impact of the long life journey that one has passed. It is suggested that suitable precautions and timely awareness as to physical and mental health results in better quality of life in old age.

REFRENCES

Allem, F. and Faruquie, D.S. (2002). "Healthy Aging—AMU, Aligarh." *Social and Financial Problems of the Aged in India*.

Bose, A. (1982). Aspects of Aging in India. *Journal of Social Action,* 32, 9–12.

Kumar, S.V. (1995). Aging in India an Anthropological Outlook. Helpage India. *Research and Deveplopment Journal,* 2, 23–29.

Ramamurty, P.V. and Jamuna, D. (1993). "Psycological Dimensions of Aging in India." *The Indian Journal of Social Sciences,* 6(4).

Sinha, A. (2004). *Helpage India Research and Development Journal, October 2004*, 10, 3, 11–22.

Tinker, A., Daly, P., Green, C., Saxenian, H., Laxminarayana, R. and Gill, K. (1994). "Women's Health and Nutrition: Making a difference." The World Bank, Washington DC.

http//www.oldadult.htm.

http//www.Population aging A Public Health Challenges.htm.

SECTION–2
Occupational Health Psychology

A Study of Type A/B Personality and Values of Academic and Management Engineers: A Health Perspective for Organizations

Kavita Kumar*

ABSTRACT

Organizations today face a dynamic and changing environment and require employees who are able to easily adjust to the changing situations to maintain a conducive and healthy environment. It is important that employees' personalities fit with the organizations culture and value system. Therefore, recruiting new employees who fit better with the organizational demands and values will definitely lead to higher employees' satisfaction and reduced turnover. In the present paper an attempt is made to explore the personality Type A/B and the value pattern of the two groups of engineers *viz.* academic and management. 50 engineers each from the two groups were selected and administered Jenkins Activity Survey Questionnaire by Jenkins *et al.* (1971) to measure personality Type A/B, and Personal Value Statement Questionnaire by Oliver, J.E. (1985) to study the five values namely: Political, Aesthetic, Social, Theoretical and Economic. The data was analyzed on the basis of t-test. Significant difference was found between the two groups of engineers with regard to their personality type A/B and the value pattern. There was a significant difference found between the personality type A/B academic and management engineers' value pattern also.

INTRODUCTION

At the advent of the 21st century, the world is witnessing a rapid growth and advancement in the scientific arena. Engineers are playing a pivotal role in controlling the reigns of a complex technological society. In other words, engineers are responsible for the growth of the society and the nation at large. Edwin Layton (1986) in his book "The Revolt of the Engineers, Social Responsibilities in the American Engineering Profession" says that an engineer is "...socially responsible for ensuring the progress and benevolence of technological change." Society is more or less 100 percent dependent on the efficiency of the engineers. It is hard to miss the obvious and tremendous responsibility contained within the engineering profession. In order to utilize the expertise of these engineers, organizations are working hard to select the best engineers suitable to fulfill their goals and objectives. They have to successfully select those who best match the job requirements.

---

*Department of Psychology, Faculty of Social Sciences, Dayalbagh Educational Institute, Deemed University, Dayalbagh Agra, UP, India. E-mail: kavita.kumars@gmail.com

Psychologists are helping both the organization and the employees to understand how they can affect and further the progress together. Psychologists are working hard to find out the right personality that may create the balance between the two. Organizations require employees who are able to readily adjust to the dynamic and changing situations to maintain a conducive and healthy environment. It is important that employees' personalities fit with the organizations culture as well. The most essential reason for leaving a job is that the jobs are not compatible with their personalities (Schneider, 1987). Therefore, at the time of hiring, recruiting new employees who fit better with the organizational demands and culture will definitely lead to higher employees' satisfaction and reduced turnover.

The study of personality types started with the work of Friedman and Rosenman (1974), to study the relationship between behavioral patterns and the prevalence of Coronary Heart Diseases (CHD). They found that individuals manifesting certain behavioral traits were significantly more at risk to CHD. These individuals were later referred to as the Coronary Prone Behavior Pattern Type A as distinct to Type B (Low risk of CHD). It has been found that patients with Type A personality are likely to have severe coronary artery disease in comparison to Type B patients (Goldband, *et al*., 1979). Many studies (Kaushik, *et al*., 1991; Bulbulian and Bitters, 1996; Mecacci and Rocchell, 1998) confirmed that Type A behavior pattern is positively associated with psychosomatic illness. Type A behavior is defined as "*Individuals, who exhibit enhanced hostility, ambitiousness and competitiveness, and are often preoccupied with deadlines and with work*" (Chesney and Rosenman, 1980).

According to Robbins (2004), individuals with Type A personality are always moving, walking and eating rapidly; feel impatient with the rate at which most events take place; strive to think or do two or more things at once; cannot cope with leisure time; are obsessed with numbers, measuring their success in terms of how many or how much of everything they acquire. Characteristics of Type B personality are that they never suffer from a sense of time urgency with its accompanying impatience; feel no need to display or discuss either their achievements or accomplishments unless such exposure is demanded by the situation; play for fun and relaxation rather than to exhibit their superiority at any cost; can relax without guilt.

Robbins (2004), inferred that in managerial positions, Type A's demonstrate their competitiveness by working long hours and, not infrequently making poor decisions because they make them too fast. Type A's are also rarely creative. Due to their concern with quantity and speed, they rely on their experience, when faced with problems. They do not allocate the time necessary to develop unique solutions to new problems. They rarely vary their responses to specific challenges, hence their behavior is easier to predict than that of Type B's.

It has also been found that Type A's do better in job interviews because they are more likely to be judged as having desirable traits such as high drive, competence, aggressiveness, and success motivation. Despite the Type A's hard work, the Type B's are the ones, who appear to make it to the top. Great sales persons are usually Type A's, while senior executives are usually Type B. This is due to the fact that Type A possesses the tendency to trade off quality of effort for quantity. Promotions in corporate and professional organizations, "...usually go to those who are wise rather than to those who are merely hasty, to those who are tactful rather than to those who are hostile and to those who are creative rather than to those who are merely agile in competitive strife," (Friedman and Rosenman, 1974).

For the growth and development of an organization, the study of values is also important because they generally influence the attitudes and behavior of the employees. There has to be a value system consistent with the growth strategy, for the soundest socio-economic program to succeed. Values not only determine the social climate and national culture but also set the pace of social change and the rate of acceleration of the growth process. By studying the value system, there is a possibility that predictions can be made for the future. In any organization, culture is also expressed in the form of values and beliefs, which are not observable but are expressed by the way people explain and justify what they do. Some values are so deeply embedded in a culture that the members are not conscious of these values.

Allport (1960), Vernon and Allport (1931) carried out important works on values. Allport writes, "A value is a belief upon which a man acts by preference." They are also by and large ego-defensive (Allport, 1954; Glock and Start, 1965 and 1966; Allen and Spilka, 1967; Allport and Ross, 1967). For several years Allport, Vernon, and Lindzey's (1960) 'Study of Values' has been used to learn about personal values and their impact on the behavior of people of organizations. Spranger's theory (1929), describes 6 basic value systems that motivate people to act as they do. They are religious, aesthetic, theoretical, economic, social and personal. According to him, the religious and aesthetic values are common instances of unifying the philosophies of life. Human values are defined as characteristics of individuals that represent what is desirable, that vary in importance, and that guide people's lives (Kluckhohn, 1951; Rokeach, 1973; Schwartz, 1992). The study of values is central to the understanding of both individual and cultures. Values have been described as ideas tied to feelings and are the organizing factors within the personality, specially related to morals and character (Garrison, 1962) Social scientists have linked values to a number of behaviors including cigarette smoking (Grube, Weir, Getzlaf and Rokeach, 1984), religious behavior (Feather, 1984) consumer behavior (Henry, 1976; Homer and Kahle, 1988; Kahle, Beatty and Homer, 1986; Kamakura and Novak, 1992; Vinson and Munson, 1976) and political behavior (Feather, 1973; Rokeach, 1973; Tetlock,

1986).When the individuals' priorities meet with the organizational goals the efficiency and productivity increases in geometric progression and the corporate objectives are achieved. Prevalence of a value system unfavorable to growth strategy hinders and retards the growth process. The planning, formulation, implementation and evaluation of the growth strategy must be correlated with the value system prevailing in that social group.

The above explanation led the investigator to study the personality Type A/B and value system of engineers working in different areas of work and also investigate the value system of personality Type A/Type B engineers.

OPERATIONAL DEFINITIONS OF THE TERMS

1. *Type A:* "Aggressively involved in a chronic incessant struggle to achieve more and more in less and less time, and if required to do so, against the opposing efforts of other things or other persons." (Friedman and Rosenman, 1974).
2. *Type B:* Type B behavior is just opposite to Type A behavior Personality characteristics.
3. *Values:* "An enduring belief that a specific mode of conduct or end state of existence is personally or socially preferable to an opposite mode of conduct or end state of existence." (Rokeach, 1973).
4. *Academic:* Engineers who are working in the field of education *i.e.,* teaching or research.
5. *Management:* Engineers who are actually engaged in managing some engineering installations other than in academics.

OBJECTIVES OF THE STUDY

The main objectives of the present study were:

1. To study Type A/Type B behavior patterns of academic and management engineers.
2. To study the value patterns of the engineers of the aforesaid two groups.
3. To analyze personality Type A group of academic and management engineers with regard to their personal value system.
4. To analyze personality Type B group of academic and management engineers with regard to their personal value system.

HYPOTHESES

1. There is no significant difference between academic and management engineers with regard to their personality Type A/Type B behavior patterns.

2. There is no significant difference between academic and management engineers with regard to their five value *viz*. Political, Aesthetic, Social, Theoretical and Economic.
3. There is no significant difference between personality Type A group of academic and management engineers with regard to their personal value system.
4. There is no significant difference between personality Type B group of academic and management engineers with regard to their personal value system.

METHOD

Sample

The sample for the present investigation was restricted to 100 engineers. Purposive sampling was conducted. 50 engineers each from academic and management areas were selected. In order to control the demographic variables such as age, sex, educational qualification and experience, engineers selected for the study were only males, between 35 to 50 years of age, having a bachelor's degree in engineering and with at least 10 years of work experience.

Tools

Two separate questionnaires were used to measure personality Type A/Type B and values of the two groups of engineers.

1. *Jenkins Activity Survey (JAS) Scale* (Jenkins, Zyzanki and Rosenman, 1971). The JAS is a paper-and-pencil, self-report questionnaire. It is a self-report multiple choice questionnaire of 52 items designed to measure Type A behavior pattern. Hand scoring was done according to the instructions provided in the manual.
2. *Personal Value Statement (PVS)* (Oliver, J.E., 1985). The PVS questionnaire contains twenty items. PVS measures five Values namely political, aesthetic, social, theoretical and economic. The respondent is asked to rank the words in the order of their importance. Five scores are computed by transferring the numerical rankings of the words provided by the subjects in the questionnaire form to the scoring sheet and summing the responses in each column on the scoring sheet. Each type of value constitutes twelve items. Thus total scores assigned to each value refer to the corresponding value pattern.

Procedure

The questionnaires were conveniently administered in a group or individually. The instructions were very explicitly given about the questionnaires. The investigator briefly explained them the purpose of the study and requested them to sincerely complete the questionnaire in one sitting and do not ask others for suggestions. They were assured that no one will have access to their responses; the data will be kept confidential and used for research purpose only. The questionnaire was collected on the same day or in a day or two.

RESULTS AND ANALYSES

The data of the present investigation has been statistically analyzed on the basis of t-tests. The results are shown in the following Tables 1–6.

Table 1: Personality Type A/Type B Engineers on JAS

Personality Types	*Academic Engineers N = 50*	*Management Engineers N = 50*
Type A	33 (66%)	38 (76%)
Type B	17 (34%)	12 (24%)

Table 1 indicates that there are more Type A personalities found in the Management group (76%) in comparison to Academic group (66%). The mean scores were analyzed on the basis of t-test as shown in Table 2.

Table 2: Mean Scores, SD and t-test of Type A/Type B on JAS

Personality Types	*Academic Engineers*		*Management Engineers*		*t-test*	*Significance Level*
	Mean	S.D.	Mean	S.D.		
Type A	272.76	46.02	284.74	42.90	1.13	p > 0.05
	(N = 33 engineers)		(N = 38 engineers)			
Type B	148.29	41.09	169.17	34.43	2.32	p < 0.05
	(N = 17 engineers)		(N = 12 engineers)			

In Table 2, the t-value calculated for personality Type A between the two groups shows that there is no significant difference between Academic and Management engineers ($p > 0.05$). On the other hand there is significant difference found between personality Type B engineers of the two groups ($p < 0.05$).

The rank order of value pattern on PVS, Personality of Type A & Type B engineers between the two groups were also analyzed as shown in Table 3.

Table 3 clearly indicated that there is difference in hierarchy of the value patterns of the two groups. The rank order of academic group was social, theoretical, economic, political and aesthetic, while that of the Management group was economic, social, political theoretical and aesthetic on PVS. Also, the hierarchy of values for personality Type A and Type B engineers of the two groups is different as shown in Table 3.

Table 3: The Rank Order of Values on PVS, Personality Type A/Type B Engineers

Groups	*Academic*			*Management*		
Values	*PVS* *N = 50*	*Type A* *N = 33*	*Type B* *N = 17*	*PVS* *N = 50*	*Type A* *N = 38*	*Type B* *N = 12*
Political	4	4	4	3	3	4
Aesthetic	5	5	5	5	5	5
Social	1	2	1	2	2	1
Theoretical	2	1	2	4	4	3
Economic	3	3	3	1	1	2

Later the level of significance for the two groups of engineers on PVS was calculated as depicted in Table 4.

Table 4: Mean Scores, SD and t-test of the Value Pattern

Values	*Group I Academic Engineers*		*Group II Management Engineers*		*t-test*	*Significance Level*
	Mean	*S. D.*	*Mean*	*S. D.*		
Political	22.26	4.17	23.74	3.90	1.83	p > 0.05
Aesthetic	21.74	3.00	21.50	2.95	0.40	p > 0.05
Social	26.52	4.47	25.50	4.15	1.65	p > 0.05
Theoretical	26.40	3.84	23.76	3.55	3.57	p < 0.01
Economic	24.72	2.52	25.96	3.09	2.20	p < 0.05

N = 50 engineers in each group.

Table 4 shows that there is a significant difference found between the two groups on theoretical value ($p < 0.01$) and economic value ($p < 0.05$). There was no significant difference found on political, aesthetic and social value.

Further the scores of Type A Academic and Management group of engineers on PVS were analyzed on the basis of t-test as indicated in Table 5.

Table 5 shows that there is a significant difference found between political ($p < 0.05$), social ($p < 0.05$), theoretical ($p < 0.01$) and economic ($p < 0.05$) values of the two groups of engineers. While no significant difference is found for aesthetic value ($p > 0.05$).

Table 6 outlines the mean, SD and t-values of personality Type B Academic and Management engineers.

Table 5: Mean Scores, SD and t-test of the Value Pattern of Type A

Values	*Group I Academic Engineers (N =33)*		*Group II Management Engineers (N = 38)*		*t-test*	*Significance Level*
	Mean	*S. D.*	*Mean*	*S. D.*		
Political	22.33	4.17	24.21	3.37	2.10	$p < 0.05$
Aesthetic	21.19	2.92	21.66	3.24	0.64	$p > 0.05$
Social	26.21	4.48	24.37	3.95	2.02	$p < 0.05$
Theoretical	26.30	3.48	23.76	3.61	3.00	$p < 0.01$
Economic	24.82	2.58	26.16	3.04	2.08	$p < 0.05$

Table 6: Mean Scores, SD and t-test of the Value Pattern of Type B

Values	*Group I Academic Engineers (N = 33)*		*Group II Management Engineers (N = 38)*		*t-test*	*Significance Level*
	Mean	*S. D.*	*Mean*	*S. D.*		
Political	22.12	4.28	22.25	5.14	0.11	$p > 0.05$
Aesthetic	21.12	3.22	21.00	1.76	0.20	$p > 0.05$
Social	27.12	4.51	27.40	4.38	0.28	$p > 0.05$
Theoretical	26.39	4.58	23.75	3.52	2.94	$p < 0.01$
Economic	24.53	2.45	25.33	3.28	1.14	$p > 0.05$

The statistical analysis on the basis of Table 6 shows that value patterns of the personality Type B engineers of the two groups is significantly different for theoretical value ($p < 0.01$). There is no significant difference found for other values of the two groups.

DISCUSSION

Engineers work in different environments like Educational, Theoretical, Research, Design, Productions, Sales, Service, Management, Technical etc. Engineers with different Personality Type may be more naturally skilled or comfortable in certain area than in others and can flourish more in that area. Keeping this in mind, organizations can look into the personality types and recruit those that best fit the job profiles. In the present study, the results have been discussed for Academic and Management Engineers with regard to their Personality Type A/Type B, and the value patterns of the two groups.

The present investigation showed that Management Engineers possess more Personality Type A characteristics than the Academic Engineers. There may be a possibility that Management Engineers show more Type A personality because they are goal oriented and success driven, which are among the few important characteristics of Type A personality. These results are also supported by Howard *et al.* (1976) study, which showed that majority of Americans are Type A, and an even higher percentage of Managers are Type A. Howard *et al.* (1976) study demonstrated that 60% of the Managers sampled were clearly Type A and only 12% were Type B. In the present study, 76% Management engineers are Type A while only 66% Academic engineers are Type A. The study by Boyd (1984) exerted that firms run by Type A executives, showed higher return on the investments than those run by Type B executives, further supports the results of the present study, that Management Engineers possess more Type A behavioral characteristics. Engineers involved in management field of work need to be highly aggressive, goal-oriented, risk seeking and competitive in pursuit of success in their endeavors.

Research indicates that employer's selection decisions on job applicants may be based on personality tests (Tross, Harper, Osher, Kneidinger, 2000). Most 'Type A's' are unable and unwilling to change and cope with their Type A characteristics (Steers, 1984; Velsor & Leslie, 1995). This should be taken into account by the organizations to take due measures to deal with this issue as change is important factor in the modern context.

The distinction between Type A and Type B raises several challenging questions for employers. Should organization consider Type A or Type B Personality employees when allocating job assignment? Should it develop training programs to help change Type A employees into Type B employees or *vice versa*? Does organization have a responsibility to provide training that will help both Type A's and Type B's cope with the work habits and expectations of the supervisors who are different from themselves?

Regarding the value system, the Academic engineers value system comprises of the Social Value at the top. Academicians lay importance to societal norms and try to conserve and maintain them through educating the masses. Thus, they tend to be kind, sympathetic and warm, and reflect a humanitarian concern and the welfare of others. Second in order is the Theoretical value for Academic engineers. This value is associated with empirical, critical, systematic and rational aspects. For Academic engineers social norms, rationality, empirical attitude, critical and intellectual pursuits are very important. They tend to value science, research, information and theory more. Therefore, it can be inferred that Educational engineers rank it at the second place. The Academic engineers ranked economic value third after the social and theoretical value. In today's hardships, money is required to fulfill both personal and professional means. But for Academic engineers it only comes after the social and theoretical values. Political value is preferred at rank fourth by Academic engineers. Political value is related to be influential, renowned and powerful. In educational group this drive is observed lower than the other two groups, where power and prestige are preferred more. Aesthetic value remains the least preferred value between the two groups of engineers.

Management engineers unlike the Academic engineers have ranked the economic value at the top. In today's materialistic and competitive world, money has become most valuable in the corporate world. Advancement and globalization in the corporate world are attracting people to work hard and accumulate more and more wealth. Therefore for them, perks and remunerations provided by the organizations have become most important. Management engineers probably believe that money can fulfill their socio-psychological needs as well as their high professional dreams and aspirations. In comparison, teachers are more focused in imparting knowledge and remain concerned about social values in the society. Teachers present themselves as role model for their students in the name of nation building. For Management engineers, second in order of rank is the social value. Having acquired monetary power, Management engineers tend to use it to gain social status. Social value follows the economic value. Next in line, for the Management engineers is the political value. Perhaps after the fulfillment of monetary and social needs, the third choice for the Management engineers is the political value. Fourth rank is given to the theoretical value by the Management engineers. Since they are involved in the decision-making and are result-oriented in the corporate world, they rate the theoretical value lower than the other three values. Aesthetic value, as already stated, has been ranked the lowest among all the five values.

In a study by Schanbroeck (1995), it was suggested that professional in arts are involved in social interactions and creativity, which are closely associated with aesthetic value. The subjects for the present study have been selected from engineering background and therefore they do not value creativity and beauty as much as individuals from arts background. This may be the explanation that in the present study also, both the groups of engineers ranked the aesthetic value the lowest.

CONCLUSION

The present study will be beneficial to both organization and employee in the following ways:

1. The study will facilitate the organization to achieve its known objectives. It will help the organization to learn about the Personality Type and Value System of their employees without bringing out significant change in its basic assumptions.

2. The organization will be able to understand their employees better and if needed may help them to change the organizational culture accordingly.
3. The research will also help the employees to better adjust in their work environment. The insight into their Personality Type and Value System will also act as a defense to their self images. This will lead to conductive and healthy environment.
4. The study will be helpful for the organization to plan intervention programs for Type A individuals. Research indicates that Type A and Type B persons react quite differently to stressful situations (Glass, 1977, Krantz, Glass and Snyder, 1974).
5. Value Personality tests are often used as a key part of the employee selection process.
6. Study of value system facilitates the growth process of the organization.
7. Values are important for the development of our Personality. They help the individual in his self- development or the moral development.
8. No research has been found that is based on the two groups of Engineers *viz.* academic and management areas of work. Thus, the present study is an attempt to investigate the difference between the two groups of Engineers with regard to their Personality Type A/Type B and Values.

Thus the findings of the present investigation may encourage organizations to be more sensitive to the needs and problems of the employees according to their personality types, value systems and determine the best approaches to be used to succeed, as well as the most effective ways to overcome problems and blind spots. The study would furnish an insight and facilitate the organizations to define the core values, differentiate them from competitors, grow in a positive manner and promote changes in a constructive way. The importance of the present study will underscore the factors that are essential for the healthy environment of the organizations also.

REFERENCES

Allen, R.O. and Spilka, B. (1967). "Committed and Consensual Religion: A Specification of Religion- Prejudice Relationships." *Journal for the Scientific Study of Religion,* 6, 11–20.

Allport, G.W. (1954). *Nature of Prejudice*. Cambridge: Addison-Wesley.

Allport, G.W. (1960). *Study of Value (*3rd edition). Boston: Houghton Mifflin Co.

Allport, G.W. and Ross, J.M. (1967). "Personal Religious Orientation and Prejudice." *Journal of Personality and Social Psychology,* 5, 432–433.

Allport, G.W., Vernon, P.E. and Lindzey, G. (1960). *Study of Values*. Boston: Houghton Mifflin Co.

Boyd, D.P. (1984). "Type A Behavior, Financial Performance and Organizational Growth in Small Business Firms." *Journal of Occupational Psychology*, 57, 137–140.

Bulbulian, R. and Bitters, D. (1996). "Blood Pressure Responses to Acute Exercise in Type A and B Females and Males." *Physiology and Behavior*, 60(4), 1177–1182.

Chesney, M.A. and Rosenman, R.H. (1980). "Type A Behavior in the Work Setting." In Cooper, C.L. and Payne, R. (Eds.), *Current Concerns in Occupational Stress,* New York, N.Y.: John Wiley and Sons.

Feather, N.T. (1973). "Value Change among University Students." *Australian J. of Psychology*, 25, 57–70.

Feather, N.T. (1984). "Protestant Ethic, Conservatism and Values." *J. Personality and Social Psychology*, 46, 1132–1141.

Friedman, M. and Rosenman, R.H. (1974). *Type A Behavior and Your Heart.* New York: Alfred A. Knopf, 84–86.

Garrison, K.C. (1962). *Psychology of Adolescence,* New Jersey: Prentice Hall, 203.

Glass, D.C.B. (1977). *Behavioral Patterns, Stress and Coronary Heart Diseases.* Hillsdale, N. J. Lawerance Erlbaum Associates.

Goldband, S., Katkin. E. and Morrell, M. (1979). *Stress and Anxiety*, 6, 351–370.

Grube, J.W., Weir, I.L. Getzlaf, S. and Rokeach, M. (1984). "Own Value System, Value Images, and Cigarette Smoking." *Personality and Social Psychology Bulletin*, 10, 306–313.

Henry, W.A. (1976). "Cultural Values do Correlate with Consumer Behavior." *Journal of Marketing Research*, 13, 121–127.

Homer, P.M. and Kahle, L.R. (1988). "A Structural Equation Test of the Value-Attitude Behavior Hierarchy." *Journal of Personality and Social Psychology*, 54, 638–646.

Howard, J.H., Cunningham, D.A. and Rechnitzer, P. (1976). "Health Patterns Associated with Type A Behavior: A Managerial Population." *Journal of Human Stress*, 24–31.

Jenkins, C.W., Zyzanski, S.J. and Rosenman, R.H. (1971). "Progress toward Validation of the Type A Computer- Scored Test for the Coronary-Prone Behavior Pattern." *Psychosomatic Medicine*, 33, 193–202.

Kahle, L.R., Beatty, S.E. and Homer, P. (1986). "Alternative Measurement Approaches to Consumer Values: The List of Values (LOV) and Values and Life Styles (VALS)." *Journal of Consumer Research*, 13, 405–409.

Kamakura, W.A. and Novak, T.P. (1992). "Value System Segmentation: Exploring the Meaning of LOV." *Journal of Consumer Research*, 19, 119–132.

Kluckhohn, C. (1951). "Value and Value Orientation in the Theory of Action: An Exploration in Definition and Classification." In Parsons, T. and Shils, E.A. (Eds.). *Towards a General Theory of Action.* Cambridge: Harvard University Press, 395.

Krantz, D.S., Glass, D.C. and Snyder, M.L. (1974). "Helplessness, Stress Level and the Coronary Prone Behavior." *Journal of Experimental Social Psychology,* 10, 284–360.

Layton, Edwin Jr. (1986). *The Revolt of the Engineers, Social Responsibilities in the American Engineering Profession.* Baltimore: John Hopkins University Press, MD.

Mecacci, L. and Rocchell, G. (1998). "Stress-related Personality Aspects." *Personality and Individual Differences,* 25(3), 537–542.

Oliver, J.E. (1985). "Personal Value Statement." *Annual Handbook for Group Facilitators: Developing Human Resources*, University Associates, 107–116.

Robbins, S.P. (2004). *Organizational Behavior*, Ed. 10th, New Delhi: Prentice-Hall of India, 101–102.

Rokeach, M. (1973). *The Nature of Human Values*. New York: Free Press.

Schanbroeck, J. (1995). "Creative Stress." *Psychology Today*, 28, 14.

Schneider, B. (1987). "The People make the Place." *Personnel Psychology*, 437–453.

Schwartz, S.H. (1992). "Universals in the Content and Structure of Values." *Advances in Experimental and Social Psychology Orlando, FL: Academic press*, 25, 1–65.

Spranger, E. (1929). *Types of Men*, J.W. Pigeons (Ed.), New York: Strobert Hafner.

Steers, R.M. (1984) *Introduction to Organizational Behavior.* Scott, Foresman and Glenview III, 518.

Tetlock, P.E. (1986). "A Value Pluralism Model of Ideological Reasoning." *Journal of Personality and Social Psychology*, 50, 819–827.

Tross, S.A., Harper, J.P., Osher L.W. and Kneidinger, L.M. (2000). "Not Just the usual cast of Characteristics: Using Personality to Predict College Performance and Retention." *Journal of College Student Development*, 41, 323–324.

Velsor, E.V. and Leslie, J.B. (1995). "Why Executives Derail: Perspectives across Time and Culture." *Academy of Management Executives*, 62–72.

Vernon, P.E. and Allport, G.W. (1931). "A Test for Personal Values." *Journal of Abnormal Psychology*, 26, 223–235.

Vinson, D.E. and Munson, J.M. (1976). *Personal Values: An Approach to Market Segmentation.* In K.L. Bernhardt (Ed) Marketing: 1776–1976 and Beyond. Chicago: American Marketing Association, 313–317.

Reduction in Anxiety of Aspirants of Campus Placement—Achieved as a Result of a Placement Workshop: An Experiential Approach

D.S. Narban*

ABSTRACT

In the competitive world of today, nothing gives one person so much advantage as to remain cool and unruffled under all circumstances. The population of professional college students, close to campus placements is at a greater risk of anxiety. The objective of the study was to reduce anxiety level of aspirants of campus placement using experiential learning approach. So, a random sample of thirty-one boy-students and equal number of girl-students was drawn and administered SCAT (Sinha's Comprehensive Anxiety Test; Sinha & Sinha, 1995). After obtaining the pre-test scores on anxiety, they were given a four-day placement training in experiential learning settings; at the end of which they were administered SCAT once again. The pre-post scores were analyzed using the Repeated Measures *t* Statistics, and the Independent Measures *t* Statistics. The results at α = .5 (two tailed) were: significant reduction in anxiety level of the students, and no significant difference between male and female students on reduction in their anxiety levels. The qualitative inputs substantiated the quantitative results. This study can be applied in reducing anxiety level in line with the aspirations and with potential of wide application in Clinical Health Psychology, Organizational Psychology, and Social Psychology.

INTRODUCTION

In the competitive world of today, nothing gives one person so much advantage over another as to remain cool and unruffled under all circumstances. It is amazing what harm anxiety can do to a person. Anxiety most generally is a vague, unpleasant emotional state with qualities of apprehension, dread, distress and uneasiness. Anxiety is frequently distinguished from fear by its being often objectless, whereas fear assumes a specific feared object, person, or event.

In techniques of Behavior Therapy following the process of Systematic Desensitization, along with Relaxation Training, the therapist and patient explore the patient's history and experiences and construct an anxiety hierarchy. First, major themes are identified (*e.g.,* fear of dog, of height, *etc.*) then particular situations are described which could produce anxiety reactions, ranging from most moderate to most extremes—in total

*Dy. Director, Amity Institute of Behavioral (Health) and Allied Sciences, Amity University, Noida, UP, India. E-mail: dsnarban@amity.edu

may be about twenty to twenty-five. The desensitization sessions follow step by step (Korchin, 1999).

The anxiety disorders are a group of psychological problems whose key features include excessive apprehension, dread, worry, avoidance, and compulsive rituals. The most prevalent anxiety disorders listed in the Diagnostic and Statistical Manual of Mental Disorders, Fourth Edition (DSM-IV; American Psychiatric Association, 1994) include panic disorder with and without social phobia, specific phobia, Obsessive-Compulsive Disorder (OCD), Generalized Anxiety Disorder (GAD), and Posttraumatic Stress Disorder (PTSD). Specific types of anxiety among children also include separation anxiety disorder (Veeraraghavan, 2006).

Causes of anxiety disorders range from biological, psychological to social and familial factors. Psychological etiology explains anxiety disorder in terms of a combination of increased internal and external stresses which overwhelm a person's normal coping ability. Social and familial factors include broken families, conflict between parents, alcoholic parent, *etc.* (Veeraraghavan, 2006). The effect of familial factors reduces with age, for example on account of an alcoholic parent it is invariably much reduced by the time one acquires middle age.

As an adolescent grows, leaves school and joins college, the first thing that strikes his mind in choosing curriculum and college is the prospect of placement. Realizing this, for past more than a decade almost all professional colleges in India hold a counseling session before admission where they entertain such questions to be answered. The students do have the placement issue in their mind throughout the course, the degree of which may vary. Medical colleges and some good colleges running psychological programmes have continuous field training spread throughout the academic programme on specified days of every week. But in most other curriculum the final term or a term before are set aside for summer training. The students suddenly experience the symptoms of anxiety as they are to get an agency to do summer training with which may or may not be their dream choice. Then comes the stage when the companies start coming for campus placement, and none may have had the experience of undergoing a selection process. This anxiety, seemingly close to social phobia, when relates to what the society will think in case not respectably placed may also be experienced by an often introvert doing a distant learning course who does not want to fall in eyes of his own future-self. While the term 'job anxiety' has been used in organizational behavior with relation to further job prospects, the anxiety related to first placement may be referred as *'placement anxiety'*.

While, being in one's own natural self is important in any selection process, anxiety tends to pull a person away from his otherwise normal self. Hence it is important to reduce this anxiety, and help aspirants of campus placement to be their own best-self while facing on-campus selection processes. For this one may conduct special workshops for reducing anxiety and inducing relaxation through certain exercises at both individual and group levels.

At this time, there is a need for a facilitator of experiential learning who can play a very effective role in making the students learn experientially to deal with intrinsic and extrinsic stressors, thereby reducing their anxiety level, and preventing them from potentially devastating effects of anxiety.

In the present study an attempt was made to conduct an experiential learning based placement workshops for aspirants of campus placement to reduce their anxiety and bring out their best-self to the forefront—experientially.

Rogers distinguished two types of learning: cognitive (meaningless academic knowledge) and experiential (significant applied knowledge). He felt that all human beings have a natural propensity to learn; the role of a teacher is to facilitate learning (Rogers, 1951, 1961, 1969; Rogers and Freiberg, 1994). Dewey focused on importance of experiential learning in natural sciences with his famous formula: Experience + Reflection = Learning (Dewey, 1938, 1939). Kolb (1971, 1975), in the world of today, gave his approach of experiential learning using four cycles of learning, *viz.*, observation of a concrete experience, its reflection on to ownself, making an abstract conceptualization, and doing active experimentation, which in itself would be a new concrete experience. Experiential Learning therefore is, the knowledge, skills, or abilities attained through observation, stimulation, or participation that provides depth and meaning to learning by engaging the mind through: activity-generated concrete experience, reflective observation, abstract conceptualization, and active experimentation.

Claimed as the core phenomenon of human activities, 'learning', is a relatively permanent change in knowledge, behavior, or understanding that results from experience. Innate behavior, maturation and fatigue are however excluded from learning.

The present research has used Kolb's approach of experiential learning, beginning with provision of concrete experience through specially innovated indoor simulations specific to the objective at hand, and taking them through the cycle of experiential learning.

Objective

The objective of the study was: *firstly,* to find out the level of anxiety amongst students who were to appear for campus placement interviews; *secondly*, to use intervention measures and bring down their anxiety level by preparing them experientially to face the selection process, and then to find out the degree to which the anxiety level has gone down.

Hypotheses

Two null hypotheses were:

1. There will be no effect of experiential learning on anxiety levels amongst the sample taken for this research.
2. There will be significant difference between boys and girls in regard to the decrease in the level of anxiety.

MATERIAL AND METHODS

Sample Size and Sampling Method

The sample consisted of aspirants of campus placement: 31 boy-students and 31 girl-students of campus placement—in all 62; selected randomly from an institute with large number of students with no involvement (bias) of the researcher in forming of this group.

Research Design

A Pre-Post research design in which the subjects were initially measured for their level of anxiety, thereafter given intervention through an experiential learning based campus placement workshop, and again at the end of the workshop the level of anxiety was re-measured. All 62 formed the experimental group.

Tools

The tool used for quantitative measurement of anxiety level of the students was: SCAT (Sinha's Comprehensive Anxiety Test) (Sinha, A.K.P. and Sinha, L.N.K., 1995). Qualitative inputs were feedback of participants and their faculty, and actual placements.

Procedure

The experiential learning based placement workshop was conducted over four days. It began with before-test, and after-test was administered at the end of workshop, *i.e.,* before first campus placement.

The workshop progressed as follows:

1. Introduction and ice breaking.
2. Free expression of the participants regarding their aspirations and expectations from the workshop.
3. Introduction to the workshop by the facilitator.
4. Experientially giving of insight into the selection process at various stages.

5. Division of participants into four groups of 15–16 each with almost equal number of boys and girls.
6. Conduct of group discussions, and facilitation experientially on being at their best.
7. Role-play of interview process for all.
8. Individual mock interviews and experientially given feedback.
9. Common feedback points to the group of 62.
10. Written feedback to the institute on all participants.

At the end of workshop SCAT was administered again as a post-test.

Results

The pre-post scores obtained on SCAT were analyzed using the Repeated Measures *t* Statistics to find effectiveness or otherwise of the workshop, and the Independent Measures *t* Statistics to find if there was any difference in variation of levels of anxiety as a result of workshop between boys and girls. The results are tabulated below:

Table 1: Effect of Experiential Learning on Anxiety-level of Aspirants of Campus Placement using the Repeated Measures t Statistics

Experimental Group									
Test/ Sub-domains	*Mean*		*Std Dev*		*Diff in Means*	*Difference*		*Std Error*	*t (df = 30)*
	Before	*After*	*Before*	*After*		*SS*	*SD*		
	$\overline{X}_{before}$	$\overline{X}_{after}$	s_{before}	s_{after}	$\overline{D}$	*SS*	*s*	$s_{\overline{D}}$	*t*
Boy-Students	30.55	24.27	6.20	2.44	–6.28	766.71	5.06	0.91	–6.92
Girl-Students	29.84	24.26	4.12	1.89	–5.58	505.38	4.10	0.74	–7.57

t(30) critical = at/beyond + 2.042 or –2.042; *p*<.05, two tails

Table 2: Difference of the Effect of Experiential Learning on Anxiety Level between Males and Females using Independent Measures t Statistics

Domain	*Sample Size*		*Difference Scores*			*SS*		*Pooled Variance*	*Std Error*	*t (60)*
	Boys	*Girls*	*Boys*	*Girls*	*Boys-Girls*	*Boys*	*Girls*			
	n_{Boys}	n_{Girls}	$\overline{D}_{Boys}$	$\overline{D}_{Girls}$	$\overline{D}_{Boys-Girls}$	SS_{Boys}	SS_{Girls}	s_p^2	$s_{\overline{x}_1-\overline{x}_2}$	$t(60)$
Anxiety	31	31	–6.28	–5.58	-0.70	766.71	505.38	21.20	1.17	–0.60

t(60) critical = at/ beyond + 2.000 or -2.000; *p<.05 two tails*

The statistical analysis indicates that:

The effect of experiential learning in reducing anxiety in male aspirants was significant: $t\,(30) = -6.92$; $p < .05$, two tails, and of the female aspirants also significant: $t\,(30) = -7.57$; $p < .05$, two tails.

The effect of experiential learning in reducing anxiety between male and female aspirants was not significantly different: $t\,(60) = -0.63$; $p < .05$, two tails.

Qualitative Results

The students during the process of workshop were seen constantly adding to their confidence level and pleasantness out of new learning directed towards their objective. Their confidence was reflective of longevity of learning beyond the placements which were to be held the following day. Feedback obtained by the concerned institute from all the aspirant participants was that they found the workshop very useful and had gained confidence. Result of placement that took place the very following day of the workshop was found very encouraging by the concerned institute. It was interesting to note that months after the workshop ended, the students continuously reported high level of confidence which was also substantiated by their faculty members.

DISCUSSION

With significant reduction in anxiety level of the students and their qualitative inputs received, both the null hypotheses were rejected which stated that there will be no reduction in anxiety and there will be difference between the effect of treatment on boys and girls.

Possibility of contribution of environmental variables in reduction of anxiety over the duration of workshop can safely be ruled out, because the students were not involved in any other activity in the institute, and in off-institute hours their routine was stable at places of stay—home or hostel, close to campus placement day.

Additionally, the study has its importance for the following:

1. It is one of the unique ways of reducing anxiety level of individuals.
2. The study was done in one of the six cosmopolitan cities of the country. Life in cosmopolitan cities is known to be more stressful and anxiety-prone. So, the approach used in the study is likely to find success in any city of the country.
3. All the campus placement aspirants in the study were of an MBA programme. So, this approach is likely to find success with any other similar professional course where campus placements are held.
4. Since the present study was done with both boys and girls, the approach used in the study is likely to find success with the student community at large.

It is said that, science never solves a problem: without creating ten more. The enumerated importance of the study also indicates the scope for further studies in areas where the present study did not do specific measurements but is suggestive of for example stress, phobia, neuroticism, introversion, and the like.

Fletcher (1971), Roland (1981), Priest and Lesperance (1985), Priest and Baillie (1987), Weil and McGill's (1989), Galpin (1989), Dulkiewicz and Chase (1991), King (1991), Bronson, Gibson, Kishar and Priest (1992), Vince and Martin (1993), Priest and Gass (1993), Bramwell *et al.* (1997), Isenhart (2000) have all been among others to measure effect of outward bound training, not inbound training, and mostly in the field of organizational team building. The present study used inbound experiential learning in line with aspirations of the participants.

Finally, as no other work was found applying experiential learning in the field of anxiety, this study with certain innovative modulations can be found having a potential of wide application Clinical Health Psychology, Organizational Psychology, and Social Psychology.

Anxiety remains a mental health challenge, and the initiative of use of experiential approach to reduce it, can be: a vision for the future.

REFERENCES

Antony, M.M. and Barlow, D.H. (1996). "Emotion Theory as a Framework for Explaining Panic Attacks and Panic Disorder." In R.M. Rapee (Ed.), *Current Controversies in the Anxiety Disorders*. New York: Guilford Press.

Arthur, S. Reber and Emily, S. Reber (2001). *Psychology*. London: Penguin.

Bramwell, K., Forrester, S., Houle, B., LaRocque, J., Villeneuve, L. and Priest, S. (1997). "One Shot Wonders Don't Work: A Causal-comparative Case Study." *Journal of Adventure Education and Outdoor Leadership,* 14(2), 15–17.

Bronson, J., Gibson, S., Kishar, R. and Priest, S. (1992). "Evaluation of Team Development in a Corporate Adventure Training Program." *Journal of Experiential Education*, 15(2), 50–53.

Dewey, J. (1938). *Experience and Education*. NY: Collier Books.

Dewey, J. (1939). *Experience and Education*. NY: Kappa Delta.

Dulkiewicz and Chase (1991). "Other Works Related to CAT/EBTD (Corporate Adventure Training/Experience-Based Training and Development)." www.xperentia.com.

Dunner, David L. (2001). *Anxiety*. NY: Wiley-Liss, Inc., 71.

Fletcher, B. (1971). *The Challenge of Outward Bound.* London: Heinemann.

Galpin (1989). "Other Works Related to CAT/EBTD (Corporate Adventure Training/ Experience-Based training and Development)." www.xperentia.com.

Isenhart, M.W. (2000). *Collaborative Approaches to Resolving Conflict.* Thousand Oaks, CA: Sage.

Jones, F. and Fletcher, B.C. (1983). An Empirical Study of Occupational Stress Transmission in Working Couples. *Human Relation,* July 1983, 881–903.

King, K.V. (1991). "The Role of Adventure in the Experiential Learning Process." *Journal of Experiential Education* 11, 2, 4–8.

Kolb, D.A. (1971). *Individual Learning Styles and the Learning Process*, Cambridge: MIT Sloan School of Management, 535–71.

Kolb, D.A. and Fry, R.E. (1975). *Toward an Applied Theory of Experiential Learning: Theories of Group Process*. London: John Wiley.

Korchin, S.J. (1999). *Modern Clinical Psychology.* ND: CBS, 341, 2.

Priest, S. and Lesperance, M.A. (1985). "Effective Outdoor Leadership: A Survey." *The Journal of Experiential Education*, 8(1), 13–15.

Priest, S. and Baillie (1987). "Justifying the Risk to Others: The Real Razor's Edge." *Journal of Experiential Education,* 10, 1, 16–22.

Priest, S. and Gass, M. (1993). "Five Generations of Facilitated Learning from Adventure Experiences." *The Journal of Adventure Education and Outdoor Leadership* 10, 3, 23–25.

Rogers, C. (1951). *Client-Centered Therapy.* Boston: Houghton Mifflin Company.

Rogers, C. (1961). *On Becoming a Person.* London: Constable.

Rogers, C. (1969). *Freedom to Learn.* Columbus, Ohio: Charles E. Merrill.

Rogers, C. and Freiberg, H.J. (1994). *Freedom to Learn* (3rd ed). Columbus, OH: Merrill/ Macmillan.

Roland (1981). "Other Works Related to CAT/EBTD (Corporate Adventure Training/ Experience-Based Training and Development)." www.xperentia.com.

Sinha, A.K.P. and Sinha, L.N.K. (1995). *SCAT (Sinha's Comprehensive Anxiety Test).* Agra: NPC.

Veerarghavan, V. (2006). *Behavior Problems in Children and Adolescents.* Delhi: NBC, 6–18.

Vince, R. and Martin, L. (1993). "Inside Action Learning: An Exploration of the Psychology and Politics of the Action Learning Model, Management Education and Development." *The Journal of Experiential Education* 24, 3, 205–15.

Weil, S. and McGill, I. (1989). *Making Sense of Experiential Learning.* Buckingham, UK: OU Press.

Modelling of Occupational Health Hazards of Glass Workers with ANN for Intelligent System

Sanjay Srivastava*[1], Yogesh K. Anand[1], Devi P. Sharma[1], Ajit[1] and Bhupendra Pathak[1]

ABSTRACT

Excessive heat in the workplace of glass/bangle manufacturing units, in general, leads to a continuum of medical problems with symptoms ranging from headache and nausea to vomiting syncope, and more severe central nervous system disturbances. We designed and implemented an intelligent system to reduce Occupational Health Hazards (OHHs) of workers of a glass/bangle manufacturing unit at Firozabad, India. We used Artificial Neural Networks (ANNs) with backpropagation learning as model free estimators to evaluate OHHs of workers for different job combinations.

INTRODUCTION

In glass manufacturing industries, studies have been conducted and there has been a general observation that working in glass industries may lead towards many Occupational Health Hazards (OHHs). Managing such hazards in an optimum manner is a challenging task. Glass/bangle manufacturing workers are subjected to high heat stresses owing to high temperature of kiln. In many indoor operations including smelting, mining, laundries, kitchens, bakeries, electrical utilities (particularly boiler rooms), foundries, glassware and ceramic operations heat stress is a pertinent problem. To address the issue, the American Conference of Government Industry Hygienists (ACGIH) and the National Institute for Occupational Safety and Health (NIOSH) have set guidelines for a safe thermal environment. Current guidelines define working environment that cause either a decrease in body core temperature below 6°C (cold stress) or an increase above 38°C (heat stress) as potentially hazardous (ACGIH, 2004). However, the effectiveness of these guidelines is limited by the individual variation among employee and variation in work practices in different industries (Gun and Budd, 1995). The least number of unsafe behaviors were observed when the Wet Bulb Globe Temperature (WBGT) was between 17° and 23°C, which is below the ACGIH threshold limit value for heat stress and strain (ACGIH, 2004). The physiological strain at the $WBGT_{crit}$ in five different clothing ensembles was investigated and the

* Corresponding author.

[1] Department of Mechanical Engineering, Faculty of Engineering, Dayalbagh Educational Institute, Deemed University, Agra–282 005 India.

E-mail: *ssrivastava.engg@gmail.com

effects of gender were observed on the level of heat strain at $WBGT_{crit}$ (Candi *et al.*, 2008). Hot conditions can give rise to cognitive decrements which may result in unsafe behaviors before harmful physiological responses are manifested (Hancock and Vasmatzidis, 1998; Enander and Hygge, 1990).

We identified four types of workers based on their job category in a glass/bangle manufacturing unit at Firozabad. Each job has its specific earning and degree of severity. Usually high earning jobs are more tedious, and perceptibly workers performing such jobs are more prone to health hazards. Another side of the coin is that workers, in general, aim at maximizing their earnings by subjecting themselves to extreme work conditions. We observed that the OHH of workers is largely determined by factors such as Working Hours (WH), duration of Rest Breaks (RB), and Working Hours between Two Consecutive Rest Breaks (WHBTRB). We propose that job-combination can be a way of reducing the OHH and yet maintaining the good earnings of workers. The most severe job (*tarwala* job) is combined with rest of three jobs sequentially resulting in three job combinations. OHH for a job combination is evaluated based on the Rate of Perceived Exertion (RPE) on a scale of 0 to 10. Since it is extremely difficult to evaluate OHH for every possible combination of WH, RB, and WHBTRB of jobs under consideration, therefore ANNs with backpropagation learning, also called Backpropagation Neural Networks (BPNNs), are used for evaluation of OHHs. Three ANNs are trained, one for each job combination, with known data set. Each trained network facilitates the estimation of OHHs for input values of WH, RB, and WHBTRB of jobs under consideration. The proposed intelligent system would act as an advisor to a worker to choose a job combination and the corresponding values of WH, RB, and WHBTRB so that the worker is within the prescribed safe limit of occupation health hazards and yet not compromising his earnings to a greater extent.

This paper is organized as follows. Basic features and architecture of BPNN is presented in section 2. Work methodology is described in brief in section 3. The simulation results obtained using BPNN based models are discussed in section 4, followed by conclusions in section 5.

BACK PROPAGATION NEURAL NETWORK

As mentioned, BPNNs are used to estimate the OHH of workers for different job combinations. BPNN is a multiple layer network with an input layer, output layer and some hidden layers between input and output layers. Its learning procedure is based on gradient search with least sum squared optimality criterion. Calculation of the gradient is done by partial derivative of sum squared error with respect to weights. After the initial weights have been randomly specified and the input has been presented to the neural network, each neuron currently sum outputs from all neurons in the preceding layer. The sum and activation (output) values for each neuron in each layer are propagated forward through to entire network to compute an actual output and error of each neuron in the output layer. The error of each neuron is computed as the difference between the actual output and its corresponding target output, and then the partial derivatives of sum-squared errors of all the neurons in the output layer is propagated back through the entire network and the weights are updated. In course of the back propagation learning a gradient search procedure is used to find connection weights of the network. The architecture of back propagation neural network employed is shown in Figure 1. It comprises two hidden layers, and six input nodes to input WH1, RB1, WHBTRB1 for *tarwala* job, and WH2, RB2, and WHBTRB2 for second job under consideration. The second job would be one of the following: *gundiwala* job, bangle formation, or bangle finishing. Therefore in total three BPNNs is employed one for each job combination.

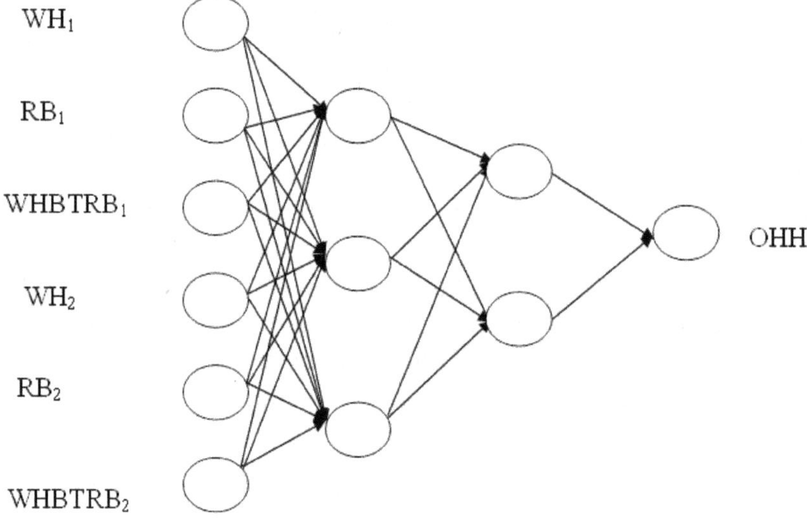

Figure 1: BPNN Architecture to Predict OHH

WORK METHODOLOGY

The following parameters are identified to be important to determine the OHHs of different jobs in Glass/bangle/bangle manufacturing unit.

1. *WH (Working Hours):* It is defined as the amount of time worker spends on a specified job per day.
2. *RB (Rest Break):* It is defined as rest time interval between continuous works. Workers take rest when they get tired after doing continuous work.
3. *WHBTRB (Working Hours Between Two Rest Breaks):* It is defined as working hours between two consecutive rest breaks.

The range of input variables for each job is set as below:

1. RB = [0 to 30 minutes with an interval of 5 minutes]
2. WHBTCB = [0 to 3 hours with an interval of 1 hour]
3. Time spent in Industry including rest breaks per day [< 14 hours].

The following procedural steps are followed:

1. Visiting glass/bangle manufacturing units to get an idea about the working conditions of glass workers.
2. Taking feedback from workers regarding their occupational health hazards.
3. Analyzing and recording the perceived discomforts of workers with respect to variation in the following factors for different job combinations: (i) rest breaks, (ii) working hours, and (iii) working hour between two consecutive rests breaks. Three exhaustive data set are generated, one for each job combination.
4. Training ANNs with available data set for each job combination.
5. Testing and validating the accuracy of ANN models with data set which has not been used in training.

SIMULATION RESULTS

Three ANNs are trained, one for each job combination. Sample training data for each ANN is shown in the following tables (Tables 1 to 3).

Table 1: Training Data Set (*tarwala* job + *gundiwala* job)

WH_1	RB_1	$WHBTRB_1$	WH_2	RB_2	$WHBTRB_2$	*OHH*
10	30	2	0	0	0	9
9	10	3	2	0	0	8
8	30	3	4	15	2	7
7	20	2	4	15	2	6
6	30	1	5	15	3	6
5	10	1	6	20	3	4
4	20	2	8	30	2	3
3	10	1	8	10	3	2
2	10	2	9	30	3	1
1	0	0	10	30	3	1
0	0	0	11	30	3	1

Table 2: Training Data Set (*tarwala* job + bangle formation)

WH_1	RB_1	$WHBTRB_1$	WH_2	RB_2	$WHBTRB_2$	*OHH*
9	10	3	1	0	0	10
8	20	2	2	0	0	8
7	10	1	3	0	0	7
6	20	2	4	15	2	6
5	30	3	5	10	3	5
4	20	2	6	15	2	4
3	10	1	7	10	2	3
2	20	3	8	20	3	2
1	10	2	9	30	3	1
0	0	0	11	30	3	1

Table 3: Training Data Set (*tarwala* job + Finishing)

WH_1	RB_1	$WHBTRB_1$	WH_2	RB_2	$WHBTRB_2$	*OHH*
10	30	2	1	0	0	9
9	10	3	3	0	0	8
8	20	2	4	0	0	7
7	20	2	5	15	2	6
6	30	1	6	15	3	5
5	10	1	7	20	3	4
4	30	3	9	30	3	3
3	20	3	9	20	3	2
2	10	2	10	30	3	1
1	0	0	10	30	3	1
0	0	0	11	30	3	1

BPNN algorithm is implemented in MATLAB. Figure 2 shows the training performance with respect to number of epochs for (*tarwala* job + *gundiwala* job), and Figure 3 illustrates the final training results of the same. Once each of the three BPNNs is trained, testing data is presented to verify the accuracy of the models. Simulation results for two testing data set are presented in Tables 4 and 5. It is found that OHHs estimated by ANNs are in close proximity with actual OHH values.

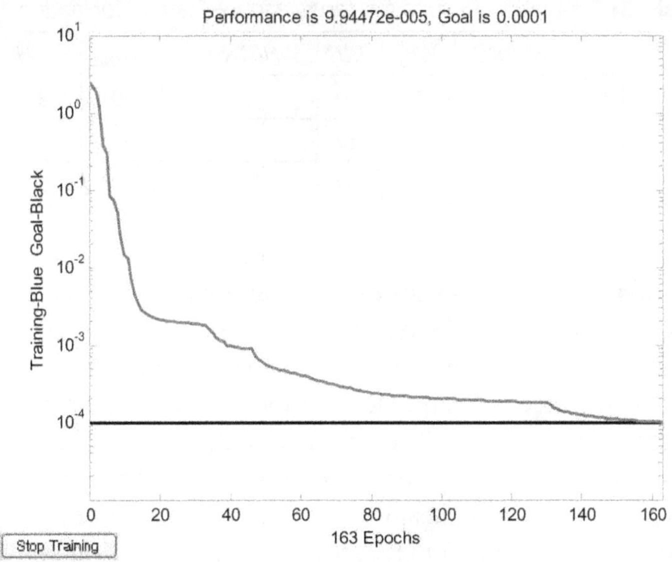

Figure 2: Training of (*tarwala* job + *gundiwala* job) Data

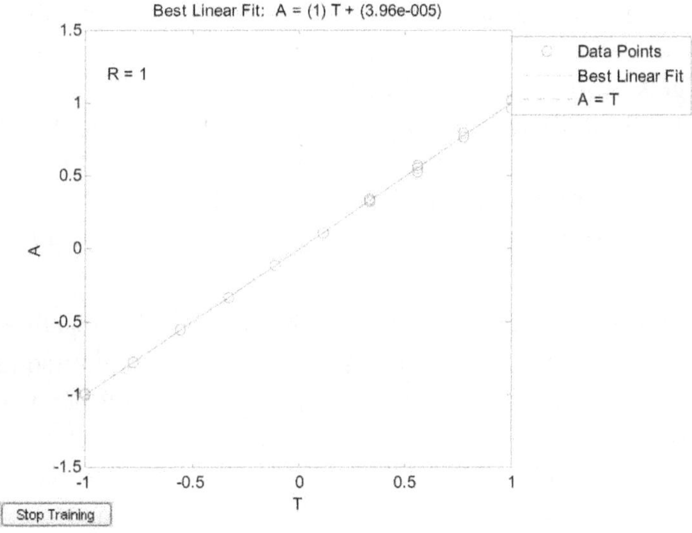

m = 0.9998, b = 3.9581e–005, r = 0.9999

Figure 3: Final Training Result of (*tarwala* job + *gundiwala* job)

Table 4: Simulation Results for *tarwala* job + *gundiwala* job

WH_1	RB_1	$WHBTRB_1$	WH_2	RB_2	$WHBTRB_2$	OHH_{ANN}	OHH
9	10	1	5	15	3	9.9997	10
6	30	1	3	10	1	5.0005	5
4	15	1.5	8	10	3	3.0008	3

Table 5: Simulation Results for *tarwala* job + bangle formation

WH_1	RB_1	$WHBTRB_1$	WH_2	RB_2	$WHBTRB_2$	OHH_{ANN}	OHH
9	10	1	1	0	0	9.0001	9
6	10	3	5	10	2	6.9996	7
2	10	1	9	10	3	2.9994	3

The above results of ANN based intelligent system help the workers in selecting a right job combination with right choices of working hours and rest breaks. We know that the stressfulness of manual activities of an occupational worker is evaluated by comparing job demands to human abilities or norms established in the scientific literature. If job demands exceed capabilities or published norms, the task is considered serious. Greater departures from the capabilities or the norms cause higher risk of occupational health disorders. Such departures are not uncommon in a developing country like India wherein labor is cheaply available and also limited job opportunities prevail for a worker. The worrisome aspect is that glass/bangle manufacturing workers, in general, desire to earn as much as they can without bothering for their health hazards and hence they subject themselves to extreme work conditions. Factors like long working hours, improper rest breaks etc. severely affect workers' health and therefore they suffer from various disorders when working beyond prescribed limits. This problem gets further aggravated due to the fact that they are usually ignorant about such health hazards until it appears in the form of some disorders at a later stage. In this scenario, the system presented in this work not only depicts the effects of extreme conditions on the health of the workers but also help in selecting a job combination which would reduce their occupational health hazards at the desired earnings.

Glass/bangle manufacturing owners face the problems of putting together and managing large number of workers while considering their absenteeism, limited time schedules, and environment uncertainties. The owners' problems get further worsened due to monopoly of workers of *tarwala* job, a high skilled job. The system presented in this work will alleviate this problem as job combination approach will make other workers getting trained for *tarwala* job. In fact the system will help in work generalization to take over work specialization. Moreover it enhances the feasibility of implementing this system as it is beneficial to both the parties—workers as well as owners. In view of these facts, the work presented here forms an important basis to effectively address these issues in health management of workers. The methods devised in this work are efficient and robust enough to solve different classes of OHH-earning tradeoff problems.

CONCLUSIONS

It is demonstrated that job combination can be a way of reducing OHHs of glass/bangle manufacturing workers without much compromise in their income. For socio-economic reasons workers are usually bound to overstrain themselves in their jobs by working for long durations with improper rest breaks. We developed a novel system to assist glass/bangle manufacturing workers to suitably decide their job combinations and work schedule in order to reduce their OHHs. As part of future work, it is intended to develop optimal profiles representing the best case scenarios of *earnings* (max. value) and *occupational health hazards* (min. values) for parameters such as duration of work, number of rest breaks, exposure time to extreme external environment etc.

REFERENCES

ACGIH (2004). "Threshold Limit Values for Chemical Substances and Physical Agent and Biological Exposure Indices". *American Conference of Governmental Industrial Hygienists*, Cincinnati, OH.

Candi, D.A., Christina, L.L., Skai, S.S., Maeen, Z.I. and Thomas, E.B. (2008). "Heat Strain at the Critical WBGT and the Effects of Gender, Clothing and Metabolic Rate". *International Journal of Industrial Ergonomics,* 38, 640–644.

Enander, A.E. and Hygge, S. (1990). "Thermal Stress and Human Performance". *Scandinavian Journal of Work, Environment and Health,* 16, 44–50.

Gun, R.T. and Budd, G.M. (1995). "Effects of Thermal, Personal and Behavioral Factors on the Physiological Strain, Themal Comforts and Productivity of Australian Shearers in Hot Weather". *Ergonomics,* 38, 1368–1384.

Hancock, P.A. and Vasmatzidis, I. (1998). "Human Occupational and Performance Limits under Stress: The Thermal Environment as a Prototypical Example". *Ergonomics,* 41, 1169–1191.

Behavioral Approach to Health and Safety of Workers

Gur Pyari Mehra*

ABSTRACT

The paper deals with the health and safety issues of workers in an engineering work shop of a Public Sector Company. The workshop, passing through a transitory phase of closing of its redundant shop floors, had started collaborating with multinational companies to meet the increasing demand of high targets, international quality standards and customer care. The key issues related to health and safety of workers were studied through interview, observation, analysis of accident data and audit reports and brain storming exercise. The study revealed following facts:

1. High cholesterol level (40%), high blood sugar level (35%), high blood pressure (50%), acidity and ulcers (35%), and various other physical problems were observed among the workers. Three of them were found acute alcoholic. Workers were not serious about their health, and were hiding their serious health problems due to fear of removal from job.
2. The casual approach to use of Personal Protective Equipments while doing accident prone operations, making short cuts (due to peer pressure) (50%), un-just demands for overtime (70%), and ego clashes with shop In-charges (20%), were the main reasons for unsafe behavior. Most of them had tendency to do minimum work, hence had the habit of raising unjustified safety related issues to delay the work.
3. Old machines, non-availability of adequate tools, poor maintenance of old cranes, and workers' absence from duty without information, hampered the team performance, delayed the work and also the safety of workers.
4. Threat of out-sourcing of jobs to external agencies, pressure to improve work quality, emphasis on use of computer in day to day work, and adherence to work-discipline were the major job stresses for the workers, who were having casual approach towards the work.
5. Need for improvement in processes; cutting down of wasteful activities; timely planning and procurement of latest and branded tools and spares; and thrust on training of workers in advanced methods and technology; were the areas revealed through Brain-Storming session, conducted for diagnosing work related problems.

Behavior Based Safety Method was applied in Fabrication shop. The steering group carried out the observations of unsafe behavior. It recorded the frequency and duration of the target unsafe behavior; and also monitored pre and post behaviors to determine the effectiveness of the programme. After one year there was a reduction of 30% in unsafe behavior. Workers became more responsible, productive, co-operative and happy on the job.

* Ex-Chief Manager (P and A), ONGC. E-mail: mehragp@yahoo.com

INTRODUCTION

Occupational Health Services in an effective organization take care of promotion and maintenance of highest degree of physical, mental and social well being of workers in all jobs. They protect workers from all hazardous risks on the job, and are involved in the maintenance of healthy job environment to increase productivity. Health of an employee has effect on his continued presence on job, commitment, efficiency, quality of work, interpersonal relations, awareness and alertness on the job. Successful companies take care of employees' health by preventive actions, *viz.*, medical examinations at Pre-employment, Pre-placement, Periodical medical examination after 40 years, Post-sickness, and Pre-retirement stages. They give importance to the training of employees in the areas of first -aid, fire fighting, and safe work practices. They arrange regular specialized trainings for up-gradation of skills of the workers. Periodical safety Drills for all, Fire Fighting demonstrations motivate employees to follow safety rules with full understanding.

An effective "safety system" is the key to good safety standards of the company. An accident is an unpleasant event which results in a great loss to the Organization in terms of:

(a) *Direct losses*—(i) Compensation to the employee, and (ii) Expenditure on medical treatment to the victim,
(b) *Indirect losses*—(i) Damage to the machinery and material, (ii) Time lost due to stoppage of work, (iii) Loss of morale of workers, and (iv) Delay in completion of work,
(c) *Social losses*—Suffering of the victims and their families.

Researches in the field of safety and health reveal that some people are frequently involved, whereas some are rarely involved in accidents. Accident proneness increases with accidents. Accidents occur due to personal negative attributes. People often behave unsafely because they never got hurt until now or immediate gains are perceived beneficial, and the negative consequences which often come late are ignored by them.

Psychologists have developed a systematic approach called Behavior Analysis to increase safe behaviors, reduce risky behaviors, and prevent accidental injuries at work. Organizations have adopted this approach, terming it Behavior-Based Safety (BBS). It grew from early research by Skinner (1938, 1953, 1974), includes a variety of processes, programmes, strategies, and tactics that apply behavioral psychological principles to change specific behaviors (Gilmore, Perdue, and Wu, 2001). Rather than try to get people to change *via* motivation or attitude, BBS programs successfully "help people into thinking differently" (Geller, 2001). In other words, they change behavior first in order to change attitude.

Over the years, Behavior-Based safety programmes have motivated workers to wear safety helmets, safety shoes, and safety gloves; thereby reducing a number of accidents. After one year of implementing BBS, the average injury rate at such sites decreased by 29%. After five years, the reduction rate averages at 72%; and after seven years, the average recorded injury rate had dropped by 79%.

SAMPLE

The present study was conducted in a workshop dealing with repair and refurbishment of heavy equipment related to activities of an Exploration and Production Oil Company. The workshop had 12 shops. Its manpower strength was 380 (comprising 200 workers and 180 officers). Average age of workers and officers was 42 years. 40% of workers were possessing diploma qualification, 50% with ITI certificate, and 10% below matriculation level. Amongst officers 50% were diploma holders and 50% were having Q1 qualification *i.e.,* Post Graduate qualification in their discipline.

METHOD AND APPROACH

(a) Discussions were held with the Shop Floor in charges, Chief of Safety and Environment, Head of the Unit, Safety in-charge of the workshop, Welfare officer and Health officer,
(b) Participation in safety and health review meetings,
(c) Participation in council meetings at shop floor attended by Welfare officer, Union's representative and safety officer in-charges of civil and electrical maintenance,
(d) Brain storming exercise to improve health, safety and to control accidents (participants-Head of unit, Group in charges, representatives from all disciplines and Union, total 30),
(e) Analysis of Reports on accidents (occurred in past), and
(f) Implementation of Behavior Based technique at shop floors.

FINDINGS

Five categories of root causes were identfied, *viz.*, Health problems, Unsafe Behavior, Work Environment, Job Stress Factors, and Industrial Relations Related issues.

Health Problems

High cholesterol level (40%), high blood sugar level (35%), high blood pressure (50%), acidity and ulcers (35%), and various other physical problems were observed. 5% were found to be acute alcoholic.

In spite of suffering from serious illnesses, workers did not want to take retirement under Voluntary Retirement Schemes or their cases to be recommended for premature retirement. Such individuals added to the number for the task but not to the productivity of work.

Workers had preference for fried snacks in the canteen and spicy food in comparison to simple and healthy items. Help from Dietician was taken to convince them for healthy snacks and food.

Symptoms of Hyper-Tension were noticed in the workers (even in those below 35 years of age). The main reasons were high aspiration to get materialistic comforts as quickly as possible, social status, desire for big cars, and furnished house *etc.*

Health awareness Educational Programs, Fire and Safety drills were attended by the workers in large number only if there was some attraction of getting gift or Souvenir/ Memento.

Unsafe Behavior

The casual approach to work, carelessness towards use of personal protective equipments while doing hazardous operations, overconfidence, following short cuts, avoiding safe methods due to peer pressure (50%), un-just demands for overtime (70%), ego clashes with shop in-charges (20%), were the main reasons for unsafe behavior. Most of them had tendency to do minimum work, hence were raising unjustified safety related issues to delay the work. They were provided safety Kits and helmets but they were not used on the pretext that quality is poor or size not correct.

Undisciplined workers (2%) were found involved in theft of wires, plugs, tools, *etc.*, which were potential for checks of accidents. They had tendency to pass on their work to the untrained contractual workers which was threat to safety. It confirms that commitment and dedication towards work are first requirement for health and safety of employees.

Work Environment

Old machines, non-availability of adequate tools, in-adequate ventilation, greasy floors, poor maintenance of cranes, and workers' absence from duty without information, hampered the team performance and delayed the work. In view of latest development in tools and technology it is necessary that old equipments are replaced in phased manner for optimum utilization of resources and manpower. With awareness they started comparing the infrastructure facilities with outside multinational companies working in their fields.

Job Stress Factors

Stress due to automation and change in Technology, online availability of performance/ progress of work.

Collaboration with multinationals force them to improve in work habits for survival of self and the company:

- Demand for Quality output in scheduled time,
- Lack of avenues for promotion to under-qualified workers,
- Computer literacy essential to carry out day to day job responsibility,
- Job contracts for repair were outsourced, resulting into less work for groups not giving quality performance.

Industrial Relations Related Problems

- Pressure from Collectives not to take any harsh actions against some habitually alcoholic workers on compassionate grounds.
- Demand for Overtime beyond permissible limits.
- Interference in implementation of placements or Transfer orders of workers due to vested interest of few Executive Members.

BRAIN STORMING

A Brain Storming Exercise conducted on a group comprising officers, workers and union representatives (total 30), helped in identifying following key issues related to safety policy, procedure and work climate in the work shop.

- Availability and presence of all group members to be ensured for performing work on a Shop Floor (System to be implemented to pinpoint habitually erring/absent individuals),
- Team Discussion along with Shop Floor In-charge is necessary for cutting down wasteful efforts, to know the broader picture and significance of own job in the group,
- General awareness of business environment, arm yourself to handle competition, Take advantage of the opportunities, and make strategies to counter threats were suggestions given by them,
- All process owners should strive for improving their processes, explore maximizing the number of simultaneous activities rather than sequential ones, and curtail activities that are not adding value for meeting the Work Targets,
- Training and exposure to established practices in the industry,
- Analyze cause of failure/accidents carefully without any prejudices and biases, immediate corrective measure, and
- Timely planning and procurement of high quality tools and spares.

APPLICATION OF BEHAVIOR BASED SAFETY

Fabrication shop was identified for implementation of above process. A steering group comprising three responsible persons from the shop (including workers representative) was given one week's training. Safety officer was made observer. They themselves developed the check list of unsafe behavior, set targets for observation and defined roles and responsibilities of each one of them. The steering group and the observer carried out the observations and recorded the frequency, duration or rate of the target behavior, monitored pre and post measures to determine how well the programme had worked.

CONCLUSION

Behavior based safety programme motivated employees to wear personal protective devices. Reinforcement from observer and support from peers altogether changed their enthusiasm and commitment to work. The programme minimized absence from work, increased team spirit and concern for the health of self and other members of the group. They became more responsible and enjoyed their jobs.

A committee consisting of Safety officer, Quality Officer, Welfare Officer, HR officer, Medical Officer along with representative of Collective was formed to conduct quarterly meetings on Shop Floors and submit the report regarding action taken and strategies formulated for improving Safety and Health of Employees.

SECTION–3

Yoga, Meditation and Therapies

Spiritual Healing

Russell J. Sawa*[1], Hugo Meynell[1], Nancy Doetzel[1], Ian Winchester[1], Debbie Zembal[1], Robbie Motta[1] and Santosh Dubey[1]

ABSTRACT

This article describes the interim findings of an ongoing study on spirituality and healing. The study included interviewing 25 spiritual healers from a wide spectrum of cultures and religions. The methodology for this study is new and unique. It involves application of the philosophy of Bernard Lonergan, a Canadian scholar. We have interviewed the healers and are analyzing the transcripts line by line to determine what we think their meaning is. After this we decided on the propositions reflected in this meaning, and came to common agreement amongst the seven of us interdisciplinary scholars as to what the propositions are. We are not at the phase of deciding what these propositions mean in the light of our values. This is a difficult dialectical process.

INTRODUCTION

Spirituality is increasingly acknowledged by Western medicine as an important aspect of Healthcare; but there is little clarity about what spirituality is, or what role it plays in health. The object of the work of our group is to make a case for the real occurrence of what may properly be called spiritual healing, and for its acceptance by the medical and scientific community, and by society at large. We mean by 'spiritual healing' that which comes about by means inexplicable to orthodox science as it is now; for example, by a sheer act of will on the part of the healer, or by prayer, or by action at a distance. Most of us do not think that coincidence and the placebo effect are sufficient to account for the phenomena in question, which seem to us quite common rather than very exceptional (One of our members is more skeptical).

Interviews have been conducted with self-claimed practitioners of spiritual healing from a wide range of cultural backgrounds. The transcripts which have been analyzed to date include interviews with an aboriginal healer, a Hindu intuitive, a Buddhist energy healer, a Catholic priest healer and exorcist, a Christian physician and healer, a shaman, and Christian healers who were closely acquainted with Voodoo culture. We are interested both in what these healers claim to do, and in their underlying beliefs and assumptions. Twenty-five persons have been interviewed and invited to tell stories about their own experience, and of those who appear to have been healed by them. Transcripts were reviewed, word for word, by the entire team, so as to gain

* Corresponding author.

[1] University of Calgary, Calgary, Alta, Canada. E-mail: sawa@ucalgary.ca

common agreement about what was meant by the interviewees in what they said. Our research team includes several physicians, a physicist and philosopher of science, a philosophical theologian, a professional intuitive, two Reiki Masters, a nurse, and an educator and researcher with a wide background in the study of spirituality within education. Ethical consent was obtained through the Health Sciences Research Department of the Faculty of Medicine at the University of Calgary.

Evidently our task is a formidable one, and seems to include the following components:

1. Collecting the data, by conducting and recording interviews with putative spiritual healers; and by speaking with members of our group who appear to be actual practitioners of the craft.
2. Determining what the interviewees or these members of our group mean in writing or speaking as they do.
3. Evaluating the material, by assessing how far our sources are honest or well-informed about what they report.
4. We then move to what we are to say ourselves about the matters in question, having assessed the material. If our informants state or assume that telepathy, precognition, or healing by the laying-on of hands, actually occur, are we to be convinced by them that they do? Or are we rather to say that the authority of the scientific attitude is compelling on these matters, and strictly implies that such events never happen at all? Or should we perhaps suggest instead that 'the scientific attitude', when coherently conceived and properly applied, would support, at least tentatively, the well-attested of these phenomena? (About ten years ago, a forensic psychiatrist deemed a man 'incurably superstitious' on the ground that he admitted that he had, on the strength of the evidence as he knew it, come to be convinced of the existence of telepathy. Was this fair? If so, why, and if not, why not?).
5. Having determined what we believe on these matters, and why, there follows the task of finding how it all hangs together, and how we are to relate it to the rest of what we know or think we know. (However strong our apparent grounds for believing in 'precognition', the fact that it gives rise to notorious philosophical difficulties should give us pause.)
6. Having come to our conclusions, and set them out in terms of a self-consistent worldview, we still have to determine how they are to be communicated to people with their various cultural backgrounds and levels of educational attainment (It may be mentioned in passing that these six steps correspond to the first, second, fourth, sixth, seventh and eighth of the 'functional specialties' that Bernard Lonergan worked out in his "Method in Theology". So far, the group has been mainly concerned with the first and second of these stages, though some attention has also been given to the third, fourth, fifth and sixth.

Plainly the beliefs and assumptions of the practitioners themselves, though not infallible- some would be so bold as to claim that the same may apply to the alleged implications of what passes for 'the scientific attitude'—are worth taking into account. All spiritual healing, assuming that it occurs, seems to exemplify the power of mind over matter. Many healers insist that they are merely God's instruments in their healing work, or that they are conduits of energy rather than acting for and of themselves. The God in question was not necessarily the Christian God; and a Buddhist healer saw her work in terms of 'focused compassion'. It was remarked by some that spiritual, including paranormal, manifestations can be mistaken for illness. A large majority insisted that, for healing to take place, the recipient must really want to be healed (cf. John 5.6; and Freud's shrewd remarks about what he calls 'the gain from illness'). Healers sometimes claim the power to see or 'envision' what is inside the bodies of their patients. (It may be wondered how far this is really a matter of the picking up of subliminal cues; as an experienced lawyer may have a hunch, which turns out to be correct, that a witness is lying, without being able to say how she comes by her hunch). Many claim that a preliminary conversation with the patient is necessary for healing to take place. Mention is occasionally made of a number of 'bodies' in which healing occurs sequentially, the spiritual, mental, emotional and physical bodies (We wonder how these correlate with the three 'bodies' which Robert Crookall (1974) had to distinguish in order to cope with the data he amassed bearing on life after death). There is also talk of a 'causal' body. Healing powers often seem to run in families; sometimes there will be the skipping of a generation. Or an experienced healer may teach her or his craft to an apprentice.

That the supposed practitioners of spiritual healing, or for that matter producers or reporters of other paranormal phenomena, are all deluded or lying, seems scarcely compatible with facts like the following. We find many of the same phenomena in reports of spiritual healing from cultures and religions all over the world; such patterns and parallels are impressive. And the survival of such practices over millennia might be thought barely compatible with their total ineffectiveness. Still, it is important that, where possible, claims as to the occurrence of the paranormal should be subjected to stringent empirical testing. The conscientious researcher, who has more interest in finding out the truth than in making a case, will be on the look-out for hidden variables; it might be, for example, that a sick person was cured not because of the spiritual powers of the healer, but because he had been induced by her to eat more healthy foods. On the other hand, it is a sad fact that, for several centuries now, many representatives of the scientific establishment, though fortunately not all, have not only refused to consider evidence on the subject themselves, but have treated with contempt or derision those who have insisted that such evidence ought to be taken into account.

Every member of our group would attest to the fascination involved in doing this work; and it is surely difficult seriously to deny its potential importance (The ever-increasing reliance on drugs on the part of conventional medicine, and the enormous costs involved, may be cited in support of this). It may easily be seen that Herculean labours still remain to be undertaken.

One of our members concludes from his own reading of and around the transcripts, that there is no good evidence that anything has occurred over and above insightful people conversing with those who are troubled, thereby relieving their anguish; in this sense, certainly, spiritual healing takes place, and those who are adept at it have an important function in society. People's spirits may be uplifted by such means, their worries may go away, and they may be enabled to live worthwhile lives in the face of chronic or terminal illness. But this is not to imply that anything which might be called 'psychic' or 'telepathic' has occurred. He recognizes that other members of the group would like to think that ordinary illnesses could also sometimes be cured by such 'spiritual' means, though he does not suppose that they would go as far as some might.

We are now analyzing the transcript of a family physician healer. This brings us face to face with the need to obtain empirical evidence of healing. We hope that it will bring us into contact with Scholars who share our interest, and with those who might be able to provide us with empirical proof of spiritual healings. We will welcome anyone who is interested in what we are doing and who might be able to lend a helping hand.

REFERENCE

Crookall, R. (1974). *The Supreme Adventure: Analyses of Psychic Communications*. Cambridge: James Clarke and Co. Limited.

Kashmir Shaivism—The Culmination of the Development of Indian Psycho-Philosophical Thought and Yoga Psychotherapy

C. Giri*[1] and Rakesh Giri[2]

ABSTRACT

The present article tries to argue the thesis that the history of Indian philosophical thought in fact is indicative of the development of Indian mind. Thus, as we start from *Charvaka* and end in Kashmir *Shavivism* via *Mimamsa, Vaisnavism, Nyaya-Vaisheshic, Samkhya-Yoga* and *Sankar Vedanta*, we find progressive evolution of Indian mind. Thus, Kashmir *Shaivism* is the culmination. Towards this view a discussion of a few characteristics of this system is undertaken and it is shown that the simplicity, unassuming nature, natural and spontaneity are free from distinctions of caste, creed, color and profound metaphysical base. Embodying the oneness of cosmos and the individual self etc. are a few features that provide a sound base *vis-a-vis* other systems of Indian philosophy—transcending the bondage and realizing the liberation which is important for real healing and psychotherapy. The uniqueness of this system is that a pious householder while enjoying tasteful worldly objects within limits can practice the yoga or *upayas-anupaya, sambhavopaya, saktopaya* and *anavopaya*—of Kashmir *shaivism*—thereby overcoming the attraction for worldly objects (*Bhukti*) leading to self-recognition and the experience of one's extensive Godhood. This is what the constitutional and operational psychotherapeutic mode of Kashmir *Shaivism* consists in.

INTRODUCTION

Kashmir's Shaivism—The Culmination of the Evolution of Indian Philosophical Thinking Process and Thought

India is well known for its rich cultural heritage. Its proof includes the development of several systems of philosophy as fundamental sciences. The history of philosophical thought contained in these systems of philosophy shows the evolution of thinking process and the thought of human mind in an effort to know and realize the real nature of human "Self" (*Atma*) and the Universal "Self" (*Parmatma*). The progression is like this: *Carvakas* school, the lowest types of thinkers in India had their goal of good health, long life, prosperity pleasures and enjoyments etc. They believed in "Eat

* Corresponding author.

[1] Training and Research Institute for Yoga and Yoga Psychotherapy, 467 Anand Nagar-A, Patiala, Punjab, India.

[2] Department of Yoga, Gurukul Kangri University, Haridwar, Uttranchal, India.

Drink and Be Marry" and such socio-political systems which could fulfill their above-mentioned goals. For them there was no Heaven, no Hell, no Piety, no Sin, no God and no Religion. For them, the truth could be perceived through merely senses in its grossest form. Then came *Mimamsakas* who believed in the existence of Heaven and Hell and thus had the concept of good and bad actions. Afterwards the *Vaisnavites* believed in a superior place named *Vaikuntha* over the Heaven. Above them are the *Nyaya* and *Vaishesic* philosophers, who believed in soul, time, space, law of *Karma*, Omniscience and Omni-potency of *Parmatman* or *Ishwar*. *Samkhya* and Yoga philosophies produced still finer exposition of the ultimate truth. Still further, on the ladder of refinement process of evolution of Indian thought, come different systems of Monism including *Shankar Vedanta* and ultimately the stream culminates in the Kashmir's *Shaivism* system of Indian philosophy.

SPECIFIC FEATURES OF KASHMIR'S *SHAIVISM*

It adopts a realistic, utilitarian attitude and approach to empirical life and life circumstances. It believes and accepts that ultimate reality is one while rest of the universe is the cosmic manifestation of that one indivisible reality in totality. The universe is not an illusion but a true reality and is the display of the glory of the Divine. It adopts an elaborate system of practices in accordance with an individual's psycho-physical instruments and the potential he is equipped with.

It should be noted that *Saiva* Yoga is not a practice in suppression of the functions of mind as taught by Patanjali. It is a practice in uniting the individual self with the universal self by means of interesting and blissful practices as taught in Saiva scriptures. In fact, outwardly one may perform the age-old, traditional or vedic rituals, but inwardly he has to seek the exact truth through some yogic practices taught in Trika System. Maintaining the semblance of an ordinary householder, he has not to make any show of the powers aroused through its practice. There is no restriction based on caste, creed, gender, etc., as regards eligibility for initiation in Saiva yoga. Even a lowest caste can become a disciple or even a preceptor if he attains sufficient success in his practice.

In short, the following are the main characteristics of the Kashmir *Shaivism* philosophy and its practices:

1. Any individual can experience and spontaneously realize the self in any state.
2. Five sense organs condemned and considered degrading in other systems are regarded as the means of self-realization. The respective sense-objects too can help liberate the practitioner from bondage.
3. The follower of this system remains established at the source of the enjoyment of these sense organs i.e. firmly established on the *Pashyanti* state of speech

without any thought construct even while dealing with worldly affairs in *Madhyama* and *Vaikhari* states of speech (Progressive relaxed states of mind in succession: *Vaikhari, Madhyama, Pashyanti* etc.).

4. There is unrestricted flow of grace of the cosmic self (*Sakti paata*)—free, independent and neutral and thus it is not linked with any sort of effort (*Sadhanaa*).
5. Anybody can join this system without any distinction of caste, creed, colour etc.
6. The system emphasizes that knowledge must always be combined with yoga and the awareness of it must be the guide on the path of salvation.
7. One needs constantly to be aware (awakened) while performing worldly actions and transforming it into practice (*Sadhanaa*). Thus, one can experience the joy and bliss of the supreme in all actions.
8. It consider the whole universe and its entities as the manifestation of the Lord.
9. The practice of exhaling and inhaling is dealt within an insightful manner in order to transcend the time.
10. Shaiva Yoga can be practiced in every situation of one's own daily life, in every move and action of the body, in each breath, by remaining aware in God—consciousness.
11. It is assumed that only the seeker who has received the grace of Shiva is blessed with the capacity to tread this path.

Therefore, we can say that Kashmir *Shaivism* is a process of discovery of individual soul as to become one with the Universal Being through a process based on:

(a) Correct knowledge of the exact nature of the ultimate reality and of the universal elements as well.
(b) Practice in *Trika* Yoga; A highly affectionate and devotional attitude towards the Absolute Reality.

THE COSMOS AND THE INDIVIDUAL HUMAN BEING—ONENESS/ WHOLENESS THEREOF

The unity between the individual and the cosmos has been taken for granted in many ancient cultures, specifically in Indian philosophical parlance where in spirit or the soul has been considered as the sole source of all things of the universe and hence of similar nature and part of the same one whole. Today, through study, effort and intricate-analysis, we have to rediscover and to rebuild the reality of that oneness which our highly vaunted modern intellect has so violently shattered.

The entire future of all modes of psychotherapy as effective healing arts lies in the rebuilding of the lost connections between modern human beings and the cosmos. If such realignment between the individual and the greater whole of which a person is a part cannot be achieved, then no real healing can take place. The achievement of possible harmony for the individual is essential. The health, as defined by Yeshi Donden—physician to Dalai Lama is, the proper relationship between the microcosm, which is man, and the macrocosm, which is the universe. In this way, the disruption of this relationship should be considered as disease. The orthodox (western) medicine and its different modes of therapy generally have no philosophy or cosmic law. While yoga is based on eternal cosmic principles, and considered as a tool for self-knowledge and self-development which is based not on new discoveries but on a deep penetration into those few ancient principles that are already known. Overtime, we come closer to understanding and appreciating the universal truth known to the Indian seers and sages, perhaps through reformulating them or redefining them instead of replacing them with the constantly changing fads of every era. Ultimately, psychotherapy needs a cosmic framework for dealing with the energy forces that enliven the child of the cosmos, which every human being is. By placing the human being in a cosmic frame of reference, the combination of Indian *Tantra* and Yoga has unique capacity for re-attuning a person's consciousness to his or her essential nature and encouraging to have an in-depth profound self-knowledge. In view of above considerations, below is given the way of progressive involution (manifestation) of the ultimate reality i.e. pure universal consciousness (God).

From Absolute Pure Consciousness (Godhood) to Human Being

Param Shiva is the ultimate reality who is of the nature of Bliss itself and is all complete in Himself. He is beyond description, beyond all manifestation, beyond limitation of form, time and space. He is eternal, infinite, all pervading, all knowing and all-powerful. In fact, this reality is ineffable and beyond all descriptions. From *Param Shiva* let us come to universal manifestation; let us have a look at this creation of our Lord. Kashmir *Shaivism* postulates 36 categories of '*tattvas*' (elements) to explain the process of cosmic involution. Let us keenly focus our attention to this process of universal involution or universal experience, i.e., from Godhood to Maya Shakti, which is the veiling or obscuring force of nature, leading to psycho-physical elements and finally to the *Panch Mahabhutas* (five great elements): Earth, Water, Fire, Air and Ether. Let us look further into this (great descent, i.e. from God-hood to Man-hood).

Shiva Tattva (Pure Consciousness)

The first outward manifestation of the divine creative energy in the process of cosmic evolution is called *Shiva Tattva*. It is the initial creative movement of *Paramashiva*. Consciousness in this condition is technically called "*chit*". It is the static aspect of consciousness or like support of all things in the manifest world. It is like the bed of a river or the canvas of a painting. It can never be seen, it can only be known by its effects. In this condition, the emphasis is on the subject without any awareness of the existence of the object. The *Shiva Tattva* is the *chit* aspect of the universal condition of *Sat-Chit-Ananda* (Existence-consciousness-Bliss)

Shakti Tattva **(Energy—the Executive Godhood)**

Since the *Shiva Tattva* represents the passive aspect of the pure consciousness, it is dependent upon the active or dynamic aspect to bring it into being. This is called *Shakti Tattva. Shakti* is the active or kinetic aspect of consciousness. Just as an artist pours out his delight in a poem, picture or song, even so the Supreme pours out his delight in this manifestation called *Shakti*. Just as *Shiva* is the *chit* aspect of the universal condition of *Sat-Chit-Ananda, Shakti* is the *ananda* aspect. When *Shakti* is predominant, supreme bliss is experienced. As Mahesvarananda puts it beautifully in *Maharthamanjari*, 'He (i.e. *Shiva*) Himself is full of joy enhanced by the honey of the three corners of his heart, viz *ICCHA*, *JNANA* and *KRIYA* (Will, Knowledge-Action) raising up His face to gaze at His own splendor, is called *Shakti*." This *Shakti Tattva* represents the force that produces a strain or stress on the surface of the universal consciousness. It polarizes consciousness into positive and negative, the aham and idam ("I"ness and "Is" ness), the subject and object. As already mentioned, Shakti or cosmic energy is said to have three principal forms to account for the three fundamental psychological steps that precede every action. Technically, the first one is called *ICHCHA SHAKTI*, the power of feeling oneself as supremely able and of an absolutely irresistible will. The second one is the *JNANA SHAKTI*, the power of knowledge or knowing of consciousness which holds all objects in conscious relations with us and also with one another. The *KRIYA SHAKTI* is the power of supreme action, creating or assuming any and every form. One follows the other in logical succession, and with the prominence of each respective form in the process of the evolution of consciousness, the three tattvas come into being. These are respectively called *Sadashiv Tattva, Ishvara Tattva* and *Shuddha Vidya Tattva* to complete the first five elements **(Tattwas).**

Maya **and Five Kancukas (Coverings)**

Now let us come to the evolution of material universe. The power of consciousness to separate and divide is called *Maya Shakti*. This is the power to perceive differences. The term '*Maya*' means illusion. Here, it is used to refer to the veiling or obscuring force of nature which creates a sense of differentiation. As such, it makes universal consciousness which is unity, to appear as duality and multiplicity. The products of Maya are the five kancukas or coverings which are *KALAA* (limitation of authorship or efficacy); *VIDYA* (limited knowledge); *RAGA* (from all satisfaction to the feeling of interest and desire); *KAALA* (from eternity to limitation in respect of time i.e. past, present and future); and *NIYATI* (limitation in respect of cause and effect). Thus, so far the elements from 7–11 in succession are covered.

Purusha and *Prakriti*

The result of *Maya* and its five coverings as referred to above are *PURUSHA* and *PRAKRITI*. Here the dual world of mind and matter is permanently established. In other words, although the Lord is absolutely free, He puts on *Maya* and her five cloaks, forgets His true nature, limits His power and reduces Himself to an individual soul which is called *PURUSHA* and its objective manifestation as *PRAKRITI*.

Buddhi, Ahamkara and *Manas*

Now, let us come to the elements of mental operation i.e. *BUDDHI, AHAMKARA* and *MANAS*. *Buddhi* is the ascertaining intelligence which can be external (i.e., a jar) perceived through eye or internal (like images built out of the impression left on mind). *Ahamkara* is the product of *buddhi*. It is the "I"-making principle and the power of self-appropriation. *Manas* is the product of *Ahankara*. It co-operates with the senses in building up perceptions, and by itself, it builds images and concepts. We are continuing to focus on the cosmic manifestations. The products of *SATTVIC AHAMKARA* are five powers of sense perception or *JNANENDRIYAS*, five powers of action or *KARMENDRIYAS* and from *TAM*.

CONCLUSION

In summary, it can be concluded that the constitutional and operational psychotherapeutic mode of Kashmir *Shaivism* are outlined on the basis of mystic philosophy. Yoga has unique capacity for attuning a person's consciousness to his or her essential nature and encourages an in-depth profound self-knowledge.

Human Psychology and Spiritual Health: Need of Wisdom Revolution

Ratan Saini*

ABSTRACT

The human being who is the *ansha* of the All-Intelligent Supreme Being, has got and entangled in the worldly objects. He has forgotten the "True Objective of Life" to get freedom from the difficulties, troubles and sorrows of this world, that is, of reaching the permanent state of utmost happiness by attaining direct communion with the Creator of the Universe. The main hindrances in the path are worldly desires and psychological defenses like pride, anger, competition, social status *etc.* As long as the activities of mind are not brought under the control the spiritual health of higher order is not attained. The religion of the world generally speaks of both, the attachment with worldly objects and of Spiritual development. A True Religion teaches that the highest aim of life for man is the attainment of true happiness for which one has to surrender himself to a person who has attained this status, and follow His instructions.

The present society which is sufferings from these ups and downs of sorrow and happiness and searching for the ways of getting rid of these sorrows to achieve state of continuous happiness will have to undergo a "Wisdom Revolution". The paper elaborates the present status and suggests a Wisdom Society which operates on the principles of better true religion, worldliness and Brotherhood of man and Fatherhood of God, wherein every individual progresses toward the True Objective of Life.

INTRODUCTION

This world is a place of action where it is necessary that there should be pairs of opposites. Thus there are two roads in human body, one takes us towards the Abode of Supreme Lord and other leads towards hell. We are free to proceed on whatever path we like. Spirit of man, after coming down from its Abode has been ensnared in three *gunas* (attributes)—*Satogun, Rajogun, Tamogun,* five *tattvas* (elements)—earth, water, fire, air and ether and four Antahkarans—mind, intelligence, understanding and ego and ten organs of sense—five of perception (eye, nose, ear, tongue, touch or skin) and five of action (hands, feet, mouth, organ of generation and organ of excretion) and it has been so bound down with the body and things of the world thus it is difficult to get separated. These three gunas are visible in people around *viz.* those who lack sense (or *Tamasik*), those who have no proper sense (or *Rajasik*) those who have good sense (or *Saatvik*). Those who are *Tamasik* live their life like vaga bonds.

* Dayalbagh Educational Institute, Deemed University, Dayalbagh, Agra, India.
E-mail: ratansaini@gmail.com

They have no set object of life, nor do they care to make themselves happy. They lie down wherever they choose. They feel happy if they get food; if they get no food they feel miserable. In short they wander about in the world. Those who are *Rajasik* construct houses for themselves but every thing in the house is topsy turvy. Whatever leisure they have, they spend it in places of entertainment and they spend greater part of their income in useless things and lead a life of trouble and misery. Those who are *Saatvik* have good sense do everything in a systematic manner and always keep in view the object of their life. They work during the day and at night they rest at home. They do hundreds of things and yet they have time and leisure at their disposal and they have minimum anxieties and worries. A combination of these three guna also make a variety of personalities and characters as depicted in Figure 1.

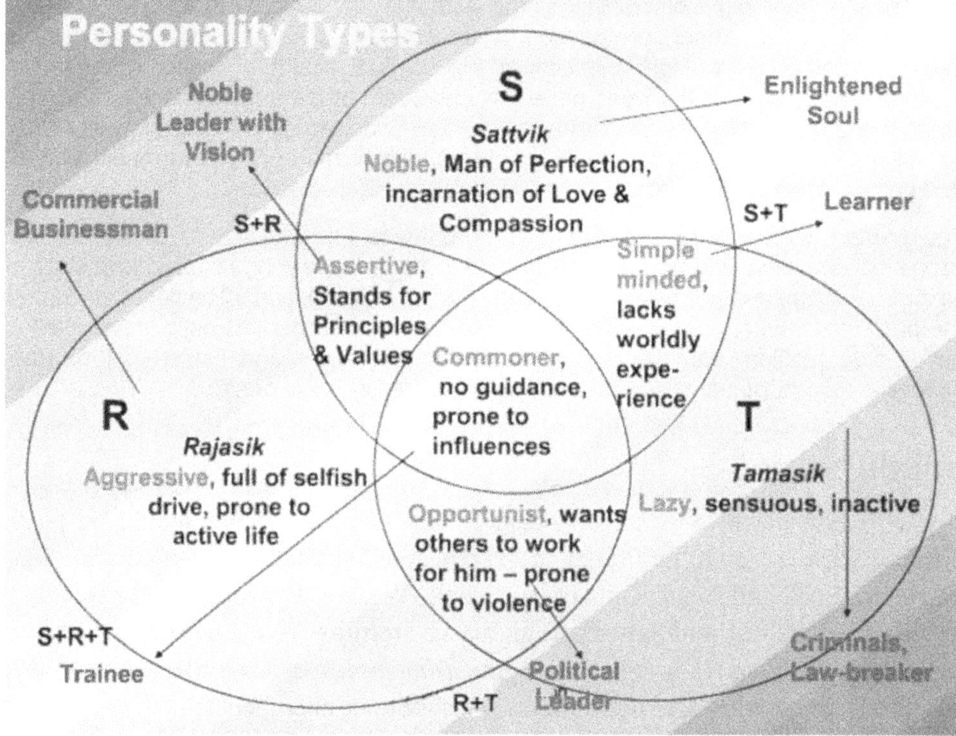

Figure 1

A true *Saatvik* person keeps his heart clean and pure. He thinks that things of the world are transient and of no value and puts them away in a corner. He discharges all his duties and yet his mind is always unruffled. As the lamp of love remains always lighted in his heart, there is no darkness within him at any time. He uses the broom of the holy name now and then, and so there is no trance of dust or dirt to be seen within him anywhere. If he gets an opportunity, he discharges his duties involving great responsibility, but he never appears to be worried. Thousands come to him and thousands go away, but he always remains detached and unaffected. At the time of leisure, he thinks of Holy Feet of Supreme Lord instead of playing with dogs and cats and instead of going to places of entertainment, he tries to see vision on higher planes of consciousness within his own self.

Thus *Tamasik* and *Rajasik people* have forgotten the "Objective of Life" and are entangled in the worldly objects. While the *Saatvik persons know the* real or true objective of life as to reach the permanent state of utmost happiness and freedom from the difficulties, troubles and sorrows of this world by attaining direct communion with the Creator of the Universe.

SPIRITUAL HEALTH AND PSYCHOLOGY

The social system or the human world is nothing but a mass of psychological defenses like pride, anger, competition, social status, victimization *etc.* which protect one in blindness, the blindness that results from an ignorance of soul or spirit. In this modern social system, human beings have lost the sense for spiritual health due to influence of social needs and desire for diversity. Psychological defense mechanisms allow psychological strategies which are used by individuals to cope with reality and to maintain self-image intact. It's all too easy to misunderstand life by confusing acceptance with tolerance, pride with holiness, and sensuality with holy love. And with the loss of spiritual health many of us today have also discarded the concept of *sin*—that is, that functional narcissism in all of us which serves the self, rather than others. So, instead of making life's decisions according to personal responsibility, one makes decisions according to personal convenience.

In the middle of the 19th century when psychology began, the concurrency of psychology was the study of the soul. The soul was seen as having a spiritual element, a mental and a physical element. An interesting study was done by psychologists in the 1980's. As they questioned, to what extent are they open to humanistic ideas? It humanized psychology. It helped create a counterpoint to the animalistic models that were coming out of Behaviorism and the very pessimistic view of human nature that was coming out of Psychoanalytic thought. Maslow identified states of being called 'peak experiences' wherein people often have spiritual experiences. He deemed them important features of human existence. Maslow's basic premise was that religiousness is central to the human psyche.

According to David Schmit, there exists a correlation between people who have religious and spiritual beliefs and mental health and physical health. Further, he says that people who have powerful spiritual, religious values, *etc.* are often times physically healthier than those that don't. For these individuals, spirituality is a living, breathing presence in their life. It's inexplicable, it's powerful, it's potent, and it's healing. So the result is they are happier and healthier! Thus, Spiritual development has close relationship with health and happiness of any person. George Bernard Shaw made a brilliant discovery: "a spiritual life is also a practical life". Therefore, if one values spirituality, what does he have to lose? Mediocrity. What does he have to gain? Everything.

The individual gets the impression of this world through the senses of eye, nose, ear, tongue and touch which give birth to intentions. The impressions on the personality also include the spiritual values one gets from observing people following a specific religion. These intentions are prioritized based on the charterer type and triggers thoughts. Thoughts lead to broader vision and selflessness and quality of actions one takes. These actions can improve the quality of the person and the attitude and thus the reaction to the action can result in improvement of the personality. This phenomenon of change of personality is represented in Figure 2.

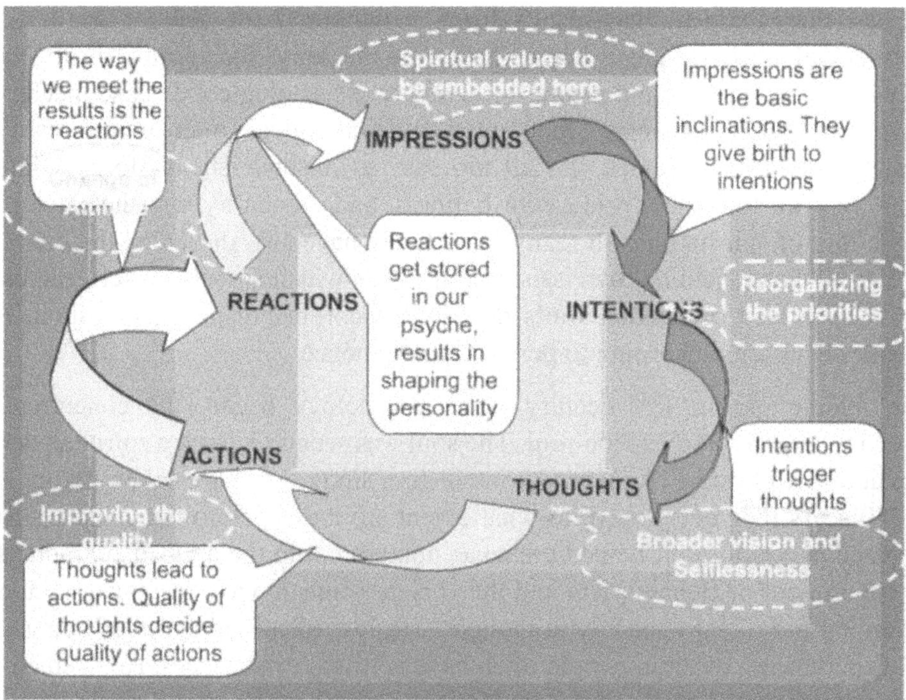

Figure 2

HINDRANCES IN SPIRITUAL DEVELOPMENT

The people of the world consider worldly progress and comforts as the object of the life and have turned away their faces from spiritual practices. Meat and wine, which are great obstructions in the performance of spiritual practices, became their normal diet with the result that in spite of there being such great prosperity, pomp and show, there is so much restlessness and unhappiness. Generally desires rule over mind. As long as the activities of mind are not brought under the control or stopped and consciousness of higher order is not attained by human being, the success in spiritual practices can not be achieved. This status of higher order consciousness can only be achieved by bringing changes within oneself by destroying the consciousness of low order so that the spirit is freed from the covers of materialism and attains self-realization.

One of the main reasons for lack of spiritual development of people in the society today is lack of knowledge of a true religion. A primary reason for the split between religion and spirituality is the increasing dissatisfaction and anger at organized religion. While there are both healthy and unhealthy forms of organized religion, it is not surprising that so many people have upset at organized religion given the atrocities which have occurred by religious groups in the past. Furthermore, many of these atrocities have been highly publicized by the media; often in less than favorable light. However, it is still problematic to generalize the sins of some organized religion to all religious groups.

Religion has become a business. People generally like such religions and such religious teachings as may help them in the fulfillment of their worldly desires. When man has wealth he becomes indifferent about the True Objective of Life. He feels that every thing can be achieved with the help of money. Thus it is extremely difficult to make rich people agree to make an effort to control their mind and senses and to engage in spiritual practice. The religion of the world generally speaks of both, the attachment with worldly objects and of deliverance that is Parmaratha, in fact, mostly with the objects of the world.

Religion has also become associated with rigidity, fundamentalism, and definitive claims at ultimate truth. Often, this gets further associated with the judgment, hate, and anger of some of these groups. As we move into the post-modern era, many people have become increasingly suspect of claims of ultimate truth and groups seeking positions of power and authority. Again, these trends are both healthy and unhealthy. It seems rational and healthy to have some caution about groups seeking power and claims of ultimate truth, particularly following many of abuses of power which have occurred in the recent past.

Religion is increasingly used to refer to the more structured and corporal aspects of faith or belief. For some, this would be may primarily be related to organized religion. For other, it may refer more broadly to the systematic or structured aspect of faith. This would include systematic theology, rituals and traditions, and views on morality and ethics.

Spirituality, conversely, is typically referring to the more relational and experiential aspects of faith or belief. For many people spirituality is closely connected with religious belief, as discussed above. For others, they work hard to distinguish the relational and experiential components of religious belief. However, if religion is viewed as the organized or structured aspects of faith, spirituality cannot be completely separated from religion. They are related to each other and spirituality would tend to flow from religion. They can be distinguished, but not separated.

To fully separate religion from spirituality, they must be defined more specifically. This typically occurs by using religion to refer to more traditional approaches to religion (Christianity, Islam, Judaism, *etc.*) while spirituality is more emergent trends in society. At other times, religion is used more broadly to include any organized approache to religion, while spirituality is referred to personal process of faith or belief which is kept separate from any particular governing organization.

Spirituality and religion are much more confusing than they used to be. Through time, these terms have evolved to be used very differently than how they were traditionally used. More than likely, they will continue to change with time. For religious professionals, professionals who work with religious/spiritual people, and people who are religious/spiritual, these trends can be particularly important.

A TRUE RELIGION AND SPIRITUAL DEVELOPMENT

Spiritual Development means ability to commune with the Creator of the Universe, the Supreme Lord by awakening the spiritual faculties. This is possible only by following the Path of Devotion under the guidance of True Guide, who has attained that ability. True peace cannot be attained merely as a result of the fulfillment of one's worldly desires, nor through engagement in charitable activities, nor even by reducing the number of desires, nor by turning away from the world. Human gets peace only when he gives up selfishness and shares the joy of others. True peace is attained when one's spiritual faculties are awakened. Such peace goes on increasing day by day with spiritual practices till a state of perfect peace is reached when no desire for anything or for any experience or any condition is left.

A True Religion teaches that highest aim of life for man is the attainment of true peace and freedom or liberty *i.e.,* man should decide that his spirit should attain complete freedom from the bonds of body and mind when this state is attained then there is no pain or suffering of any kind that would touch that person. He becomes absolutely free from all physical and mental troubles *i.e.,* hunger, thirst, sickness, old age, desire, anger, greed, attachment *etc*. Also he has no desire left for anything else. To attain this condition, one should surrender himself to or become the disciple of a person who has attained this status, and follow His instructions.

The religion of Saints deals only with deliverance that is secret and glory of the Lord and it describes the mode of reaching His Holy feet by performing the practice of Spiritual Sound Meditation.

That person alone can attach proper importance to *Parmaratha i.e.,* True Objective of Life whose receptacle is sufficiently large and who is always wide awake and who is not affected by the feelings of worldly loss and gain and whose heart is always filled with yearning for the vision of Supreme Lord. Human can understand the True Objective of Life only when the Supreme Lord showers His Special Grace on him. The person thinks about this only when he turns away from the world because of his old deeds and seeks betterment.

The person who desires to have grace of the Lord should behave with truth and honesty with Him. The easiest and most effective way to obtain the Grace of the Supreme Lord is to offer thanks in all sincerity now and then, for the grace and mercy received in the past. As soon as one thinks of the past mercies and wishes to thank the Lord, his mind sincerely becomes humble, his connection with Supreme Lord gets internally established.

To get success in spirituality what one need is:

(a) the special grace of Supreme Lord,
(b) real interest and eagerness to achieve the object and
(c) he must have the help of True Satguru.

To improve the psyche, one should bear in mind the following:

1. One should not take food prepared by everybody or food touched by everybody. Food produces a great effect on one's body and mind. Should take care that people whose ideas and actions are bad and people who are dirty do not touch, see or cook your food.
2. One should associate with those people who are superior and who are trying to further improve themselves. In their association one should be able to cover the distance of months within days.
3. One should perform spiritual practices, daily, to enable the awakening of dormant spiritual faculties; on getting success all the weaknesses and complaints will be removed.

The above needs can be fulfilled when wisdom is available.

WISDOM REVOLUTION

The present society which is suffering from these ups and downs of sorrow and happiness and searching for the ways of getting rid of the sorrows to achieve state of continuous happiness will have to under go a "Wisdom Revolution". The Wisdom

Revolution in the society is necessary to remove all sorts of misconceptions from the minds of the people around the world. The Wisdom Revolution would transform the prevailing thinking strategy and the state of mind of all individuals in the world, from the state of ignorance to know the right and wrong in absolute terms to the state of total clarity as to what is right and what is wrong (Saini, 2003).

The transformation to the state of Wisdom Society has to follow a path of systematic approach of development of all individuals in the society through enrichment of knowledge, adherence to cohesive social goals, complete truthfulness leading to development of the social ethics and moral values. For instance, the basic concepts of living, working and social and individual development must be transformed to a state of highest level where every member of the society respect each other and have perfect coordination in thought and action. Ideally, this process of transformation would be such that there is total active support in all the activities and there is no resistance from any individual or group in the society. To achieve the status of a Wisdom Society, the members of the society would be willing to adopt the new concepts and will be ready for any change in their present philosophy about the life. The Wisdom Society would formulate a set of recommended actions including the methods and procedures to reach the state where every member of the society is satisfied with his daily routine as well as progressing internally as an individual towards the Real Objective of his life *i.e.,* to reach a purest state where any entity, activity of this world and his personal ills and deficiencies do not trouble him in his communication with the All mighty. This will lead to absolute synergy of thought and attainment of Real Objective by all the people in the society.

Thus, a Wisdom Society will be one where all the individuals carry the same real objective of achieving a state of absolute contentment and real happiness by achieving a form of Purified Human, who is free from bondages of the worldly joys and sorrows, felt by the senses of body and the mind. To achieve this real objective, all the members of the society perform every routine activity of life, which is necessary to survive in this world, without any attachment for any object or entity of the world. Once, the transformation of the Wisdom Society is complete; all the individuals in the Society will be able to achieve the Real Objective of Life.

REFERENCES

http://www.guidetopsychology.com/spirit.htm

http://drsanity.blogspot.com/2005/12/psychological-defense-mechanisms.html

http://en.wikipedia.org/wiki/Defense_mechanism

Ratan Saini (2003). "Need for and Transformation to a Wisdom Society", DEI Magazine.

Yoga Psychotherapy around the World

Ganesh Shankar*

Psychotherapy is experiencing a strong fresh impetus all over the world, as it has reached a level of development that predestines it for the treatment of a large number of emotional disturbances. Worldwide neuroses is increasing, headed by depression, numerous fears and psychosomatic complaints. But likewise the treatments of psychiatric illnesses and prophylaxis in psycho-social conflict constellations have developed into important scopes of work for psychotherapists.

On one hand psychotherapy is a young science (which can be dated back to the systematization of psychoanalysis by Sigmund Freud and his collaborators around 100 years ago), on the other hand all cultures of this world have, since time immemorial, known methods and professions, that dealt and are still dealing with the reduction of mental suffering. That is the reason why we have to take into account, in modern psychotherapy, not only western, but also different cultural influences. Only then it can really count as a scientific method. Psychotherapy is not only confined to the therapeutic context. Psychotherapists are also asked to intervene in psycho-social conflicts such as the mediation of partner conflicts or in politics regarding ethnic conflicts or in managing refugee movements.

In fact, Indian culture as a whole has psychological orientation and has strong and mature traditions of profound psychotherapy. Thus, India can make a distinctive contribution to western system of psychotherapy for a comprehensive treatment of the fundamental problem of integration of personality from the comparative standpoint of yoga and depth psychology.

Yoga should not be considered as an antiquated myth of yesterday because it has as much validity and value now as it had ever before and can offer guidance and help to the modern man. There is genuine and urgent need today to integrate yoga concepts into the main stream of modem psychotherapeutic thought and be made an essential integral part of the global culture of tomorrow.

In order to fulfill the above-mentioned idea, I would like to draw the attention of all of you towards the works of three illustrious Indian exponents to study and understand their views in the context of modern psychotherapy. These are Standard English Commentaries on Patanjali's Yoga Sutras (father of yoga psychotherapy), Yoga of

*Faculty of Human Consciousness and Yogic Science, Sagar University, Sagar-470003, MP, India. E-mail: ypai_yoga@hotmail.com

Sri Aurbindo and Dr. A.K. Mukhopadhyaya's two latest scientific volumes *i.e.,* Conquering the Brain and the Millennium Bridge dealing mainly with consciousness and its newly emerged psychotherapeutic paradigm along with the western works of Freud (father of psychoanalysis) Adler, Jung, Assagioli, Maslow and Sorokin.

THE SYSTEM OF YOGA

It is true that yoga is ancient. In fact, its origin is shrouded in antiquity. No one really knows when Yoga was first developed or who gave it to man. There are many historical conjectures which even suggest that the Gods themselves taught yoga to man. The fact is that yogic practices were unknown even in the Vedic times, and references to yoga abound in the Vedas, in particular the Rig Veda, and in the Upanishads and Bhagawad Gita. That they only prove how ancient yoga is and consequently how much they evolved it, is the growth of Indian culture. Indian Rishis of old, recognised the unalterable fact of life, namely that man is not a mere body, not a mere mind, but a body-mind complex in which one reacts on the other end in which one can not be separated from each other. No modern educationist or thinker could possibly disagree with such a comprehensive view of man. Yoga even emphasizes that mind influences the body more than the body influences the mind. The knowledge of yogic practices was handed down through the ages from generation to generation by word of mouth and by example through unbroken chain of devoted guru-chela relationship until around 200 years before the Christian era or over 2000 years age, Patanjali, the founder of what is known as classic yoga or Patanjala yoga first systematised and codified the then existing knowledge of yoga into 194 aphorism or sayings and gave it to the world the yoga sutras.

The yoga system of Patanjali which is also known as Raj Yoga, is a world view, a way of life and a set of practices for regulation of mind to achieve the highest goal of yoga *i.e., Kaivalya.* The celebrated text, yoga sutra of Patanjali virtually presents a psychological system. Gardner Murphy once remarked that the systematic development of yoga by Patanjali "constitute one of the great psychological achievements of all times", (Murphy and Murphy, 1968).

Patanjali has prescribed an eight-fold path for achieving the goal of *Kaivalya. Ashtanga* yoga involves: *Yama* (Restraints), *Niyama* (Discipline), *Asana* (Body Attitude/ Postures), *Pranayama* (Breath Regulation), *Pratyhara* (Detachment of Sensory Activity from the External Objects), *Dharana* (Concentration), *Dhyana* (Yogic Meditation) and *Samadhi* (Spiritual Absorption). Patanjali describes the first five limbs as the external form of yoga and that they are preparatory, the last three as internal and essential aspects. The foundations of yoga practice lie in *Abhyasa* (Practice) and *Vairagya* (Detachment). The Yamas are: *Ahimsa* (Non-injury), *Satya* (Non-lying), *Asteya*

(Non-stealing), *Brahamachara* (Sexual Abstinence) *Aparigraha* (Non-possession). The *Niyamas* are: Sauch (Cleanliness), *Santosh* (Contentment), Tapas (Asceticism), *Swadhyaya* (Self Study) and *Ishwarpranidhan* (Devotion to God). Asana is a body posture that is stable and comfortable. Patanjali devotes only one verse to it. The important point about *asana* is that it gives the body stability reducing physical effort to a minimum, which may be distraction to meditation. *Pranayama* is a discipline of respiration. Patanjali devotes only three verses to it. It is the arrest of the movement of inhalation and exhalation, which is practised after mastering the asana. Pratyahara, the withdrawal of senses from external objects is the final stage of the external yoga. The core of yoga practice lies in *Dharana* (Concentration), *Dhyana* (yogic meditation) and *Samadhi* (Absorption). Concentration involves attention to a single object or place, external or internal, like a lamp, the space between the eyebrows, the tip of the nose or thought (Like God or *Mantra*). The continuous concentration is called *Ekagrata* (On a Single Point). When the mind flows towards the object of concentration uninterruptedly and effortlessly, it is the stage of meditation when it happens for a prolonged period of time, it leads to *Samadhi*. *Samadhi* is a state of absorption in which the subject/object distinction is lost. The state of Samadhi is believed to be characterised by the comprehension of the true nature of reality, which ultimately emancipates the individual. Patanjali has described a variety of stages in *samadhi*. In modern times, the meditative practices like trancendental meditation (T.M. of Mahesh Yogi, 1963), Benson's technique (Benson, 1975) and Carrington's clinically standardized meditation (Carrignton, 1977) among others are based on the system of Patanjali.

***Hatha* Yoga**

Techniques of yoga have been practised for thousands of years mainly for the sake of the final goal of liberation from the cycle of rebirths and the pain associated with it. These techniques were intended to influence the mind more than the body. With the Hathayogins who flourished in comparatively later times in the history of yoga (may be about the 15th century A.D.), there was greater emphasis on the body. Their ultimate aim was also the same namely, attainment of the state of samadhi. But their means were more suited to the abilities of the common man. Gorksha Sataka of Gorakhnath (Briggs, 1973) of 10th century A.D.; Gherands Samhita of 12th century (Vasu, 1974), *Hatha Yoga Pradipika* of Swatmarama (Brahmanda, 1989) of 15th century are three important texts of Hatha yoga school. Hatha yoga as a holistic system does not consists of mere kriyas, asanas, pranayamas, bandhas, mudras and meditation *etc.* but lays great stress on control of diet social attitude and personal habits so as to bring about beneficial changes in the whole of the metabolic process. It is truly an integrated approach, treating man as a whole (Kuvalyananda and Vinekar, 1971).

YOGA THERAPY

Strictly speaking, therapy is not the proper field of yoga. However, Patanjali mentions "Vyadhi" meaning disease, which he considers as a hindrance to personality integration. But he never refers to the treatment of diseases simply because of his approach is wholistic rather than analytical that is, he prefers to integrate rather than occupy himself with the symptoms of disintegration. The modern trend towards systematic yoga therapy really began in 1920. Early scientific investigations were made by Swami Kuvalyanada, the disciple of Madhavadas Maharaj and the founder of Kaivalyadhama Yoga Institute.

Swamiji's discoveries and attempts to put yoga on a scientific basis were made public in 1924, when he started his Yoga Mimamsa Journal. At the Kaivalyadhama Institute Swami Kuvalyananda started treating patients with various complaints resorting only to yogic techniques. Throughout the many years of research into yoga therapy at Kaivalyadhama, many discoveries were made about the therapeutic effects on certain ailments. Later attempts were made by many organisations and individuals, both in India and abroad. "Yoga Therapy: Its Basic Principles and Methods" by Swami Kuvalyananda and S.L.Vinekar was published by Govt. of India in 1961. It was distributed in several countries including socialist and was even translated into Polish.

RESEARCH STUDIES IN YOGA THERAPY

Throughout Yoga's long history, there have been many misconceptions which shrouded it in mystery until proper scientific research began in the beginning of 20th century. In India, people became aware of the need to revive old traditions and sciences which might otherwise die out and scientific research into yoga was one of the areas which generated a lot of interest. Many western scholars too realized the utility of yoga and made efforts to study its significance from scientific point of view. They made some longitudinal studies in this area and their research findings are available to us for further work in this area (Kuvalyananda, 1925, 1928; Behanan, K.T., 1937; Bagchi, B.K. and Wenger, M.A. 1957; Hirai, T., 1960; de Vries, H.A. 1961; Giri, C., 1966; Wallace, R.K. 1970; Joseph C. *et al.*, 1987; Meti, B.L. *et al.*, 1989; Joseph, S. *et al.*, 1993; Meti, B.L. 1995). Swami Kuvalyananda reported sub-atmospheric pressure in the various internal cavities during Uddian Bandha and its extension of nauli. He also took X-rays to demonstrate the movements of the diaphragm during uddiyana bandha. A pupil of his, Behanana, undertook further research leading to a doctoral thesis of Yale University in 1937. He estimated the oxygen consumption during pranayama practice and reported an increase during Ujjai, Bhastrika and Kapapbhati. He also brought different types of pranayama on to kymographic record. The ability of yogis to voluntarily stop the beating of the heart was considered—a fascinating feat, and aroused the interest of scientists in India and elsewhere. In 1936 an article by the French cardiologist, Brosse, reported studies on subjects of both Hatha and Raj yoga, the former showing the more significant results. Bagchi and Wenger (1957) studied practitioners of Rajyoga in India. They found a lower respiratory rate and raised G.S.R. (Galvanic Skin Resistance) with no consistent alterations in heart rate or blood pressure during meditation. During meditation, the EEG showed an increase in alpha wave amplitude and activity and in some of the yogis there was a loss of the alpha blocking response to all external stimuli. Around 1960, Maharishi Mahesh Yogi introduced Transcendental Meditation to the world. This technique is neither a religion nor a way of life. It is a natural effortless technique, which aims at improving all aspects of life. Adapted from ancient Indian technique, it gained in popularity and has spread all over the world. In 1968, R.K. Wallace undertook an investigation of physiological effects of TM, for his doctoral thesis, entitled, "The physiological effects of TM: A proposed fourth major state of consciousness". In this as well as in later studies by him (Wallace *et al.*, 1971) the practice of TM was found to be associated with changes in the EEG. In some of the subjects during meditation, there was an increase in alpha wave amplitude, associated with a slowing of the frequency. In some cases, there were brief periods of about 2.5 seconds during which theta waves predominated. There was also an increase in GSR, decrease in heart rate, decrease in oxygen consumption and carbondioxide elimination, along with a reduction in both rate and volume of respiration. Blood lactate levels were also reduced after meditation. This led to TM being called a "Wakeful Hypometabolic State". The changes were interpreted a sign of a functional trophotropic state, chiefly mediated by increased parasympathetic and decreased sympathetic discharge, rather like other assimilatory processes such as sleep and digestion. Kasamatsu (1973) categorised the EEG changes in Zen meditation as four stages. The first is the appearance of alpha rhythm in spite of the eyes being open. In the second stage, there is an increase in amplitude of persistent alpha frequency and finally, in the fourth stage the appearance of rhythmic theta train was observed. During the last 3–6 decades, the Hatha yogic practices have been evaluated for their efficacy in the management of diabetes and found useful (Udupa and Singh, 1972; Malkote, 1973; Sahay, 1986; Gore, 1988).

One may wonder how yoga can affect all these responses. The practice of *asanas* may send a volley of nerve impulses from muscles and joints, spine and other receptors located on the surface as well as inside the viscera. It can influence the homodynamic mechanism improving blood circulation to vital organs like brain, heart, lungs, liver, kidney, pancreas *etc.* it may also act through the neuro-endocrine axis. Scientists like Anand, B.K. (1961) strongly feel that yogic practices may modulate the cerebral cortico-limbic system of the brain and strengthen the inhibitory components of the nervous system. More documentary evidences are required to consolidate these claims and assumptions. Whatever be the mechanism involved, it is established beyond doubt that regular practice of yoga certainly has many beneficial effects on the human physiology, biochemistry and psychology.

Psychoanalysis and Yoga

With the emergence of transpersonal psychology as a distinct force within humanistic circles, the spiritual aspects of psychotherapy and the psychotherapeutic value of spiritual practices have been a matter of serious consideration among some psychotherapists (*e.g.,* Frankl, 1975; Vaughan, 1991; Tart and Deikman, 1991). Some secular methods which have been developed from the spiritual systems, such as Benson's technique and Carrington's Clinically Standardized Meditation (CSM) have also become popular *e.g.,* Benson, 1975; Carington, 1977). Meditation techniques like Zen and T M have come to be used as adjuncts to psychotherapy (*e.g.,* Goleman, 1971; Deatherage, 1975; Engler, 1984). Striking parallels have also been shown by a number of thinkers between some schools of psychology and spiritual systems (*e.g.,* Harvey, 1976, 1980; Ballentine, 1980; Neurenberger, 1980; Rama, Ballentine and Ajaya, 1976, Ajay, 1980). Swamy Rama, a spiritual leader of distinction has inspired some of his disciples to develop and practice a system of psychotherapy based on classical Indian thought at the International Institute of Yoga Science and Philosophy in U.S.A.

YOGA AND PSYCHOTHERAPY

The Evolution of Consciousness (1976) of Swamy Rama, Ballantine and Swamy Ajay and Psychotherapy East and West: A Unifying Paradigm (1984) of Swamy Ajay, presented a full fledged system of yoga therapy based on *Smakhya* Yoga, *Hatha* Yoga, *Advita Vedanta* and *Tantra*. The system encompasses a wide variety of body, mind and behavior techniques. Swami Ajaya also pointed out in his book, sticking similarities between current psychotherapies and classical practices. Those of us who are looking for a conceptual framework and a set of procedures, which are not alien but close to the Indian mind, would certainly find yoga therapy as very handy.

It is very interesting to note that historically it was the psychoanalytic writer Geraldine Coster who in the classic, Yoga and Western Psychology (1934) first appraised the therapeutic potential of yoga and presented an elaborate comparison of Freudian Psychoanalysis and Patanjali's yoga. In a sense she anticipated the contemporary interest in yoga as a psychotherapeutic system.

It would be refreshing for those of us who are interested in yoga or psychoanalysis to look at some of Coster's observations, especially in the context of an overwhelming contemporary interest in yoga. In the background of Freud's sceptical attitude towards the mystical experience, which he tended to regard as regressive and pathological in nature (*e.g.,* Freud, 1961) it will be instructive to juxtapose yoga and psychoanalysis.

According to Coster, Yoga contains the clue needed by the West if the psychoanalytic method and theory is to reach its fullest scope as a regenerating and recreating factor in modern life. If salvation is understood as the security of genuine happiness, poise determined by one's own inner life, self-knowledge of the analytic kind and the Eastern kind might supplement each other. For some people it may even give an experimental proof of the reality of the world beyond the drop curtain.

The majority of people who seek an analyst are those who are ill in the body and mind or ill at ease with life, the self and the world. Most often these are the people who could not be helped by other methods. The students of yoga are also likely to be those who are deeply dissatisfied with their own adaptation to life and to the external world.

In analysis there is always an analyst and in yoga there is always the teacher (Guru). The analyst and the teacher differ in the degree of their directive ness. The latter tend to be more directive than the former. In both analysis and yoga the first step consists in the letting go of old automatisms of thought and feeling. The analyst and the disciple are given training to loosen the rigidities of thinking and feeling which were consequence of their experiences, education and environment.

The yoga practitioner and the seeker of analysis, both look for an interior solution to their problem, however different their approach and working hypotheses may be. While the former goes by a belief system which subscribes to the transcendental embedded in ones own self, the latter is guided by the hypothesis that self-knowledge is worth attaining. Both are contemplative unlike the active out-ward directed tradition of the West. Coster, however, does not point out the antagonistic attitude of psychoanalysis towards religion and assumes that analysis provides a method of interior approach for the agnostic as well as for the religious type of mind.

The description of mental functions and the state of the mind of a beginner of yoga practice as described by Patanjali is strikingly similar to the descriptions of the analysed in psychoanalytic literature. Confused thinking and identifications characterize them both. It is the viewpoint of both the yoga teacher and the analyst that "nothing can be done unless the person is willing to alter the entire habit of his mind and emotions from the group up".

While considering the preliminary limbs of Ashtanga Yoga, namely *Yama* (Restraints), *Niyama* (Observances), *Asana* (Body Posture), *Pranayama* (Breath Regulation) and *Pratyahara* (Sensory Withdrawal) Coster remarks that whereas *Yama* and *Niyama* are forms of moral and spiritual training which are familiar to the West, the value of breath regulation, sustained poise and sensory withdrawal are yet to be recognized as techniques to deal with neurosis among psychotherapists. She further states in anticipation of yoga psychotherapy that "if however the whole matter of moral and social discipline, relaxation, breathing, and control of thought by meditation were approached by psychotherapists in the non-religious and scientific attitude of the student of yoga, it might well be that this would lead to the discovery of new and valuable psychotherapeutic methods".

It is with a comfortable posture that both meditation and analytic sessions begin in order to deal with the mind. While the expression aloud of thought *i.e.,* free association is the primary technique the analysed masters in course of his analytic practice, the yoga practitioner attempts to control his mind by attending to a chosen object, the obstacles to progress in Yoga-ignorance (*Avidya*), Self-Esteem (*Asmita*), Desire (*Raga*), Aversion (*Dvesha*) and Attachment to Life (*Abhinivesha*) are also the obstacles to analytic development. The lack of knowledge of the source of distress, narcissism *etc.* shows that this is also fundamental to analytic treatment. Accepting life as it comes rather than demanding from it what one expects is a mark of "free psyche" and also "liberation". Such an attitude comes out only of relentless pursuit. However, Coster states that the yogi's idea of liberation goes far beyond the analyst's conception of a free psyche and that they are not easy to compare. Further she says that yoga is an ancient and mature discipline and we are left with only speculation as to the future directions of the young experiment of psychoanalysis. She also notes the ethical values preached by yoga are not yet in the domain of analytic treatment. It ought to be, in future, if analysis is to be more comprehensive.

The approach of yoga, encompassing moral and social discipline, relaxation, breathing and control of thought by meditation *etc.*, may well provide many valuable psychotherapeutic methods if approached by the analysts. Coster states with conviction that the ideas on which yoga is based are universally true for mankind and the yoga sutra of Patanjali contain the information that some of the most advanced psychotherapists of the present day are ardently seeking. No wonder that Swamy Rama, Swamy Ajaya, Ballantine, Neurenberger and others in their scholarly pursuits and therapeutic work developed a holistic therapeutic system based on yoga.

CONCLUSION

Indian tradition, scientific research and clinical experience, all point out that yoga practices are probably the most important and effective self-help tools available to man. The importance of yoga is coming into light in the west in the comparative analysis of different systems by psychologists to find out meaningful answers to some problems of life. We seem to be very close to a behavior technology and self reliance in the domain of yoga. The main principle of yoga therapy is that it seems to establish the homeostasis in the organism as a whole. These endeavours have been leading to the development of principles and procedures separating yoga more or less from its mystical and metaphysical spheres and perfecting it on secular and scientific grounds.

As yoga embraces all aspects of human life and also provides techniques for the regulation of the mind body complex, it is up to the researchers and clinicians to develop an indigenous psychotherapeutic system out of it, which would be comprehensive enough to deal with the complexities of modern life and its cultural values. It appears that the Indian practitioners of psychotherapy, who have been looking for a conceptual framework and a set of procedures which are not alien but intimate to the Indian mind would definitely find an alternative in yoga. It is evidenced in the writings of Geraldine Coster, Swamy Rama, Ajay and several other thinkers of East and West.

It is hoped that this paper will encourage some of the Eastern and Western Psychologists and Psychotherapists to incorporate yogic techniques in their therapeutic work and also to develop new and more effective integrated methods of psychotherapy from the system of yoga.

REFERENCES

Ajaya, Swami (1984). *Psychotherapy East and West: A Unifying Paradigm,* Honesdale: Himalayan International Institute of Yoga, Science and Philosophy.

Akhilanad, S. (1952). *Mental Health and Hindu Psychology.* London: George Allen and Unwin.

Ananda, B.K. and Chinna, G.S. (1961). "Investigations on Yogies Claiming to Stop Their Heart Beats." *Ind. J. Med. Res.*, 49, 82–94.

Bagchi, B.K. (1936). "Mental Hygiene and Hindu Doctrine of Relaxation". *Mental Hygiene*, 20, 424–440.

Bagchi, B.K. and Wnger, M.A. (1957). "Electrophysiological Correlates of Some Yogic Exercises." *Electroencephaclin Neurophysol.*, 7, 132–149.

Behanan, K.T. (1937). *Yoga: A Scientific Evaluation.* New York: Dover Publications.

Benson, H. (1975). *The Relaxation Response*, New York: McMillian.

Bhaba, Brahmananda (Tr.) (1989). *Hathayogapradipika.* Bombay: Sacred Books of Hinds.

Briggs, G.W. (ed. and Tr.) (1973). *Gorakhnath and the Kanphata Yogis,* Delhi: Motilal Banarsidas.

Carrington, P. (1977). *Freedom in Meditation.* Garden City, New York: Doubleday.

Coster, G. (1934). *Yoga and Western Psychology: A Comparison.* London: Oxford University Press.

Dasgupta, S. (1975). *A Histroy of Indian Philosophy.* Vol. 2, Delhi: Motilal Banarsidas.

De Vries, Herbert (1961). "Prevention Muscular Distress after Exercise." *Research Qr.*, 32, 177–185.

Deatherage, G. (1975). "Clinical Use of Mindfulness Meditation Technique in Short Term Psychotherapy", *Journal of Transpersonal Psychology*, 7, 133–143.

Eagan, G. (1982). *The Skilled Helper*. Monterey: Brooks/Cole Publishing Company.

Eliade, M. (1969). *Yoga: Immortality and Freedom*. Princeton: Princeton University Press.

Engler, J. (1984). "Therapeutic Aims in Psychotherapy and Meditation: Developmental Stages in the Representation of Self." *Journal of Transpersonal Psychology*.16, 25–61.

Frankl, V.E. (1975). *The Unconscious God: Psychotherapy and Theology*. New York: Simon and Schuster.

Freud, S. (1961). *The Future of an Illusion*. New York: Double Day.

Garbe. R. (Ed. and Tr.) (1985). *Samkhya-pravachna Sutra*, Cambridge, Harvard.

Giri, C. (1966). "Yoga and Physical Fitness with Special Reference to Atheletes" *IATHPER Qr. Jour*. 2: 6.

Goleman, D. (1971). "Meditation as Meta Therapy: Hypothesis Towards a Proposed 5th State of Consciousness." *Journal of Transpersonal Psychology*, 31, 1–26.

Gore, M.M. (1987). *Anatomy and Physiology of Yogic Practices*. Kaivalyadhama, Lonavala: Kanchan Prakashan,.

Harver, R.J. (1976). "Behavior Therapy and Yoga". In Swami Ajay (Ed.) *Psychology East and West. Honesdale:* The Himalayan International Institute of Yoga Science and Philosophy, 50–75.

Harver, R.J. (1980). "Behavioral Principles Cast in the Non-reductionastic Context of Classical Yoga Psychology." *Annual Convention of the American Psychological Association*, Montreal, Canada.

Hirai, T. (1960). *Electroencephalographic Study on Zen Meditation*. Folia Psychatr Neurol, Japan, 62, 76–105.

Horney, K. (1937). *Neurotic Personality of Our Times*. New York: Norton.

Joseph C., Shankar, Ram, A. Kulkarni, D.D. and Ramchandra, T. (1987). "Post Meditational Effects of Brankmkumari (BK) and Transcendental Meditation ™ on Computer Averaged Event Related Evoked Potential Components Recorded in the P 300 Congnitive Paradigm" *Ind. J. Physiol. Pharmac,* 31, 5, 49.

Joseph, S., Sridharan, K., Patil, S.K.B., Kumar, M.L., Selwamurthy, W., Joseph, N.T. and Nayen, H.S. (1981). "Study of some Physioligical and Biochemical Parameters in Subjects Undergoing Yogic Training" *Ind. Jour. of Med. Res.*, 14, 120–124.

Kasamatsu, A. and Hirai, T. (1960). "An Electroencephalographic Study on Zen Meditation": In *Altered States of Consciousness*. Tart, C. (Ed.). New York: John Wiley and Sons.

Krishna Rao, P.V. (1995). "Yoga: Its Scientific and Applied Aspect" *Jour. of Indian Psychology,* 13:2, 1–11.

Kuppuswamy, B. (1985). *Elements of Ancient Indian Psychology*. New Delhi: Vani Educational Books.

Kuvalyananda, Swami (1925, 1928). *Cited in Papers on Yoga*, Swami Digambar Jo (Ed.), Kaivalyadhama, Yoga Institute.

Kuvalyananda, Swami and Vinekar, S.L. (1963). *Yogic Therapy* Central Health Education Bureau, Ministry of Health, Govt. of India, New Delhi.

Melkote, G.S. (1973). *Concise Report of Work Done at Yoga Research Institute*, Hyderabad, *Presented at First Scientific Seminar, CCRIMH,* New Delhi.

Meti, B.L. (1995). *Sleep Pattern Abnormality in Dysthnic Syndrome*. *ANCIPS,* Patana, 36.

Murphy, G. and Murphy, L.B. (Eds.) (1968). *Asian Psychology*, New York: Basic Books.

Nuernberber P. (1976). "Yoga Encounter Groups". In Swami Ajay (Ed.) *Psychology East and West*. Honesdale: The Himalalyan International Institute of Yoga Science and Philosophy, 75–102.

Nurenberger, P. (1986). "Mind Meditation and Emotion", In Ballentine, R.M. (ed.) *The Theory and Practice of Meditation*. Honesdale, Pennsylvania: Himalayan International Institute, 67–89.

Ram, Swami, Ballentine, R. and Ajay, Swami (1976). *Yoga and Psychotherapy: The Evolution of Consciousness*. Honesdale: The Himalyan International Institute of Yoga and Philosophy.

Sahay, B.K. and Sitaram, Raju *et al.* (1986). "Glucose and Insulin Levels in Obese Non-diabetics," *JAPI,* 34, 6.

Satyananda, D. (1972). *Dynamic Psychology of the Gita of Hinduism*. New Delhi: Oxford and I B H.

Singh, H.G. (1977). *Psychotherapy in India*. Agra: National Psychological Corporation.

Tart, C.T. and Deikman, A.J. (1991). "Mindfulness, Spiritual Seeking and Psychotherapy". *Journal of Transpersonal Psychology*, 23(1), 29–52.

Udupa, K.N. and Singh, R.H. (1972). "Scientific Basis of Yoga", *Jour. of American Medical Asso.* 220, 1365.

Vasu, Sris, Chandra (Tr.) (1914). *Gheranda- Samhita.* Allahabad: Sacred Books of Hindus.

Vaughan, F. (1991). "Spiritual Issues in Psychotherapy." *Journal of Transpersonal Psychology,* 23(23), 105–121.

Vijaylakshi, S., Vindhya Sudhakar, U. and Kalpana Rao, V. (1986). "Role of a Counsellor in the Indian Context". *Journal of Indian Psychology*, 5, 76–82.

Wallace, K.W. and Benson, H. (1972). "The Physiology of Meditation". *Scientific American*, 226, 846.

Wallace, R.K. (1970). "Physiological Effects of Transcendental Meditation", *Science*, 167, 1751.

Werner, K. (1977). *Yoga and Indian Philosophy*. Delhi: Motilal Banarsidass.

Woods, J.H. (Ed and Tr.) (1924). *The Yoga System of Patanjali.* Harvard Cambridge

Yogic, Mahesh (1963). *Transcendental Meditation.* New American Library, New York.

Meditation—Panacea for Afflicted Souls

Renu Josan*[1] and Agam Kulshreshtha[2]

ABSTRACT

Life of the modern man is characterized by stress, anguish, conflict and depression due to the cut-throat competition, desire to reach the top within the shortest span possible, anxiety to meet the set target and above all, materialistic attitude. Technology and scientific innovations have provided man with all the material comforts but have not evolved anything for the well-being of his mental and spiritual health. The modern man is desperately in search of a remedy that will calm his mind, soothe his nerves and provide relaxation to his body. The psychologists and researchers in mental health have zeroed in on the practice of meditation as an effective therapy. Meditation in, one form or the other, has been practiced in most of the religions of the world; but, whereas, the eastern religions have tended to concentrate on meditation as a means of realizing spiritual enlightenment, in the west many people regard meditation as a tool for stress management and good health. The eight parts of yoga described in *Patanjal Darshan* are *Yama, Niyam, Aasan, Pranayam, Pratyahar, Dharma, Dhyan and Samadhi.* Meditation is not a technique but a way of life. It describes a state of consciousness, when the mind is free of scattered thoughts and various patterns. This idea has been conveyed more succinctly in the following *Shloka* from *Yogsutra 3/2* "*- Tatra Pratyayektanata Dhyanam.*" A range of disorders can be cured with regular meditation, as it helps in promoting physical, emotional and mental health, focused and clear thinking, more equanimity in the face of challenges and finally an improved sense of spiritual fulfillment and awakening. There are many different ways to meditate, such as using a mantra, looking at an object or focusing on the breath. Meditation is also looked upon as an effective therapy for diseases of the modern age, such as cancer, AIDS or psychological conditions caused by the stress and strain of daily life. It has been rightly said in *Shwetashvataropanishad-2.12* "*Na Tasyarogo Na Jara Na Mrityu PraptasyaYogagnimayam Shariram*". The *Shloka* means that a person practiced in the art of meditation gains control on both the physical or mental working of his body. Thus the effort of the paper lies in the exploring how the modern man wallowing in the fiery gulf of anxiety, stress, alienation, insomnia and mental anguish, can redeem himself through the practice of meditation.

INTRODUCTION

Life of the modern man is characterized by stress, anguish, conflict and depression due to the cut-throat competition; desire to reach the top within the shortest span

*Corresponding author.

[1]Department of English, Faculty of Arts, Dayalbagh Educational Institute, Deemed University, Dayalbagh, Agra, UP, India.

[2]Department of Sanskrit, Faculty of Arts, Dayalbagh Educational Institute, Deemed University, Dayalbagh, Agra, UP, India.

possible, anxiety to meet the set target and above all, materialistic attitude. The way of life has changed tremendously over the last hundred years or so. The social system and other systems have undergone drastic change over the passage of time. Technology and scientific innovations have provided man with all the material comfort but have not evolved anything for the well-being of his mental and spiritual health. Man has lost his equilibrium and harmony in every sphere of existence. Man is so engaged in materialistic pursuit that he has failed to realize the precarious situations which he has been creating for himself. No wonder the renowned astrophysicist, Stephen Hawking posed a very relevant question "In a world that is in chaos politically, economically and environmentally, how the human race can sustain another hundred years?"

Within the last century or two, diseases have sprung up with new dimensions and manifestations. Medical science has brought to an end the epidemics of the past but we are now faced with a new epidemic of stress related disorders caused by our inability to adapt to the highly competitive pace of modern life. Psychosomatic illnesses such as diabetes, hypertension, migraine, asthma *etc* arise from tensions in the body and mind. The dreadful disease like cancer and heart disease also stem from tension. The medical science has been tackling such problems but has not been very successful because the real problem does not lie in the body but in man's changing ideals, his way of thinking and feeling. When there is dissipation of energy dispersion of ideas, how can harmony of body and mind be achieved? The psychologists and researchers in mental health have zeroed in on the practice of meditation as an effective therapy.

Mediation in one form or the other has been practised in most of the religions of the world like Christianity, Buddhism, Hinduism and Islam. Earlier religions have focused on meditation as a means of attaining spiritual enlightenment and this also includes many health promoting practices. In the west, meditation is practiced for both the reasons although most of the people regard it as a tool for stress management. The word meditation is derived from the Latin word; meditari (to think, to dwell) and mederi (to heal). The eight parts of yoga described in ***Patanjal Darshan*** are *Yama, Niyam, Asan, Pranayam, Pratyahar, Dharna, Dhyan and Samadhi*. Defining meditation it is said in Yoga Sutra 3/2—"*Tatra Pratyayektanata Dhyanam*" (Goswami 36), which means that when there is absolute concentration on the object of contemplation and there is no other extraneous influence to suppress it, then it is called meditation.

Meditation is one such unparalleled technique of physical mental, moral and spiritual discipline, through which complete control over body, mind and soul can be attained. Besides this, it also helps in the realization of truth, thereby, aiding one in detaching himself from all kind of attachments. *Dhyan* is one of the parts of yoga and it is based on the pre-knowledge of the mysteries of body and mind, minute working of the important organs, bones of the brain and spinal cord and the conscious, subconscious and unconscious states of mind.

Meditation is not a technique but a way of life. It refers to that state of consciousness when the mind liberates itself from the scattered thought and various patterns and all the activity of the mind is reduced to one. The idea is beautifully conveyed in the following *shloka* from *Siddha Siddhanta Padyati* 5/31 "*Yadi Chek Nirantaram Sarvasnam/Kimu Shedeshi Manav Sarvasamam*" (SSP 60). This means that during meditation, the mind of the meditator is freed from all extraneous influence thereby attaining the state of self realization.

There are different ways in which one can meditate. Some of them are:

(a) *Breath Concentration*—In this technique one consciously notices the movement of air in and out of one's nostrils.

(b) *Clearing the Mind*—A person pushes aside any stray thought and allows thoughts to move in and out of awareness.

(c) *Looking at an Object*—One focuses the attention but not necessarily his thoughts on the shape, sound and texture of an object.

(d) *Using a Mantra*—One repeats a word or phrase over and over either loudly or silently.

Meditating everyday can help to develop a regular habit and make it easier to attain deeply meditative states. The life of the modern man is engulfed in the stream of many psychological and mental illnesses, leading to such dreadful disease like cancer and maladies of the nervous system. Modern medicine has started investigating different methods of treatment to cure such conditions and restore good health to people. Many modern doctors admit that as the mind controls the body's performance so it can only provide the cure for body's illness. Learning how to meditate can improve both body and mind, bringing improvement to the health at the same time. Now-a-days treating disease depends on science and technology but in Thailand, Dr. Sathit Inthara Kamhaeng has started holistic treatment which lays stress upon understanding how nature works in our lives and learning how to meditate. Dr. Sathit once stated, "Actually living a holistic life doesn't only mean eating a natural diet. It also means changing and correcting our life style by learning how to meditate, learning how to reduce stress in every day life…." (Cheowit, 1988, p. 37).

The Buddhist precept teaches that rust which comes from iron can destroy that same iron. Human minds are the same. If we learn how to meditate and be filled with positive thoughts then the bodies will also be healthy. Dr. Sathit stated, "It is bad thinking which damages us. To take a particular example; if a cancer patient keeps having bad thoughts then eventually these thought will be like the rust that corrodes, allowing death to destroy the patient even quicker…..because such thoughts are one of the causes of cancer". Dr. Simonton of the cancer care centre in California U.S.A has demonstrated the effectiveness of the meditation in treating cancer. He states, "Although meditation and visualization are used for releasing tension and attaining spiritual fulfillment, they can also be used as a first step to setting up changes in one's life and health." Dr. Benson of the Harvard Medical School has worked on the effects of meditation on the health and body. He has found that depression, hopelessness, loneliness, despair and other psychological conditions can be cured with meditation.

Duangjai Gasandigun (1986) carried out research on how the moods affect mental health. He experimented on the effect of meditation on 156 people between 15–25 years and measured their level of depression both before and after meditation. The average score showed that depression was lower after meditation. So, meditation relives stress and enhances the ability to analyze, understand problems and alleviate the cause of depression. It has also bee a useful complementary therapy for treating chronic pain and insomnia.

There are a number of Yoga Asanas which help in the development of mental and physical powers. Practising Pranayam only makes the body spirited and provides mental peace and happiness. It is said in *Shwetashvataropnishad "Na Tasyarogo Na Jara Na Mrityu/Praptasya Yogagnimayam Shariram*" (Shwet. Up. 2.12). This means that one who is practiced in the art of yoga neither falls sick, nor becomes old nor dies. In other words he can will his own death.

Through meditation we are not only relaxing but restructuring and reforming our whole personality from within. We are shedding off old habits and tendencies in order to be endowed with a new personality. The inner tensions of the individuals contribute to collective psychological tensions which manifest in unhappy family life, chaos and disorder in social life, and aggression and warfare between communities and nations. Religions, law, government have been unable to establish harmony among men as peace can only be found within and not without. Therefore in order to create a peaceful world and provide an answer to Hawkings question, each individual must first learn to relax and harmonize his own body and mind through meditation which can be the only panacea for all the maladies and afflictions plaguing man today.

REFERENCES

Goswami, Surakshit (2005). *Patanjalyoga Evam Nathyoga*. New Delhi: Satyam Publishing House.

Saraswati, Satyananda Swami (1982). *Yoga Nidra*. Monghyr: Bhihar School of Yoga.

Siddh Siddhanta Padhyati (2003). Chowkhamba Sanskrit Sansthan.

www.buddhanet.net/sangha-metta/medhealth.html.

Relaxation Value of Meditation in Coronary Heart Disease Patients

Sunita Gupta*

ABSTRACT

The present study examined the psycho-physiological responsiveness to meditation in coronary heart disease patients. 80 heart patients served as subjects. The subjects were assigned randomly to two conditions namely, control (40 subjects) and experimental (40 subjects). The subjects in the experimental group were exposed to meditation for 20 minutes daily for 20 days. Pre-Post design was used for recording psycho-physiological assessments. The meditation was found to have relaxing and soothing effect on heart patients.

INTRODUCTION

Coronary Heart Disease is a general term that refers to illness caused by atherosclerosis, the narrowing of coronary arteries, the vessels that supply the heart with blood. The narrowing of these vessels leads to partial or complete obstruction of the flow of oxygen and nourishment to the heart thereby resulting in heart attack (myocardial infarction). Two of the predominantly involved psychological risk factors in CHD are anxiety (Watkins *et al.*, 1998; Sehgal, 2000) and depression (Musselman and Nemeroff, 2000; Miller *et al.*, 2003; Pasic, *et al.*, 2003). Both anxiety and depression have been found to be predominant psychological risk factors for CHD (Priscilla *et al.*, 2002).

Anxiety is central to most psychiatric illness and is one of the potent precursors of sudden cardiac death (Watkins *et al.*, 1998). Billing *et al.* (1980) in their study on pre- and post- myocardial infarction patients found that 17% to 51% of the patient samples were rated to be seriously anxious. Blatt (2007) reports that higher anxiety levels lead to higher rate of heart attacks.

Depression has been found to be a major independent environmentally determined risk factor for CHD (Wulsin and Singal, 2003; Lett *et al.*, 2004). A strong link between depression and heart failure has been reported in other studies too (Singh and Chowdhary, 1999; Williams *et al.*, 2002; Porter, 2003). Thus there is ample evidence suggesting that depression is associated with increased mortality and morbidity in patients with cardiovascular disease and a significantly higher proportion die of cardiovascular diseases relative to non-depressed individuals.

* Department of Psychology, Guru Nanak Dev University, Amritsar, Punjab, India.

Since the role of medication is not very effective, the Behavioral Medicine can play a very important role, which emphasizes the role of psychological factors in health. This includes biofeedback, meditation and yoga and many other behavioral medicine techniques.

According to Seaward (1999), meditation is focused concentration and increased awareness of one's being when the mind has been emptied of conscious thoughts, unconscious thoughts can enter the conscious realm to bring enlightenment to our lives. Meditation can improve strength and flexibility, help in the management of physiological variables such as blood pressure, respiration, heart rate and metabolic rates and improve over all exercise capacity (Raub, 2002). Delmonte (1985) also reports that the practice of meditation promotes an immediate decrease in oxygen consumption, heart rate, blood pressure and muscle tension and increase in EEG alpha waves and skin conductance thereby having a soothing effect.

OBJECTIVES

Not even a single study has been conducted on heart patients in Indian context so far that has tried to investigate the effects of meditation on physiological measures namely EEG frequency, muscle action potential and blood pressure (Systolic and Diastolic) and psychological measures which assess anxiety in terms of its four components namely cognitive, somatic, behavioral and feelings and depression. The present study is a step in this direction.

HYPOTHESIS

Meditation will reduce anxiety and depression in heart patients.

METHODOLOGY

Subjects

80 male indoor and outdoor heart patients in the age range of 21–40 years diagnosed from Escorts Heart Care Hospital, Amritsar served as subjects. The subjects were classified into 2 groups (40 in control group and 40 in experimental group on the basis of random assignment).

Materials

- *Physiological Measures:* (1) Alpha EEG Apparatus was used for recording alpha EEG brain-wave pattern. (2) EMG Bio trainer Apparatus was used to measure the muscle action potential. (3) Sphygmomanometer was used to measure both systolic and diastolic blood pressure.

- *Psychological Measures:* (1) Four Systems Anxiety Questionnaire—FSAQ (Koskal and Power, 1990) was used to assess anxiety on four components; somatic, cognitive, behavioral and feeling. (2) The IPAT Depression Inventory (Krug and Laughlin, 1976) was used to assess the depression level of the subjects.

Design

Pre-post experimental design was used for the assessment of all the dependent variables.

Procedure

The blood pressure (systolic and diastolic) of each subject was noted down. The alpha EEG measurements were taken using alpha EEG apparatus; the electrodes were placed on the occipital, parietal and frontal regions of the head. The muscle action potential was measured using the EMG apparatus; the electrodes were placed over the fore-finger. The measurements were automatically recorded in terms of Micro-volts per second.

After the EEG, EMG, and blood pressure recordings, the FSAQ and Depression Inventory were administered on each subject. A gap of 5 minutes was given in between all the assessments whether physiological or psychological. For pre- and post- treatment assessments, each subject was tested individually, asked to relax in the testing room for five minutes and then tested on the physiological and psychological parameters mentioned above.

The subjects in the meditation group were first kept on meditation practice for one week. The subjects were instructed to sit in the lotus position, close their eyes with their hands in '*Gyan Mudra*'. The subjects were instructed to inhale deeply but slowly and then exhale slowly while chanting 'Om'. The subjects were instructed to focus on the movements of abdomen during the whole process.

After one week's practice, the meditation procedure was continued for 20 minutes daily for 20 days before breakfast after emptying the bladder and bowel. The pre-treatment testing was done a day before commencement of the meditation treatment, while the post-treatment testing was done a day after the meditation treatment was over. The subjects in the control group were simply tested for physiological and psychological assessments and retesting was done after 20 days.

RESULTS

The results of the present study are reported in Table I in which the means and standard deviations for scores on physiological and psychological measures under various groups and conditions are given.

Table 1: Means, Standard Deviations and Significance of Differences between Means by t-test for Various Groups and Conditions

Measures	*Control Group*			*Experimental Group*			*Post-test Comparison Control vs. experimental group t-Ratio*
	Pre-test	*Post-test*	*Comparison Pre vs. Post t Ratio*	*Pre-test*	*Post-test*	*Comparison Pre vs. Post t Ratio*	
Alpha EEG	16.12 (8.13)	17.02 (7.72)	3.094*	4.86 (3.77)	18.52 (9.59)	14.13***	9.23**
EMG	26.05 (8.69)	27.71 (8.29)	5.78*	31.34 (10.12)	11.86 (3.85)	18.05***	11.28***
Blood Pressure (Systolic)	189.39 (15.78)	190.56 (16.62)	1.42	183.80 (17.48)	148.66 (13.48)	21.89***	13.01***
Blood Pressure (Diastolic)	99.02 (11.25)	98.66 (11.68)	0.64	90.10 (13.19)	72.94 (7.27)	13.007***	12.29***
FSAQ							
Feelings	79.08 (5.75)	80.99 (3.89)	2.89*	82.32 (2.16)	22.24 (8.53)	47.86***	37.81***
Cognition	80.69 (5.94)	82.11 (2.65)	1.44	82.63 (2.22)	12.61 (7.17)	64.13***	5.52**
Behavioral	79.17 (7.49)	81.95 (2.31)	2.57*	82.29 (1.47)	12.99 (6.85)	71.52***	58.5***
Somatic	72.88 (5.67)	73.69 (4.93)	1.06	70.35 (7.39)	25.90 (8.52)	28.88***	4.89**
Anxiety Composite Score	77.65 (5.97)	79.66 (2.25)	2.31*	79.37 (2.21)	18.47 (3.72)	108.89***	6.26**
Depression Score	68.41 (7.36)	68.68 (7.70)	0.62	75.68 (2.65)	23.18 (5.13)	64.84***	32.05***

SD's are given in parentheses
* = $p < .05$ level
** = $p < .01$ level
*** = $p < .001$ level

The significance of differences between means was tested by the t-test; two types of comparisons were made: intra group comparison *i.e.,* pre- *vs.* post-treatment comparison for the control as well as the experimental group, and inter-group comparison *i.e.,* control *vs.* experimental group comparison for the post-treatment condition.

Intra Group Comparisons

For the control group, the pre- *vs.* post-comparisons yielded increase in psycho-physiological parameters of anxiety. The subjects in the control group were therefore not responding to medication.

The pre-post comparison for the experimental group provided statistically significant results for all the psycho-physiological measures *i.e.,* reduction in EMG, blood pressure, all the components of anxiety and depression and increase in alpha EEG thereby revealing clear cut soothing effects of meditation in the experimental group.

Inter Group Comparisons

For the control *vs*. experimental group post-treatment comparisons, the results clearly revealed highly significant and beneficial effect of meditation on physical and mental status of heart patients.

CONCLUSIONS

The practice of meditation for 20 minutes daily for 20 days leads to:

(a) Significant reduction in all components of anxiety, depression, EMG and blood pressure (Systolic and Diastolic).

(b) Significant increase in alpha EEG thereby producing the relaxing and soothing effects on heart patients.

REFERENCES

Billing, E., Lindell, B., Sederhohm, M. and Theorell, T. (1980). "Denial, Anxiety and Depression Following Myocardial Infarction." *Psychosomatics*, 21, 639–645.

Blatt, C.M. (2007). "Anxiety Worsens Prognosis in Patients with Coronary Artery Disease." *Journal of American College of Cardiology,* 49, 2021–2027.

Delmonte, M.; Psychologia (1985). *An International Journal of Psychology in the Orient*, 28(4), 189–202.

Koskal, F. and Power, K. (1990). *Journal of Personality Assessment*, 54, 534–544.

Krug, S.E. and Laughlin, J.E. (1976). *Manual of Depression Inventory*, Institute for Personality and Ability Testing, America.

Lett, H.S., Blumenthal, J.A., Babyak, M.A., Sherwood, A., Strauman, T. and Robins, C. (2004). "Depression as a Risk Factor for Coronary Artery Disease: Evidence, Mechanisms and Treatment." *Psychosomatic Medicine,* 66, 305–315.

Miller, G.E., Freedland, K.E., Carney, R.M., Stetler, C.A. and Banks, W.A. (2003). "Cynical Hostility, Depressive Symptoms and the Expression of Inflammatory Risk Markers for Coronary Heart Disease." *Journal of Behavioral Medicine,* 26, 501–516.

Musselman, D.L. and Nemeroff, C.B. (2000). "Depression Really does Hurt Your Heart: Stress, Depression and Cardiovascular Disease." *Progress in Brain Research,* 122, 43–59.

Pasic, J., Levy, W.C. and Sullivan, M.D. (2003). "Cytokins in Depression and Heart Failure." *Psychosomatic Medicine*, 65, 181–193.

Porter, V. (2003). "Depression and Stress Hit Hard on the Heart." *Medscape Cardiology,* 7(1), 1–6.

Priscilla, S., Paul, E. and Cherian K.M. (2002). "A Psychological Evaluation of Cornary Artery Disease Patients for Life Style Modification: Preventive Cardiology." *Journal of Personality and Clinical Studies,* 18, 73–78.

Raub, J. (2002). *Journal of Alternative Complementary Medicine*, 8(6), 797–812

Seaward, B. (1999). *Managing Stress*. Boston: Jones and Bartlett Publishers, 308–328.

Sehgal, M. (2000). "Anger, Anxiety and Type A Behavior as Determinants of Essential Hypertension and Coronary Heart Disease." *Journal of Indian Academy of Applied Psychology*, 26(1), 33–39.

Singh, L.N. and Choudhary, S.D. (1999). "Replication of Symptom Questionnaire: Indian Standardization Data." *Disabilities and Impairments*, 13(1), 65–72.

Watkins, L.L., Grossman, P., Krishnan, R. and Sherwood, A. (1998). "Anxiety and Vagal Control of Heart Rate." *Psychosomatic Medicine*, 60, 498–502.

Williams, S.A., Kasil, S.V., Heiat, A., Abramson, J.L., Krumholtz, H.M. and Vaccarino, V. (2002). "Depression and Risk of Heart Failure among the Elderly." *Psychosomatic Medicine*, 64, 6–12.

Wulsin, L.R. and Singal, B.M. (2003). "Do Depressive Symptoms Increase the Risk for the Onset of Coronary Disease?" Systemic Quantitative Review. *Psychosomatic Medicine*, 65, 201–21.

Modification of Sitting Posture among Primary School Children

Surila Agarwala[1], Shellyka Ratnakar*[2] and Priyanka[3]

ABSTRACT

The study aimed to modify sitting posture among primary school children. A sample of 50 children with defective sitting posture was taken from primary schools of Agra. The defects observed in these children were: forward neck posture, rounded shoulders, scoliosis, lordosis, kyphosis, tightness of back muscles, and swayback posture. Pre and post design was used. After pre measure of defects, an intervention of one hour per day for fifteen days was given. Modeling technique was used for intervention. Post measure of defects in sitting posture was taken. Results show significant reduction in the identified defects in sitting posture during intervention, in post measure, and in follow-up data.

INTRODUCTION

Posture is a position or attitude of the body, the relative arrangement of body parts for a specific activity, or a characteristic manner of bearing one's body. Posture is a composite of the positions of all the joints of the body at any given moment, and static posture alignment is best described in terms of the positions of the various joints and body segments. Posture is essentially the position of the body in space. Optimal posture is state of muscular and skeletal balance that protects the supporting structures of the body against injury or progressive deformity, whether at work or rest. Correct posture involves the positioning of the joints to provide minimum stress on the joints of the body. Conversely, faulty posture increases stress on the joints and strong muscles can become weak. Poor posture may cause fatigue, muscular stress, compression of blood vessels and pain. In addition, faulty posture can affect the position and function of major organs.

The main types of defects in sitting posture are Scoliosis, Lordosis, Kyphosis, Forward Neck Position, Rounded Shoulder, Tightness of Back Muscles and Slouched Posture.

---

* Corresponding author.

[1] Department of Psychology, Dean, Faculty of Social Sciences, Dayalbagh Educational Institute, Dayalbagh, Agra-282005, India. E-mail: surilaagarwala@gmail.com

[2] Saran Ashram Hospital, Dayalbagh, Agra-282005, India.

[3] Department of Psychology, Faculty of Social Sciences, Dayalbagh Educational Institute, Dayalbagh, Agra-282005, India.

Scoliosis is defined as lateral curvature of spine with fixed rotation of the vertebrae. Lordosis is defined as increase in lumbosacral angle of spine with increase in anterior pelvic tilt. Kyphosis is abnormal posture characterised by increase in thoracic curve accompanying forward head flexion and rounded upper back. Forward Neck Posture is characterised by forward flexion of lower cervical vertebrae and backward flexion of upper cervical vertebrae. Rounded shoulder is characterised by protraction of scapulae accompanying forward head flexion. Tightness of Back Muscles is defined as over-tension of back muscles due to stress and tension. Slouched Posture is also known as swayback and relaxed posture seen in children with weak muscles.

Good posture is a good habit that contributes to the well-being of the individual. The structure and the function of the body provide all the potentialities for attaining and maintaining good posture. Conversely, bad posture is bad habit and unfortunately is of rather high incidence. Postural faults have their origin in the misuse of the capacities provided not in the structure and function of the normal body. Posture is very important both at home and the school. Back-friendly posture is a valuable component of preventing or managing back pain while performing any activity. Incorrect posture while standing for long period of time, sitting in an office chair, and driving are all common causes of back pain. Posture is important for sitting in school chairs and at a work station. Many of us spend hours in front of computers, resulting in back pain or neck pain. Much of this pain may be avoided by combination of adopting a user friendly work station by adjusting the school chairs, computer, and desk positioning. Many people sit towards the front of their chairs and end up hunching forward to look at their computer screen. The better seated posture is to sit back in the chair and utilize the chair's lumber support to keep the head and neck erect. Taking stretch breaks and walking breaks if sitting in school chairs for long periods of time is good.

A biochemically incorrect body position is largely responsible for the adverse effect of prolonged sitting. Poor body position can also originate from an unsuitable study time that requires students to sit continuously for longer than one hour. The duration of sitting, along with the shape of the body in a sitting position is the most critical risk factor in work in a sitting position. A poorly designed or improperly selected chair will resist all attempts to achieve proper posture. An unsuitable workspace that prevents students from sitting in a balanced position can cause poor body position. The workstation may be unsuitable because the chair is too high or low with respect to the table height for a student's body size and shape. Improper or inadequate training can also lead to in-appropriate body positions. Students may be unaware of the health hazards of sitting posture because they are not as apparent as those of physically strenuous tasks. As a result, students may not know which work practices to avoid and which one's to adopt.

For each major body part such as hips, knees, shoulders, elbows and wrists, there are ranges within which every person can find comfortable positions. These positions should not interfere with a person's breathing or blood circulation, impede muscular actions or hinder the normal functions of the internal organs. Varying these positions frequently is the essence of healthy sitting work. Hence, a good sitting position is one that allows students to change their body position frequently and effortlessly when they want without being restricted by the workstation design (Sharan, 2004).

We are not proactive enough at this early stage of our children's formal education in preventing bad posture habit from forming. A lot of our children are sitting at our dining room tables or kitchen tables and are sitting on chairs which are simply not built for children. Most parents have experiences of the constant frustration of trying to get their children to "sit properly at the table". Wrong posture may cause many problems as strain, stress, fatigue etc. (Murphy, 2001). These problems affect the physical health, mental health, quality of work life and academic performance. One problem leads to another problem and the individual faces problem of adjustment in one's personal as well as social and occupational life. Right posture adopted by individual may prevent these problems. Children are the future of society. It is necessary that they should be healthy physically as well as mentally. Hence, early identification of defects in sitting posture and their correction is a great responsibility of psychologists, teachers and parents. The present study is undertaken with an objective to create awareness among parents and teachers that correct sitting posture is extremely important for child's future mental and physical well being and posture defects can be corrected by applying simple behavior modification techniques.

METHOD

Aim

Modification of sitting posture among primary school children.

Sample

The initial sample consisted of 100 children with defective sitting posture taken from primary schools of Agra. Defects in sitting posture were identified with the help of a qualified physiotherapist. Children having any other physiological or psychological disorder have been excluded from the sample. In the final sample, 55 children who had defects in sitting posture were included.

Design

Pre and post design was used.

Tools and Techniques

Observation method and modeling technique have been used. Defects in sitting posture were identified with the help of observation. Modeling technique was used for the correction of these defects.

Procedure

Baseline measure of defects in sitting posture of children was taken with the help of physiotherapist. Observation technique was used to measure defects in sitting posture of children. After establishing baseline, intervention for correction of defects in sitting posture was given with the help of physiotherapist. Modeling Technique was used for intervention. One hour intervention was given daily for fifteen days. After intervention, post measure of defects in sitting posture of children was taken.

Follow-Up

Three follow ups at the time interval of 3 days were done to ascertain the maintenance of gains by intervention.

Analyses of Data and Results

After the post measure of defects analysis of data was done to analyze the effects of intervention on defects in sitting posture among subjects. Table 1 and Figures 1–8 show the number of reduced defects as the results of intervention. The total intervention program was divided into three parts: pre-interventions, intervention and follow up.

Table 1: Children with Defective Sitting Posture

Pre-intervention	*Days*	*FNP*	*RS*	*K*	*S*	*L*	*TBM*	*SBP*	*Total*
		14	*14*	*4*	*2*	*5*	*7*	*9*	*55*
Intervention	1	8	7	4	2	4	7	6	
	2	9	6	4	2	3	5	6	
	3	6	6	3	1	2	5	6	
	4	2	5	2	1	3	5	5	
	5	2	4	2	1	3	4	5	
	6	2	4	2	0	2	3	2	
	7	3	4	1	0	2	3	1	
	8	2	3	3	0	2	2	1	
	9	3	3	1	1	2	4	3	
	10	2	2	1	0	2	4	3	
	11	1	3	0	0	1	2	2	
	12	1	3	0	0	1	1	1	
	13	1	3	0	0	0	0	1	
	14	1	2	1	1	0	1	0	
	15	0	2	0	0	0	0	2	
Post Intervention		0	2	0	0	0	0	2	4
Follow Up		3	2	0	1	2	0	2	10
		3	2	0	1	1	2	2	11
		3	4	1	0	1	1	1	11

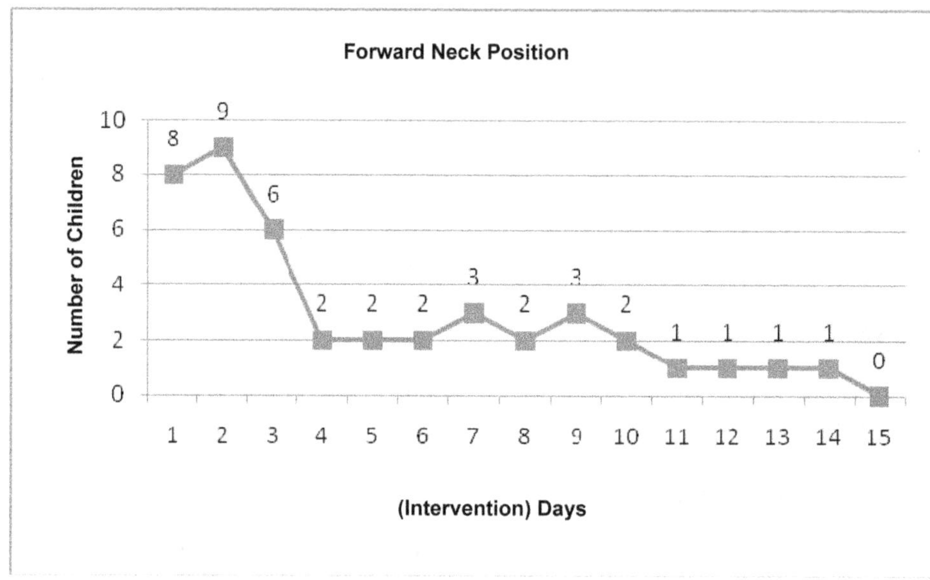

Figure 1: Frequency of Subjects with Forward Neck Posture during Intervention

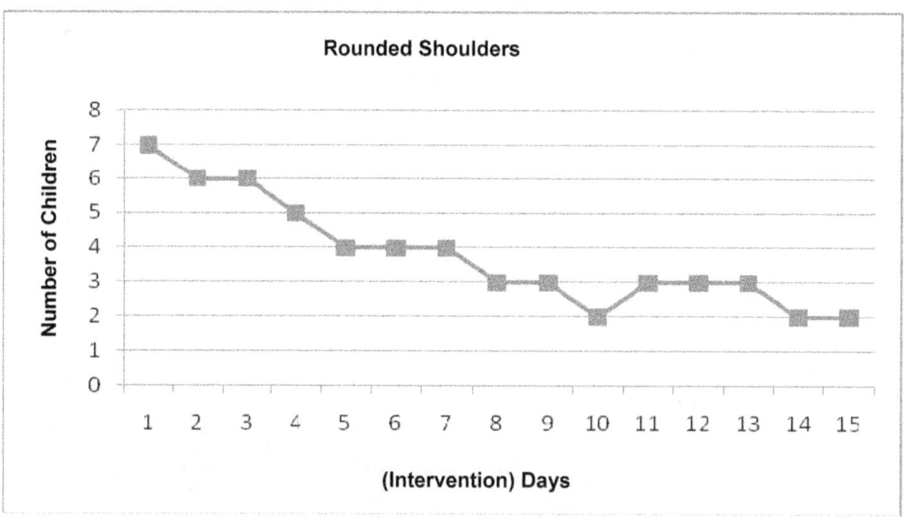

Figure 2: Frequency of Subjects with Rounded Shoulder during Intervention

The Table 1 shows the number of children with various types of defects in sitting posture in pre-intervention measure and reduction in these defects during intervention, in post intervention measure, and during follow ups. It can be further observed from Data Table 1 that 55% students showed defects in sitting posture during pre-intervention measure. Forward neck position and rounded shoulders defects were observed in maximum numbers of students (14%). Next, most common defect in sitting posture is swayback posture found in 9% students and tightness of back muscles was found in 7%

students. Other types of defects in sitting posture were observed in 2–5% students only. It can be further observed from Table 1 that in pre-intervention measure total no. of children with defects in sitting posture is 55 which reduced to 4 in post intervention measure. Moreover, downward trend i.e., reduction can be observed in case of each defect in sitting posture during intervention as well as in post measure.

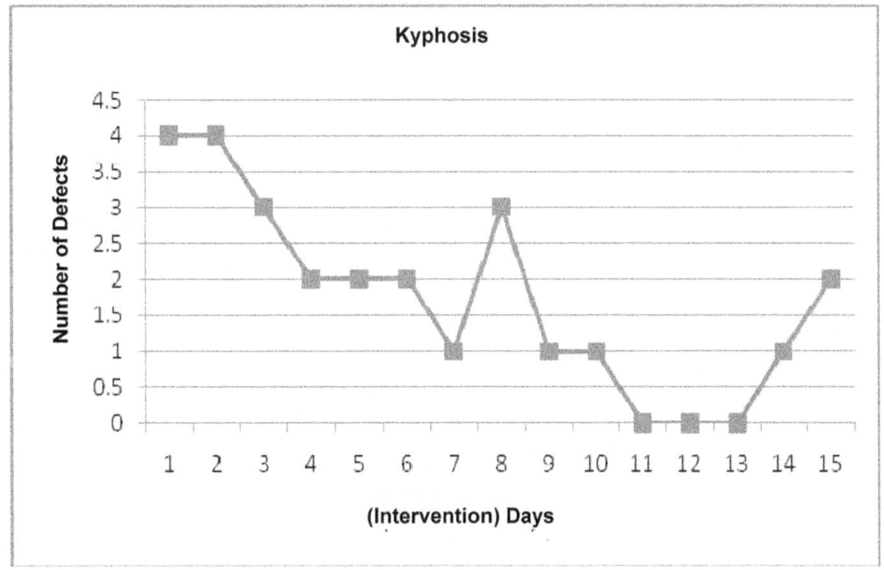

Figure 3: Frequency of Subjects with Kyphosis during Intervention

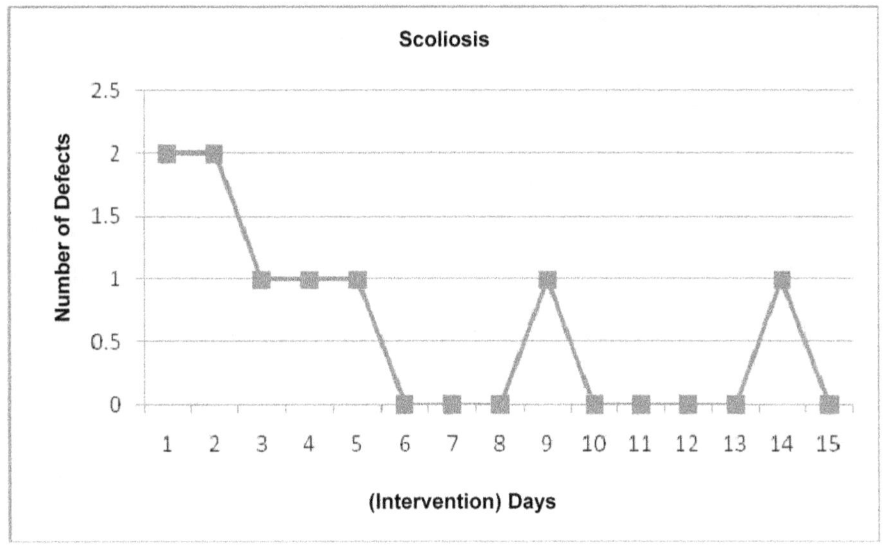

Figure 4: Frequency of Subjects with Scoliosis during Intervention

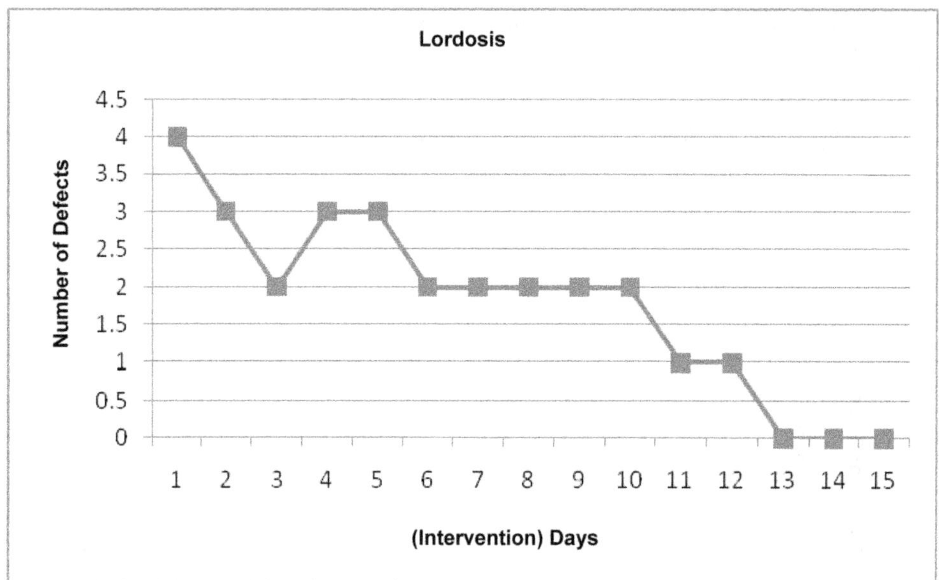

Figure 5: Frequency of Subjects with Lordosis during Intervention

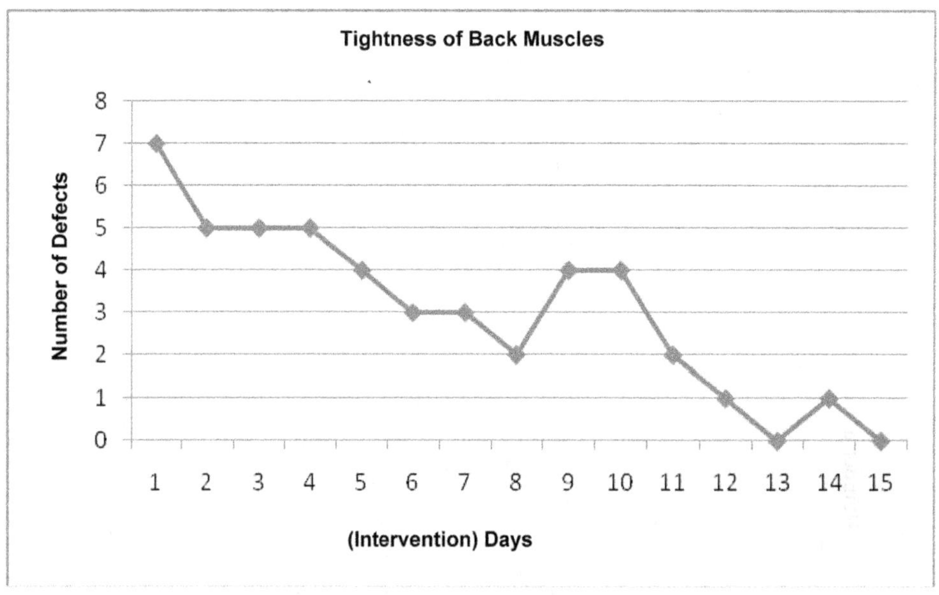

Figure 6: Frequency of Subjects with Tightness of Back Muscles during Intervention

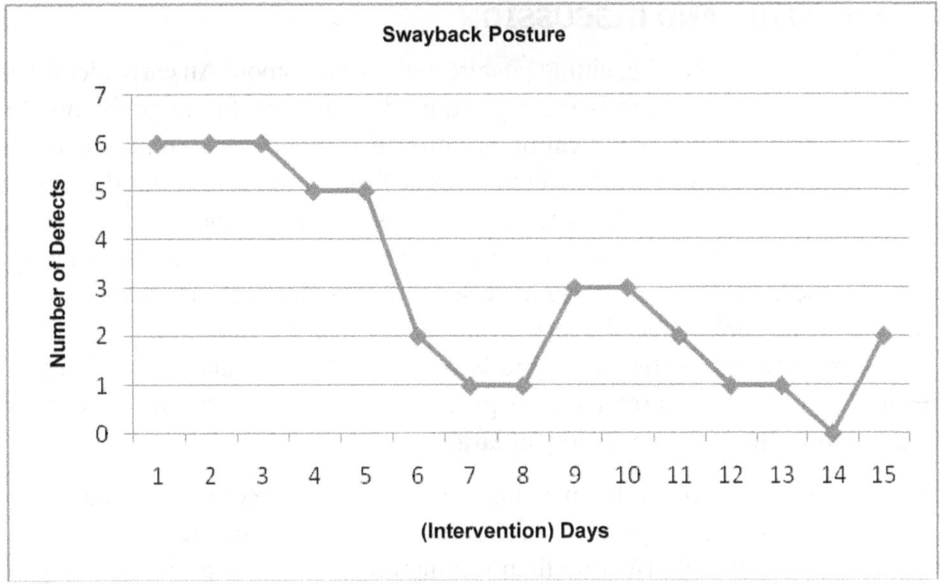

Figure 7: Frequency of Subjects with Swayback Posture during Intervention

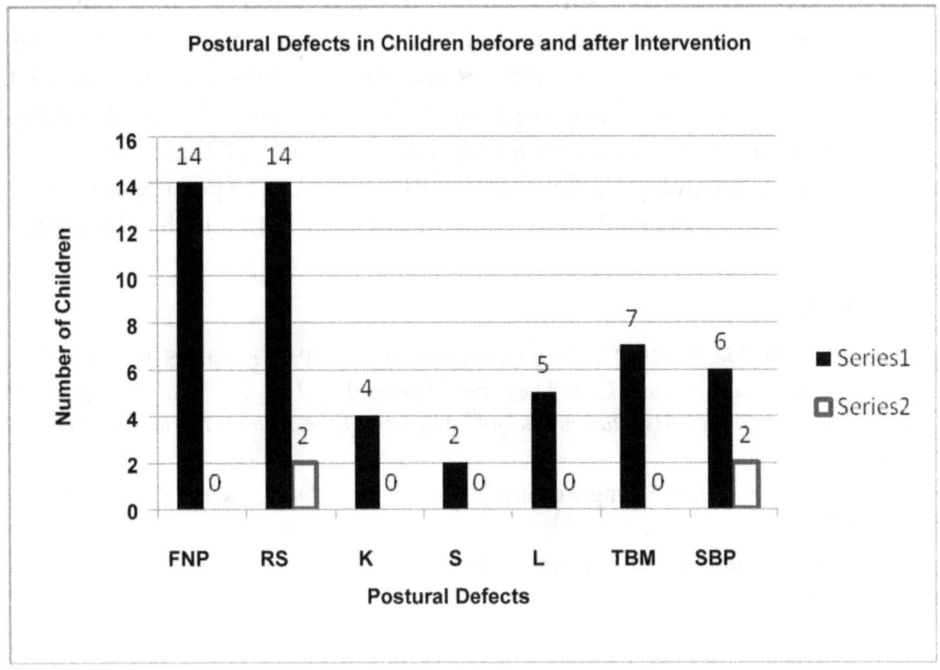

Figure 8: Number of Children having Various Postural Defects before and after Intervention

INTERPRETATION AND DISCUSSION

The study reveals that defects in sitting posture are quite common. An early identification and correction of such defects is greatly required to prevent future problems due to these defects. Psychological intervention has proved to be effective in the modification of defects in sitting posture. In fact, there is very little awareness about the defects in sitting posture and their consequences among most of the people, however educated they are. Through psychological intervention an awareness is created among the students that these defective postures have serious consequences. They are also taught and motivated to correct the defects in sitting posture by modeling of the correct posture. Correct sitting posture is naturally more comfortable and hence there is self motivation also to adopt correct sitting posture. Thus, the results of the study have important implications for the society at large.

Sharan (2004) has pointed out that maintaining balance or correct posture and becoming aware of body position irrespective of where one is sitting and for what purpose is much more important and effective than relying on furniture to do it. He has given a tip of the day, "recruit for work place neighbour as your posture consultant. Ask him or her to let you know when you slouch. Do this each for each other till maintaining good posture becomes a habit." Sitting jobs require less muscular effort, but that does not exempt people in desk jobs from the injury risks. Various studies have shown that 25%–75% of clerks, assembly-line workers and the data entry operators suffer from back and neck pain. Students have to sit for studies for long and they also complain of stiffness of neck, back etc. Considering the seriousness of these problems, it is imperative to create an awareness for the need of correct sitting posture among people and the results of the present study have a significant contribution in this direction.

REFERENCES

Murphy, S.D. and Buckle, P. (2001). "The Occurance of Back Pain among School Children and the Risk Factors in Schools: Can They be Measured?" *The Triennial Congress of the International Ergonomics Association and 44th Meeting of the Human Factors and Ergonomic Society*, 549–552.

Sharan, D. (2004). "Balanced Sitting Posture." *The Times of India,* Retrievd from http://www.thetimesofindia.com.

Sharan, D. (2004). "How to Sit Properly." *The Times of India,* Retrievd from http://www.thetimesofindia.com.

Be Aware! Complete Awareness is the Beginning of Fulfilling Your *Dharma*

Miodrag B. Milovanovic*

ABSTRACT

One of the basic principles in the Gestalt therapy is Arnold R. Beisser's (1971) "The Paradoxical Theory of Changes": He says, "The change comes out when someone accepts himself that he/she is, not when he/she tries to be someone that he/she is not". That means that the human being has to become completely aware about him/her self in the beginning, in order to change and overcome his/her problems. In other words, awareness is used to restore awareness, and this restoration can be facilitated by establishing a dialogic context. Awareness techniques teach clients how to correct their interrupted contacting. Healing and growing through the restoration of the awareness are an expression of the transcendental possibilities of human existence. The paper deals with the implications of Gestalt therapy and the author has provided demonstrative example using Gestalt therapy.

INTRODUCTION

In this text, the author would like to share with the readers his point of view of awareness and its place in yoga and psychotheapy, especially in Gestalt therapy. Gestalt therapy is one of the most popular psychotherapy approaches in the western world nowadays. *Das Gestalten* is a German word. It is sometimes translated as "shape, form or figure", but it is defined also as interaction of the particles opposite to the amount of the component part". It can not be simply translated, so the same word has been used in all other languages all over the world. Gestalt therapy is used in a variety of situations, with multiple aims: individual, couple, group, in business, within different organizations, etc.

Gestalt therapy was developed by Friedrich (Fritz) Pearls. His first book: *Ego, Hunger and Aggression* was published in South Africa in 1942, and the first edition was sub-titled: "A Revision of Freud's Theory". The birth of Gestalt therapy represents Pearls's book *Gestalt Therapy* published in 1951. In the beginning, genious Pearls in his therapeutic approach, used the term: 'Concentracion Therapy'. The aim was to reach again—the feeling of oneself. He used to say: "I invented nothing, all I did, was rediscover what was always there".

---

*General Hospital, Prijedor, Republic of Srpska. E-mail: mmichael@spinter.net

The role of awareness is at the central position (some Gestalt therapists use the word contact instead of awareness) in the Gestalt therapy approach. In fact, it is difficult to discuss Gestalt therapy without discussing awareness. Awareness, or global consciousness, in Gestalt therapy approach means that the therapist has to be constantly aware of the complete figure and background, as well as complete external and internal processes between him and the client. In addition, he uses all possible interventions to make the unconscious clients processes—conscious in the inter-subjective therapeutic field. In fact, basic contact and full awareness processes are preconditions for any dialog and intervention.

One of the basic principles in the Gestalt therapy is Arnold R. Beisser's (1971) "The Paradoxical Theory of Changes": He says, "The change comes out when someone accepts himself that he/she is, not when he/she tries to be someone that he/she is not". That means that the human being has to become completely aware about him/her self in the beginning, in order to change and overcome his/her problems. In other words, awareness is used to restore awareness, and this restoration can be facilitated by establishing a dialogic context. In this reference, contact can be used to restore contact. Awareness techniques teach clients how to correct their interrupted contacting. Healing and growing through the restoration of the awareness are an expression of the transcendental possibilities of human existence.

Very often sentence in the Gestalt therapy work may include: "I am now aware of …" the client may be often asked to complete such sentences. Gestalt therapists often ask questions like: What are you doing now? … What are you feeling now? … What do you want now? … What do you avoid now? … What do you expect now? … so on. One of the reasons for asking such questions is that the process in Gestalt therapy is similar to the peeling off the onion. In this way, the therapist helps the client to enlarge his own consciousness, there and then. That's why Gestalt therapy is also known as "now therapy".

In fact, Pearls believes that a Gestalt therapist does not use any technique. A Gestalt therapist applies whatever professional skill and life experience he has accumulated and integrated to a situation. Therefore, there are as many styles in Gestalt therapy as there are therapists and clients. They discover each other and together build their relationship.

The great leader *Mahatma Gandhi* has aptly said:

"Be that alteration that you want to see..."

These days, we witness that most of the western people are trying very hard to be conscious through some kind of body relaxation. In order to be relaxed, they are doing different relaxation activities, for example exercise, listening to some soothing music or visiting different places to enjoy the nature. Yet they are constantly in tension. A consequence thereof, that they are not at all aware of their real self. The minds are wondering in the expectation of some miracle to take place. The strongest enemies of most of the western men are—pride and greed. They are so egoistic, proud and material oriented that they think that the highest aim in the life is to be "Mr. Dollar". So, we have to look again towards the wisdom of Yoga, and regain awareness of self.

But, to become a completely new, well aware person who is living in "here and now", can not be an automatic process. There is a way of the renunciation, and happiness leading to good health. According to World Health Organization, "Health is not the absence of illness or of infirmity, but as a state of complete physical, mental and social well-being....." To reach a state of new awareness, it is necessary for a person to be free of emotions, expectations and self. It is necessary for the person to be aware of "here and now", who he is, what he thinks, what he feels, what he wants, what he is doing, what he is avoiding, and what he expects.

There are a lot of different projecting techniques, and one of the most valuable in Gestalt therapy is a process leading to imagination. It is called as—an experiment.

(The following Experiment was conducted by the author/therapist with a client) "The rose bush": Please, sit comfortably, and relax yourself. … Slowly and gently close your eyes, and please don't open it until you are told to do so. … Relax yourself. ... Feel your body. ... from the top of your head to your toes. ... Relax, ... relax, ... relax. ... Now, imagine ... that you are—*a rose bush*. ... Be aware of the shape, ... be aware of the type, ... and be aware of the sort of rose. ... You are a rose bush. ... Be aware: what is the ground under you? ... Is it wet, or is it dry? ... Is it hard or is it soft? ... Be aware: do you have one trunk, two, three, or you have a lot of them? ... Be aware: how tall are you, ... Do you have any flower? ... If you do, ... what is the colour of the flower/ flowers? ... Are there big or small flowers? ... Be aware of your leaves. ... Now, be completely aware of your surroundings. ... Where is this rose bush growing? ... How do you like being in this surrounding? ... Now, move your rose bush. ... Go directly to the top of the mountain. ... How do you feel living there? ... And now, ... go to the valley, ... there is the small river running through this valley. There are a lot of trees around you. ... How do you like being here? ... And now, ... go to your favourite place! ... Be aware: what is that—to make this place your favourite? ... How do you like being here? ... Now, it is winter. ... It is very cold winter, it's snowing. ... How do you feel? ... Slowly, a spring is coming. ... It is hot, and it starts raining. ... How do you feel now? ... And than, it becomes more and more hot, and there is less rain, ... summer is coming. ... How do you feel? ... Now, the temperature is slowly going down, and there are rains again. It is autumn. ... How do you feel? ... Be aware: what is the season that you like best? ... Be again in that sesaon. ... What is that you like in your favourite season? ... Enjoy in that season. ... And now, I want you to be aware: how do you like being a rose bush? ... Be aware of the good and the bad points. ...

And now, slowly, I want you to separate from your rose bush . ... Get out of the role of the rose bush ... and become again yourself. ... Your rose bush is behind you. ... Turn around, and look at the rose bush once more, and—be aware what do you feel for this rose bush. ... Come closer to it! ... If you want to do something—do it now, ... and then, say: good bye to the rose bush, ... turn around slowly again, ... leave the rose bush, ... and ... when you are ready ... slowly, ... come back to *here and now*, ... be again yourelf—at this place and this time, ... here and now ... and slowly, ... when you are ready ... open your eyes.

This kind of the projecting experiment can be very useful for making the client aware of his impasses, fears, and the unconscious borders which the client develops towards the whole external world. In conclusion, a correlation between Gestalt therapy and the yoga way of overcoming the problem will help in achieving the state of awareness.

Every individual has his own *dharma*. During the life span if the man protects his dharma, the dharma will also protect him. If the man does not protect his dharma, the dharma will not be in possibility to protect him. He will then be left to his karma. So, the process of reaching the complete awareness is the beginning of man's magnificent journey of fulfilling his own dharma. There are a number of old yogic stories which are suggestive of the above-stated fact.

Expressive Arts Therapy: Does it Matter? Art and Therapy: The Best of Both Worlds

Ralitza M. Vladimirov*

ABSTRACT

Art is the universal language, which opens the multicultural borders of this world, which awakens the spiritual force within the human kind, allowing in, the most natural way of mental, emotional, and spiritual expression. It holds on a mystery where the conscious and subconscious parts of the self meet in the perfect place, moment and time; achieving stages of awareness and fulfillment. Where is Art placed? Is it towards the being or doing? This is probably one of the most contrast differences between the Eastern and Western way of experiencing life. The paper deals with the 5 major forms of art: Music, Dance-Movement, Drama, Art and Poetry. Today, numerous possibilities of expressing thoughts, emotions, and feelings through these forms of art are becoming powerful ways of affecting the physical, mental, emotional, and spiritual self by effecting levels of healing. It is not about adapting or becoming part of the art; instead, the expressive art therapists seek to help the patient to live more creatively. The uniqueness of the creative process facilitates new levels of self-integration allowing an outstanding diagnostic and therapeutic technique to look at the human being as "a spirit having human experience, not as human being having a spiritual experience". Thus, it facilitates in discovering the multi-dimensional reality of the individual consciousness and sub-consciousness.

INTRODUCTION

Art is the universal language, which opens the multicultural borders of this world, which awakens the spiritual force within the human kind, allowing in, the most natural way of mental, emotional, and spiritual expression. It holds on a mystery where the conscious and subconscious parts of the self meet in the perfect place, moment and time; achieving stages of awareness and fulfillment.

Where is Art placed? Is it towards the being or doing? This is probably one of the most contrast differences between the Eastern and Western way of experiencing Life. In the process of art making, we allow ourselves to merge within and without, giving not taking; forming a continuous dance on the stage of realization of who we are and who we would like to become.

The 5 major forms of art are Music, Dance-Movement, Drama, Art and Poetry. Numerous possibilities of expressing thoughts, emotions, and feelings through these

*Lesley University, Harvard, Boston, USA. E-mail: tzgallery@yahoo.com

forms of art are becoming powerful ways of affecting the physical, mental, emotional, and spiritual self by effecting levels of healing. It is not about adapting or becoming part of the art; instead, the expressive art therapists seek to help the patient to live more creatively. The uniqueness of the creative process facilitates new levels of self-integration allowing an outstanding diagnostic and therapeutic technique to look at the human being as "a spirit having human experience, not as human being having a spiritual experience". Thus, it facilitates in discovering the multi-dimensional reality of the individual consciousness and sub-consciousness.

One of the fundamental differences between art psychotherapy and the traditional psychotherapy is the limitations in the verbal way of expression: possibilities in verbal manipulation, reflecting printed models of thinking. The hidden and subconscious parts of the individual come naturally through the performed method of creativity, where verbalization is not necessary. Some times even processing and verbalization is "Let go" due to its decreasing power in relation to the experience.

Art therapy is performed by using methods of fine and visual art (painting, drawing, sculpting, and many other techniques using alternative materials provoked by the physical reality). In the early 20th century, Carl Jung/Sigmund Freud ascribed the ability of the visual images to reflect patient's subconscious state. Initially, *Art therapy* was considered the integration of art and therapy in the Western world. What becomes essential in the analysis is not the final materialized object but the process itself. This is where the "active imagination" unfolds and lays out new sensations, emotions, feelings, and associations. Symbolism and metaphor become a way of expressing the inexpressible and transforming the impossible into possible. The materials used have their specific power and become the channels through which the creative energy opens the expressive flow. Composition, line, shapes and forms, texture, space and integration within an artwork become the observed and analyzed existence in understanding the individual.

On other side, *Dance-movement therapy* proposes that the physical body is the outer image of the inner self, emotional, mental, and spiritual, the existence of links and connections between thoughts-emotions-actions. The sensual rhythmic response aroused by dance and music may be used as ways of bypassing the conscious mind and making contact with the inner emotional world. To do this, patients explore a range of movements and learn to overcome physical limitations and cope up with their disabilities. Mirroring, authentic movement, creative movement, bouncing, etc. facilitates in both one-to-one and group sessions. The physical body and its language are perceived to be an outer expression of the inner level of being and disharmony.

Music therapy offers deepest soulful connection and becomes the most powerful of all arts. It is a powerful alternative to verbal communication. It enables the expression of emotions that may be too profound or primitive for words. Variety of techniques can be used ranging from listening, making music through different instruments, voice sounding, singing, and improvising. Facilitating conditions in which an individual to go through self-toning and resonating with their spiritual identity. This experience never repeats every time but has a new and unique universal meaning.

Drama therapy includes the use of drama techniques as a way of facilitating self-expression, developing self-awareness: inside and outside of the patient, such as psychodrama, role-playing, "improve" creative drama, imaginary theater, story-telling, performance, etc. with no limitation. In the center of drama therapy, we witness "in action" the inner dynamics, which is powerful in realizing the multi dimensional perspective of life experiences. Here the duality of existence can also be underlined.

The integration of the arts and merging their healing power without separating them creates completeness and wholeness, something that are essential in the changes that require new ways of feeling, thinking and acting.

According to Beinsa Duno

"Art is one of the most powerful and unique ways
for self-realization and spiritual growth"

"Silent Walk"

Look up in walk and sleep
Even if you fall…lose yourself
Because, everything is perfect in its imperfection
Be tender as the clouds move in their dancing stillness.
Speak in silence and let the silence speak to you, to the world.
Wonder floating.
Breathe in every little piece of air,
Embrace the moments to come and be.
Just be…just be in your endless spirit…
Let the magic opens its doors
And enter with peace and joy
Because, fear does not exist in the heart of eternity
Just be…just be in your endless spirit…
In every little corner beauty is waiting to unfold,
Caring hope, belief and green…
Undress the impurity of your self
And let the naked truth come out in love…
Just be…just be in the mystery of the spirit.

Systemic Constellations

Stefan Reiter*

ABSTRACT

Systemic Constellation work is a relatively new discipline. Although many aspects are included in other therapeutic approaches, the method of working with constellations embodies some essential differences. A system is a number of elements that are connected to one another in continuously changing relationships. With any change in one of the element there is a simultaneous change in all the other elements. The unconscious is not only in, but rather between individuals. Within a system, we are all connected to one another. The whole is more than the sum of its parts. In systemic constellation the goal is not to uncover the myriad of connections in systems, but rather to look for the most powerful entanglements which maybe hindering the client and restricting his strength. With an 'inner' request we start the constellation work. We don't use the members of the system; we work mostly with representatives for only the necessary members or structures. The representatives are aware of feelings and relationships and body postures of someone they don't know and still they don't give any information. The client places all of them in the same room, one by one the client touch them and give them a position from his inner feeling and an inner collectedness. The energies in the field (constellation) guide the representatives, taking over and causing reactions which are often surprising and inexplicable. All of them are tuning in and get in resonate of so-called morphogenetic (gestalt forming) field. We recognized that the personal conscience and the collective conscience are energies of self regulation and healing forces. In systemic constellation we are looking for different dynamics and a right intervention for a 'movement of the soul'.

INTRODUCTION

Systemic constellation work is a relatively new discipline. The method of working with systemic constellations embodies some essential differences with other therapeutic approaches. It is based on family therapy. 50 years ago therapists' discovered that illness symptoms especially in children are deeply connected with the family situation or imbalance between the parents or the grandparents.

After 1980 a German priest and therapist Bert Hellinger, who works with Gestalt therapy and NLP (Neuro-Linguistic Programming) developed in depth the constellation work. In 1993 he published *Love's Hidden Symmetries* and *Love's own Truth* and got a breakthrough in the worldwide therapy scene. In a constellation, the goal is not to uncover the myriad of connections in the family, but rather to look for the most powerful entanglements which may be hindering the client and restricting his strength.

---

*Naturopath specialist in Craniosacral Osteopathy Constellation Work, Kathmandu, Nepal. E-mail: systemicstefan@yahoo.com

In constellation work we don't work with the real family members, mostly one member comes with a special issue. In individual sessions certain steps are undertaken; which are mostly useful as a preparation for a later constellation work in a group. In a seminar we work with representatives, which the client chooses for himself and the necessary family members as the representatives. The representatives are aware of the feelings and relationships and body postures of someone they don't know and still they don't get any information. The client places all of them in the same room. One by one the client touches them and gives them a position according to his inner feelings and inner collectedness. The energies in the field (constellation) guide the representatives, taking over and causing reactions which are often surprising and inexplicable.

In many therapeutic approaches, particularly in humanistic psychology, each encounter between therapist and client is a new and idiosyncratic meeting. The therapist responds directly and spontaneously to each situation based on inner collectedness, mindfulness, centeredness and without any intentions! Staying in the moment, we called it—proceeding phenomenological. We open the field, hold the energy, invite the authentic movement of the soul, listening and observing, following the inner guidance of the systemic constellation.

The representatives are very helpful, because they can speak, feel and move and if the process goes on well then all of them are in resonance. Rupert Sheldrake (engl. biologist) writes of morphogenetic (gestalt forming) fields which rigidify over time. The process is like flowing energy. if it comes to an end; it means the energy is much focused and powerful, where an independent inner growth will go on. It is often that the client has an unconsciousness inner image of his family, some stuck and stagnated movements, some take over feelings, patterns or unreleased emotions or responsibilities. Through the constellation work the image will be changed and transformed to a powerful and authentic picture.

Imbalance will usually be redressed by a member of a later generation in the family. When one member has been unjustly excluded, someone else later will assume that fate and live a similar life. When a member doesn't accept personal responsibility, or represses their feelings, then a member of a later generation will take over and express those feelings rather than his own.

Over the years through systemic constellations work the author has recognized some basic principles like natural orders or Orders of Love:

- Every member of a family belongs equally to the family and is respected in the same way.
- Whoever comes first is in the first place, and the other follows in order. An older sister comes before his younger siblings. A first wife comes before a second. Each person is respected equally.

- Each member of the family has his own fate. Each person has to carry his fate completely and also has to carry personal responsibility.

Another point is to look for the balance between:

- Giving and Taking
- Membership (respect, appreciation, be valuable), the need to belong
- Connected relationships (authentic feelings, unconditional love, order).

In constellation work the author recognizes that the personal conscience and the collective conscience are energies of self regulation and healing forces. Still above this the author recognizes a conscience of a "Greater Whole."

There are many paths of the truth. It is quite remarkable that there are so many composers, and none have discovered the same melody as the others. Each person has an individual insight, each melody is different, and each is beautiful in its own way.

With systemic constellation work the therapists' can look into different systems:

- Individual constellations or couple constellations or family constellations.
- Constellations of organizations or companies.
- Constellations of feelings, personal characteristics, objects, structures.

Last but not the least the author looks for the different dynamics in constellations and tune in, what is the right intervention for a movement of the soul.

BASIS

Every craft has an underlying foundation and basic approach. A carpenter has to have respect for his wood as a living material, and only with this attitude can he put his tools to work smoothly and appropriately. In addressing the art of family constellation, it is also necessary to look first at the underlying foundations of the work. Without such a foundation, the practice of the work is limited and quickly becomes mechanical. Based on a solid foundation, it can unfold and continue to develop.

Despite the different orientations, the various forms of effective therapy have a lot in common. For example, in every therapeutic approach, good contact with the client is necessary for the therapy to have a positive effect. It is also true that in every therapy the therapist's own blind spot will have a negative influence on the whole processes. There are many important aspects of the family constellation work which are also meaningful in other therapies. Yet, there are two cornerstones of the family constellation work which set it apart from other therapies. The first is the concept of the 'in forming field' and the other is the basic 'phenomenological' stance.

Before addressing these issues, for those who are new to this work, a brief outline of the structure of a family constellation workshop is outlined below:

Structure of a Family Constellation

The open workshops are offered for participants who are interested in setting up a constellation of their own family. For most part, they come alone, as it isn't necessary to have other members of the family present for this work. Sometimes a participant will be accompanied by a brother or sister, or a parent will come with a child, or a couple may come together. A workshop normally runs for two to five days, which is sufficient to allow each participant to do a family constellation. There are basically two possible constellations for each person: the family of origin, or the present family, including partners and children.

The practical course of events is as follows: The person doing the constellation chooses a representative for each important member of his or her family, including a representative for him-or herself. Without any prior plan, and without speaking or explaining, the client then places the representatives in a spatial relationship to one another, showing them which direction to face, but nothing more. When all the representatives have been placed, the client is again seated and remains a spectator from this point on, observing the action and words of the course leader and the representatives. The course leader asks the representatives to pay attention to the impact of their positions on their feelings, thoughts or sensory awareness. After a short while, the course leader asks each representative for a report of their experience. Tensions in the family are revealed through the reports of the representatives. The leader then searches for a resolution for this individual family, with continual feedback from the representatives as things change in the constellation. These resolutions seem to reflect certain order, or patterns, which Bert Hellinger has documented over many years with this work. There are specific sentences, reflecting these patterns, which have proven helpful in the resolution of entangled family situations. A constellation normally takes between 20 and 45 minutes, although it may be longer or shorter than this.

In constellation involving the family of origin, the goal is not to uncover the myriad of connections in the family, but rather to look for the most powerful entanglements which may be hindering the client and restricting his or her strength. Especially significant are the connections with those in the family who have died early, or those who have been shut out of the family in some way.

In a constellation involving the present family, the aim is to assure the place for former partners and to clarify the relation of two primary partners to each other and to their children.

Often, there is a particular placement which seems to put everything in order where all the representatives feel at ease. The constellation can end at this point. The client takes in this new image, often by standing in the constellation in place of his or her representative.

THE IN-FORMING FIELD

In constellations we are confronted with the phenomenon of representatives having access to knowledge or awareness that actually belongs to the people they are representing. In other words, the representatives are aware of feelings and relationships of someone they don't know. Without this key concept as an underlying assumption of the work, a family constellation would be inconceivable. An example is demonstrated below:

> "The client is taking a family constellation because he feels unsure of himself in his role as a man. From the five male participants in the workshop, he chooses one for his father, and one for himself. He then chooses a woman to a place within the working space.
>
> He places his father's representative facing away from the others. Upon being asked, this representative reports feeling weak and drawn away from the family. In response to the therapist's questions, the client reveals that his father's brother was killed in the war. When a representative is added for his dead uncle, the father's representative beams at him happily and feels drawn towards him. The son's representative is also happy and relieved to see his dead uncle."

Anyone taking part in a constellation for the first time can only marvel at what happens. How can a representative experience such sensations and reactions? Can it possibly be real? Is it perhaps, just the representative's imaginations? However, what the representative's feel is not always lovable, nor is it ever possible to predict in advance.

Yet, clients have repeatedly affirmed that what representatives express is, in fact, really true. What we hear over and over again is, "That's exactly the way things are in my family." Occasionally, a representative even uses exactly the same words typical of that family member, or adopts the same posture or gesture, or exhibits symptoms of the person's illness. These things occur although the representatives have no information about the person they are representing.

The placement in the constellation seems to have a power of its own, so that anyone who stands in that place has a similar reaction. When something unexpected is said, generally the other representatives in the constellation do not find it unusual, or react with any surprise. The comments seem to be appropriate to those within the constellation.

This phenomenon appears in every constellation and has been described as a "field of wisdom" by Albrecht Mahr (1998). Bertold Ulsamer has chosen to call this the "in-forming field" because it is the field which forms the connection and also reveals the form and dynamics of the system, i.e. it forms and informs as well. It is which connects the representatives to the people they represent and which broadens to include all those present during the constellation. Through this phenomenon, the conflict within a family come to light and resolution may be found. Rupert Sheldarke speaks about morphogenetic fields as a biologist.

Other therapeutic approaches have also come to the conclusion that family members absorb certain energy from their own families. The effects of fateful events in a family can extend over generations, even if the children have no knowledge of these things. This is astounding but not as astonishing as what happens in a family constellation workshop, when complete strangers, within a very short period of time, come to know things that are known only to the real family members, who are elsewhere. Anyone who wishes to assess this work critically has to confront the occurrence of this phenomenon.

Some common questions asked are:

Is it Necessary for a Constellation Leader to have any Particular Personal Capability?

Probably everyone who has ever done a constellation had doubts prior to begin the first one, about whether they could do this work, thinking perhaps that the in-forming field is dependent upon certain personal abilities or special inner power.

Soon you discover that the in-forming field emerges independently of any particular person. The therapist, however, require a certain concentration or inner calm, which is often described as "being collected". The leader of constellation work must create a space within which this collectedness is possible.

Is There Some Particular Procedure, which acts as a Stimulator for this Field?

As a rule, the client chooses representatives for family members and leads them to a position in the constellation area, touching them physically on the arm or shoulder. Is this perhaps the action required to activate the field? No, the client chooses representatives for the core members of the family, the parents and children. Later, if other representatives are needed, the therapist adds himself. For example, when an uncle who died young is needed, it is quiet sufficient for the therapist to choose a representative, give him a place in the constellation and say, "You are the mother's brother who died young. Feel your way into the position." Suddenly, he gains access to feelings in this role. The mother's representative and others in the constellation also react directly to this new person.

Is There a Basic Methodology Necessary for a Constellation?

Family constellation is within a minimum of information, as opposed to methods such as psychodrama or family sculptures. This is why the reactions and the awareness of the representatives are particularly clear and visible. But the field also has an effect in other areas and other connections which are less noticeable.

What Does the Field Show? The Truth?

The representatives give information about their inner state and whatever they notice about their relationships to the other family members. They often have an urge to change their position in the constellation, for example.

Constellations are an appropriate source of establishing facts about reality. For example a report of a participant goes like this:

> "According to a woman's report, her first constellation had revealed that her mother's husband, whom she had regarded as her father, was not her biological father. Her representative in the constellation had experienced no connecting to her father. An additional representative was added for a possible father, and the child and the new man felt a great love for each other. The woman didn't leave the results of the constellation at that. Her father was still living, and she asked him to have a blood test to determine paternity. The surprising result was that he was indeed her father, but confessed to her that her mother had many lovers before her pregnancy and, in fact, he had always had some doubt about his own paternity."

Constellations merely shows energies which exist in a family. It is tempting to draw conclusions about facts in the family from what appears in the constellations, but the therapist and the client are treading on thin ice in such an attempt. A constellation can never serve a reliable test of paternity, for example. Someone who needs to be certain about fatherhood will have to undergo a medical test.

It is essential to distinguish between facts and constellation energies. In this regard, another example is given herewith:

> In the constellation, a participant had a clear feeling of having been abused by her father. The father's representative concurred. After the constellation, however, the woman, herself, denied any truth in this. Two weeks later, a phone call from the woman came, who had visited her sister and described what had happened in the constellation. Her sister burst into tears and admitted that she, in fact, had been sexually abused by their father.

This reflects that there was energy of abuse in the family. In the constellation, the wrong person noticed the energy, namely the sister who had not been abused. A constellation brings us into contact with a deeper level of forces at work in the hidden reality of a family.

Are the Representatives Playing Roles, Like Actors?

The answer is yes and no. No, because the representatives are not "playing." This is different from an actor who is performing a predetermined role. The energies in the field guide the representative, taking over and causing reactions which are often surprising and inexplicable, even for the representatives themselves.

The answer is yes, in the sense that the representatives experience their actions as those of a stranger whose place they are taking for the duration of the constellation. The representatives experience this as a role in so far as they, like actor, continue to be aware of their own thoughts and feelings, parallel to those of the person represented. For example, the representative may be in touch with his or her own doubts, objections, agreement, etc.

Does the Client have to be Present in Order for the Field to have an Effect?

No. Therapists can set up a constellation in supervision group for the family of a client without the client being present. The room fills up with the same powerful intensity that occurs when client setup his own constellations.

Does a Constellation Represent a Particular Situation or Particular Period of Time?

Constellations are basically timeless. What is experienced while standing in a particular place in a constellation, has nothing to do with a particular period of time, but rather, with a basic inner image. If you attach a particular period of time, you're not touching the absolution depths possible in a constellation.

A client described the situation and was ready to set up a constellation, and then suddenly asked, "should I set it up as it is now, or as it was back then?" Hellinger broke off the whole procedure at that point, because the client did not yet have the collectedness necessary for the work.

Does this Field have an Effect only in Constellation of Families and People?

No. The field is not limited to the family. In constellations of organizations, individuals or even departments can be represented. The representatives' awareness reflects the situation of those affected in the organization. Additionally, the field has effects in many other kinds of constellations.

Actor and acting coach Johannes Galli develops a typology for actors consisting of seven negative character types which he calls, 'slowpoke' or 'slowcoach', 'wow', 'sharp-tongue', 'swank', 'slut', 'skinflint', and 'nobody'. Although he is not familiar with family constellation, he uses these characteristics as advisors. When some one is stuck with problem, he chooses a representative for each of these characteristics and places them in a certain order next to each other in two rows. Then they are asked for advice, and each answers spontaneously according to his role. It is quite amazing how different the answers are, depending on who asks the questions.

In actual practice, abstract concepts such as 'home' or 'death' or even objects can be represented in a constellation. The individual representatives always have clear, sometimes very strong feelings.

The client describes her fear of becoming drug dependent. Constellation is set up for her and drugs [for whom the client choose a female representative]. The woman is looking straight ahead, and the representative for the drugs is standing behind her. Both of them are asked to pay attention to any impulses they feel from within, and to follow these impulses without speaking. Both stand motionless for a minute, then the woman turns around slowly. The representative for the drugs gazes at her lovingly and opens her arms. The woman closes her eyes and moves into an embrace, where she remains for a long, long time. This provided a glance into the depths at a level underlying her fear of drugs. The field includes much more than just what we see in a family constellation. It is on which all kinds of constellations rest.

Guidance from the In-Forming Field: "Movements of the Soul"

The therapist normally takes an active role in a family constellation, although a resolution comes from the representatives.

In the final image of a constellation, a son is standing in front of his father. The therapist suggests a resolving sentence for him to say, as well as an accompanying bowing down before his father. The son's representative expresses a need to bow down all the way to the floor. As he does this, the tension which has been present in the relationship between the son and his father dissolves.

Hellinger has begun to develop a form of constellation which reduces the intervention of the therapist to a minimum. He calls this process "movement of the soul." When the client has chosen and set up the representatives, the therapist simply instructs them to follow their way into their parts and notice any impulses towards movement. They are to follow these movements without speaking. The therapist remains watchful at the edge of the constellation, mostly without intervening. When it seems appropriate, the therapist stops constellation and releases the representatives from their roles.

> "The client had a difficult relationship with her mother. She placed the representatives for herself and her mother far apart, facing in opposite directions. The two representatives stood still for almost two minutes before the first tentative movements began. Then, the mother turned around slowly and looked at her daughter. Another minute passed before the daughter cautiously turned around. The daughter took a few steps towards her mother, slowly and hesitantly. The mother also moved a step towards her daughter. Eventually they stood facing each other and looked at each other for the first time. Then, the daughter moved to her mother, who opened her arms to embrace her child."

Systemic Constellation also works in single session. Then instead of representatives the client chooses pillows in different colors or different gems or even different chapels.

For example:

A 14-year old boy, bedwetting since early childhood, tried a lot of therapies without success. The boy was offered by the author to do a constellation work to find out any deeper dynamics. The mother and he agreed. In the session he was alone with the therapist. They decided to choose 4 pillows. One pillow for the mother, one for the father, one for him and another one for the symptom. He chooses the pillow one by one, gave them to the therapist and placed him with each pillow in the constellation area. Father and son were opposite facing in opposite direction. In short the therapist tuned in the mother first (I stand on the place and see and feel what I pick up) basically a kind of overprotected energy. The symptom was a feeling of wall and closing or protecting issue. Father was in a relative dark corner, facing the wall, nearly without any feelings, son feels well and easy going, looking through the window. *No contact* towards the father was observed, he could see his mother over the shoulder with respect and interest.

Intervention: First the therapist gave the mother a more distance place from the son, looking at him and saying: *Now he is nearly growing up, he can protect himself, if you separate him from the father, he will be just like him.* Then he turned the father around, so he was looking at his son. He got more and more alive and was friendly and interested in what was going on in his "family". Then the therapist asked the son to turn slowly around his father. He refused; suddenly he got very angry and shouted at his father. He never looked after me, I don't want to see him, and he doesn't like me. (He had never met his father, after the mother got pregnant, father ran away. There were stories about him like drug addiction, crimes, and times in jail etc.). The therapist went to the son became friendly and put his arms around him, supporting the process. The boy got even more aggressive (a kind of catharsis), slowly he turned around and suddenly he started crying for nearly 10 minutes. The therapist tuned in the father role and spoke from his heart to him. They moved from 5 meters distance apart to two meters. The son still wanted a line drawn between them, but finally he was willing and able to look at each other deeply in the eyes. Very weak and with fever, the young boy left the session after 55 min. His bed was never wet again, now already after 2 years.

SECTION–4

Inter-Disciplinary Approaches

Management of Characteristic Features of Personality Type A: Synthesis of *bis*-Epoxide for the Preparation of *m*-(Substituted Aminohydroxypropoxy)phenylethanolamines as β-Blocker Drugs

Surat Kumar*[1] and Kavita Kumar[2]

ABSTRACT

β-Blockers are known to be administered in the clinics in the management of various CNS-CVS disorders. A novel *bis*-epoxide was prepared as an important intermediate for the preparation of aryloxypropanolamines and arylethanolamines as potential β-blockers. The β–blocking activity of these novel compounds was potentially increased as they have features of both aryloxypropanolamines and arylethanolamines. The present paper describes the synthesis of β-blockers drugs for the management of hypertension. We have made an attempt to correlate the medicinal chemistry approach to modify the Type A behavior as reported by several studies. The beta blockers have demonstrated the ability to modify beta adrenergic reactivity, which is perhaps an important physiological characteristic of Type A persons. The central effect of beta blockers influences both physiological responses such as BP, HR, and cardiovascular reactivity, as well as overt behavior. Studies have reflected that personality Type A individuals are supposed to consume more β–blocker agents.

INTRODUCTION

Personality characteristics have long been associated with essential hypertension (Alexander, 1939). Reviews of the earlier empirical literature concluded that neuroticism (Davies, 1971), hostility, and difficulties in coping with anger were associated with hypertension (Diamond, 1982). The type A behavior score predicted a greater increase in left ventricular mass index in men ($P = 0.018$) but not in women. The 24 h mean systolic blood pressure was associated with a greater increase in left ventricular mass index in women ($P < 0.001$) but not in men (Munakata *et al*., 1999). Reviews of the earlier empirical literature concluded that neuroticism, hostility, and difficulties in coping with anger were associated with hypertension (Diamond, 1982). Several reports have linked personality types with hypertension and cardiovascular disorders

*Corresponding author.

[1]Department of Applied Sciences, Faculty of Engineering, Dayabagh Educational Institute, Deemed University, Dayalbagh, Agra, UP, India. E-mail: kumar.surat@gmail.com

[2]Department of Psychology, Dayalbagh Educational Institute, Deemed University, Dayalbagh, Agra, UP, India. E-mail: kavita.kumars@gmail.com

(Verrier and Mittleman, 1996; Muller and Verrier, 1996; Verrier *et al.*, 1992; Miller *et al.*, 1979; Kidson, 1973). Type A behavior is involved in the pathogenesis of coronary atherosclerosis, but only in younger age groups (Williams *et al.*, 1988). Social and personality factors were associated indirectly with the progression of atherosclerosis (Whiteman *et al.*, 2000). Personality type A, has been implicated in the pathogenesis of cardiovascular disease. Abnormal sympathetic responses to stress may help explain the link between certain behavior patterns and cardiovascular disease. Type A personality characteristics are associated with exaggerated heart rate, pressor, and sympathetic nerve responses to mental and physical stress (Schroeder *et al.*, 2000).

The current design does not allow commenting on how long the effects of exercise will last in patients taking α-blockers. However, it was recommended that patients keep exercising moderately and under proper supervision, as long as they are being treated with β-blockers (Michael *et al.*, 2002). Pharmacological interventions using thyroid hormone analogues, beta-adrenergic receptor antagonists, and novel metabolically active compounds is currently under clinical use for the treatment of uncompensated cardiac hypertrophy and heart failure (Zarain-Herzberg, 2006). Adrenergic-inhibiting antihypertensive drugs, most notably the β-blockers have been shown to influence a variety of Central Nervous System (CNS) and Cardiovascular System (CVS) functions (Rosen *et al.*, 1985). Beta-blockers decrease the cardiovascular morbidity and mortality in persons with atherosclerotic heart disease (Arch Intern, 1997).

There are two types of drugs arylethanolamine (I) and aryloxypropanolamines (II) that are used as β-blockers in the clinics.

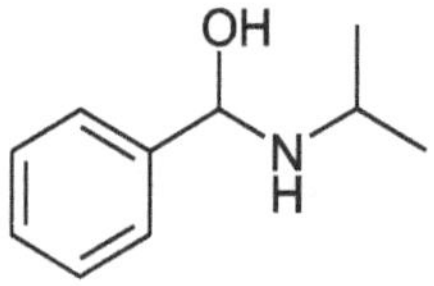

OH N H

I

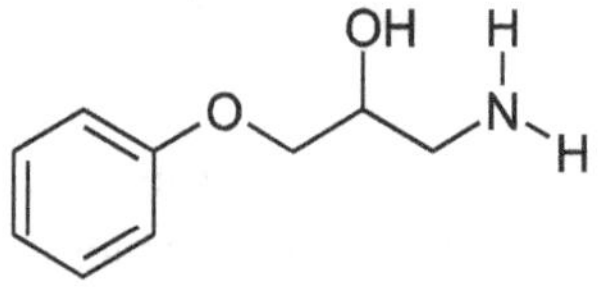

OH H O N H

II

There are a number of drugs of both types (I) and (II) used in the management of hypertension and cardiovascular disorders. These are atenolol, isoproterenol and methoxamine of type I and propranolol, nadolol and metoprolol of type II β-blockers. All these drugs are commonly used in clinics or sold on prescription by medical doctors for the management of hypertension and cardiovascular disorders.

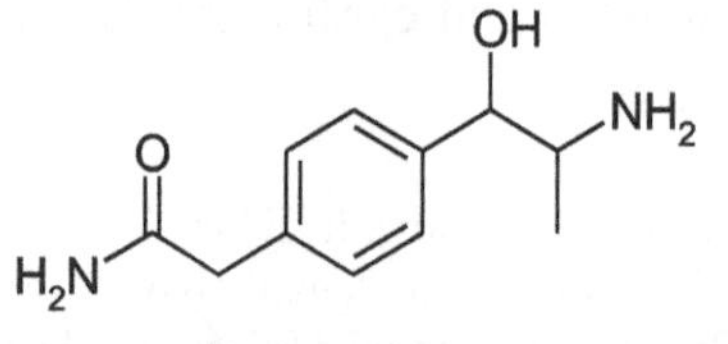

O OH NH_2 H_2N

Atenolol

OH HO H N HO

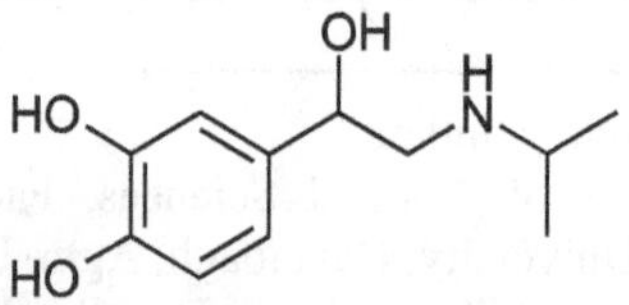

Isoproterenol

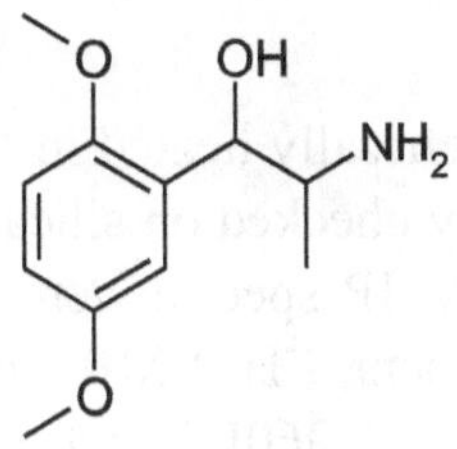

Methoxamine 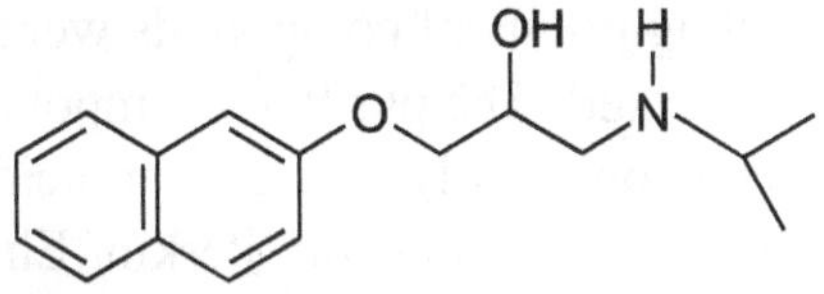 **Propranolol**

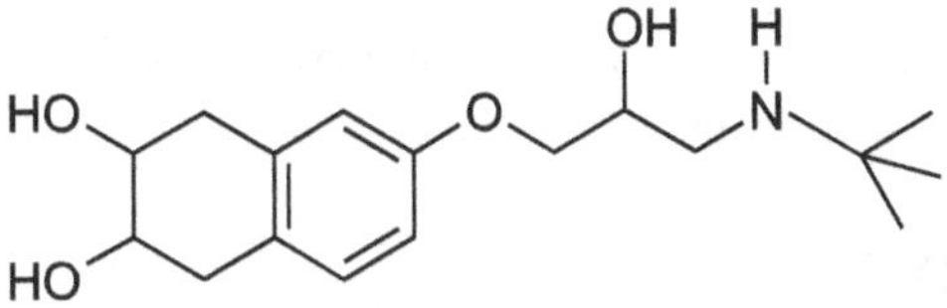

Nadolol 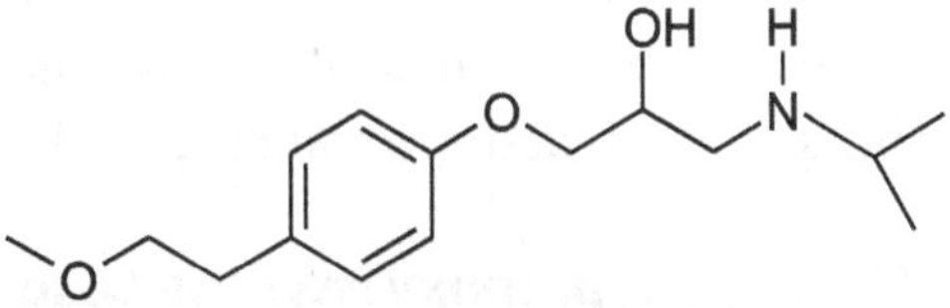 **Metoprolol**

From the structures of these two types of β-blockers, we designed a new class of β-blockers, which have the features of both arylethanolamins and aryloxypropanolamines. Thus we proposed to prepare *m*-(substituted aminohydroxypropoxy)phenylethanolamines (3–4) as title compounds. In order to synthesize these compounds, we need to prepare an important intermediate i.e. *bis*-epoxide (2).

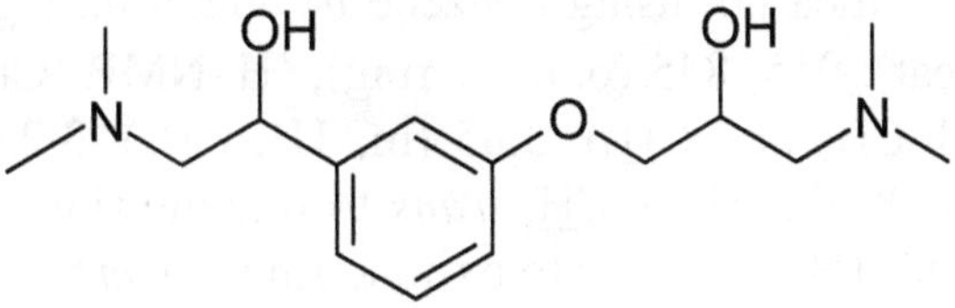

3. 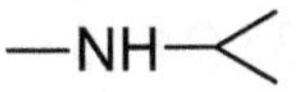 —NH—

4. 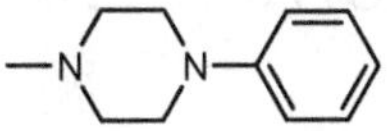 —N N—

This epoxide (2) was prepared by the reaction of a novel reagent trimethyloxosulphonium iodide on benzaldehyde compound (1) as reported (Corey *et al.*, 1965).

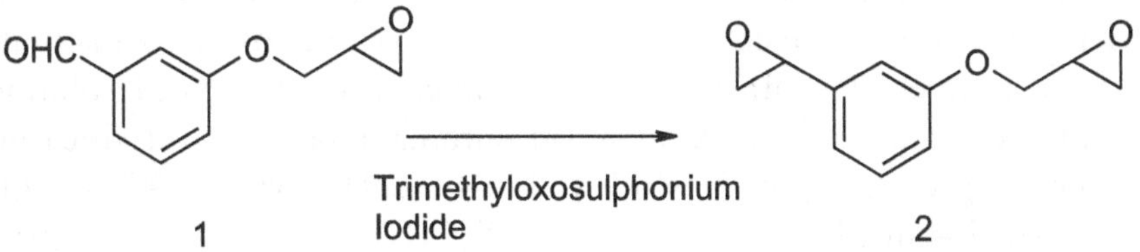

OHC

Trimethyloxosulphonium Iodide

1 2

MATERIALS AND METHODS

The melting points of compounds were taken in an electrically heated instrument and are uncorrected. The purity of compounds was routinely checked on silica gel G TLC plates developed in I_2 vapours and acidic $KMnO_4$ spray. IR spectra were recorded as neat or in KBr films on Perkin Elmer 157 instrument. ^{1}H–NMR spectra were recorded on Perkin Elmer R-32 (90 MHz) or Varian EM 360L spectrometer using TMS as internal reference and chemical shifts were expressed in δ units. Mass spectra were run on Jeol JMS D-300 spectrometer using a direct inlet system. All compounds have shown elemental analyses within ± 0.5% unless stated otherwise. Table 1 includes physical and spectral data of all these compounds.

m-(2, 3-Epoxypropoxy)styrene Oxide (2)

NaH (0.12 g, 50% dispersion) was washed with pet. ether to remove traces of oil and further evacuated to remove pet. ether. To it was added trimethyloxosulphonium iodide (0.55 g, 2.5 mmole) and dry THF (30 ml) under N_2 atmosphere. It was stirred for 2 hr. At 60° until the evolution of H_2 gas ceased and then a solution of *m*-epoxypropoxy-benzaldehyde (1, 0.35 g, 2.0 mmole) in THF (10 ml) was added under stirring. The stirring continued at 60° for 2 hr. The solvent was distilled off; residue treated with water, saturated NaCl solution, dried (Na_2SO_4) and concentrated. The residue was chromatographed over silica gel using benzene to obtain 0.31 g of styrene oxide as oil, yield 82%. IR (neat): 915, 845 (oxirane ring); ^{1}H–NMR ($CDCl_3$ and in δ scale): 2.5–2.95 (m, 3H, CH–$C\underline{H}_2$ and $C\underline{H}_a$), 3.05 (m, 1H, $C\underline{H}_b$), 3.27 (m, 1H, $C\underline{H}$–CH_2), 3.75 (m, 1H, $C\underline{H}_c$), 3.88 (dd, 1H, $OC\underline{H}$, *trans* to oxirane ring, *Jgem* = 11.5 Hz and *Jvic* = 5.5 Hz), 4.15 (dd, 1H, $OC\underline{H}$, *cis* to oxirane ring, *Jgem* = 11.5 Hz and *Jvic* = 3.5 Hz), 6.7–7.0 (m, 3H, Ar–H), 7.14 (d, 1H, Ar–H, *m* to OCH_2, *J* = 8.5 Hz). Ms (m/z): 192 (M^+) 193 ($M^+ + 1$), 191 ($M^+ -1$), 135 (M^+–57), 134 (M^+–58), 191 (134–CH_3) 107 (tropylium ion), 77 (C_6H_5), 57 (C_3H_5O) Found C, 68.76 and H, 6.34. $C_{11}H_{12}O_3$ requires C, 68.75 and H, 6.25%.

1-[*m*-(3-Isopropylamino-2-hydroxy-propoxy) phenyl]-2-isopropylaminoethanol (3)

A solution of 2 (0.38 g, 2.0 mM), water (1 drop) and isopropylamine (0.24 g, 4.0 mM) in MeOH (20 ml) was refluxed for 8 hr. Solvent was removed by distillation and residue taken in ether (10 ml) washed with water, saturated NaCl solution, dried (Na_2SO_4) and concentrated. The residual oil chromatographed over silica gel using chlorobenzene to give 0.52 g of 3 as oil, yield 84 %. ^{1}H–NMR ($CDCl_3$): 1.0[d, 12H, 2 × $(CH..CH_3)_2$, J = 6Hz], 2.4–3.0 [m, 8H $(HN.CH_2)_2$, 2 × OH], 3.15–3.65 [m, 2H $(N–CH–)_2$], 3.9 (bs, 3H, OCH_2CH), 4.5 (t, 1H, $ArCHN_3$, J = 6Hz), 6.7–7.4 (m, 14H, ArH). Found C, 66.02; H, 9.41 and N, 9.03. $C_{17}H_{30}N_2O_3$ requires C, 65.8; H, 9.67 and N, 9.03%.

Similarly, phenylpiperazinylhydroxypropoxyethanolamine (4) was prepared from styrene oxide (2). ^{1}H–NMR ($CDCl_3$): 2.3 [m, 12H, 2 × $N(CH_2)_3$], 3.1–3.35 [m, 8H, 2 × $CH_2)_2$, N.Ph], 4.7 (t, 1H, ArCHOH, J = 4.6Hz), 6.7–7.4 (m, 14H, ArH). Found C, 72.44; H, 7.36 and N, 10.36. $C_{31}H_{40}N_4O_3$ requires C, 72.09; H, 7.75 and N, 9.03%.

RESULTS AND DISCUSSION

As documented by several behavioral scientists that personality Type A is associated with hypertension and cardiac disorders. It is also very well reported and practiced by physicians that β–blockers are effective treatment in the management of hypertension and vascular disorders. So it was proposed to generate a new class of β–blockers, which have the structural features of both arylethanolamins (I) and aryloxypropaolamins (II), the most commonly used types of β–blockers. An important intermediate *bis*-epoxide (2) was prepared from substituted benzaldehyde (1) by the reaction of trimethyloxosulphonuim iodide.

Once this epoxide (2) was prepared, it was further derivatized by the reaction of isopropylamine and N-phenylpiperazine amines to get title compounds *m*-(substituted aminohydroxypropoxy)phenylethanolamines (3–4), as reported (Kumar and Rastogi, 2007). We have prepared these target compounds 3 and 4 for the management of hypertension. In the pharmacological activity testing, compound 3 and 4 were found to have ALD_{50} values of 56.2 and 316 mg/Kg respectively. Compound 3 was found to have some depressant activity. Beside this, compound 4 showed some hypotensive and diuretic activity in mice.

The use of β-blockers i.e. arylethanolamines (I), aryloxypropanolamines (II) and the title compounds (3 & 4) can help in controlling the symptoms of hypertension and CHD. In turn, β-blockers designed in this study may effectively assist in the health management of Type A Personality disorders.

ACKNOWLEDGEMENTS

Authors acknowledge their most humble gratitude for Most Revered Prof. P.S. Satsangi Sahab, Chairman, Advisory Committee on Education, Dayalbagh for the constant inspiration for carrying out this research work. Prof. V.G. Das, Director, Dayalbagh Educational Institute, Dayalbagh, Agra cordially thanked for consistent support and a Major Research Project funded by UGC (to SK) is also duly acknowledged.

REFERENCES

Alexander, F. (1939). "Emotional Factors in Essential Hypertension". *Psychosom Med,* 1, 173–179.

Arch Intern Med (1997). "The Sixth Report of the Joint National Committee on Prevention, Detection, Evaluation and Treatment of High Blood Pressure", 157, 2413–46.

Corey, E.J. and Chaykovski, M. (1965). "Dimethyloxosulfonium Methylide ((CH_3)2SOCH_2) and Dimethylsulfonium Methylide ((CH_3)2SCH_2): Formation and Application to Organic Synthesis". *J. Am. Chem. Soc*, 87, 1353–1364.

Davies, M.H. (1971). "Is High Blood Pressure a Psychosomatic Disorder? A Critical Review of the Evidence". *J. Chron Dis.*, 24, 239–258.

Diamond, E.L. (1982). "The Role of Anger and Hostility in Essential Hypertension and Coronary Heart Disease". *Psychol Bull*, 92, 410–433.

Kidson, M.A. (1973). "Personality and Hypertension". *J. Psychosom Res.*, 17, 35–41.

Kumar, S. and Rastogi, S.N. (2007). "Synthesis of *m*-(Substituted Aminohydroxy-propoxy) Phenylethanolamines as Potential Biodynamic Agents". *Int. J Pure Applied Chem.*, 2(3), 313–318.

Michael, S., David, B. and Ehud, G. (2002). *Medicine in Sports and Exercise*, 587–591.

Miller, C.L., Stein, R.F. and Grim, C. (1979). "Personality Factors of the Hypertensive Patient". *Int J. Nurs Stud*, 16, 235–251.

Muller, J.E. and Verrier, R.L. (1996). "Triggering of Sudden Death: Lessons from An Earthquake". *N Engl J. Med.*, 334, 460–461.

Munakata, M., Hiraizumi, T, Tomiie, T., Saito, Y., Ichii, S., Nunokawa, T., Nobuhiko, T.F., Yamauchi, Y. and Yoshinaga, K. (1999). "Type A Behavior is Associated with an Increased Risk of Left Ventricular Hypertrophy in Male Patients with Essential Hypertension". *J. of Hypertension*, 17(1), 115–120.

Rosen, R.C. and Kostis, J.B. (1985). "Biobehavioral Sequellae Associated with Adrenergic-Inhibiting Antihypertensive Agents: A Critical Review". *Health Psychology*, 4(6), 579–604.

Schroeder, K.E., Narkiewicz, K., Kato, M., Pesek, C., Phillips, B., Davison, D. and Somers, V.K. (2000). "Personality Type and Neural Circulatory Control". *Hypertension,* 36, 830–833.

Verrier, R.L., Dickerson, L.W. and Nearing B.D. (1992). "Behavioral States and Sudden Cardiac Death". *Pacing Clin Electrophysiol.*, 15, 1387–1393.

Verrier, R.L. and Mittleman, M.A. (1996). "Life-threatening Cardiovascular Consequences of Anger in Patients with Coronary Heart Disease". *Cardiol Clin.*, 14, 289 –307.

Whiteman, M.C., Deary, I.J. and Fowkes, F.G.R. (2000). "Personality and Social Predictors of Atherosclerotic Progression: Edinburgh Artery Study". *Psychosomatic Medicine*, 62, 703–714.

Williams, R.B., Jr., Barefoot, J.C., Haney, T.L., Harrell, F.E., Blumenthal, J.A., Pryor, D.B. and Peterson B. (1988). "Type A Behavior and Angiographically Documented Coronary Atherosclerosis in a Sample of 2,289 Patients". *Psychosomatic Medicine*, 50(2), 139–152.

Zarain-Herzberg, A. (2006). "Regulation of the Sarcoplasmic Reticulum Ca[sup2+]-ATPase Expression in the Hypertrophic and Failing Heart". *Canadian Journal of Physiology and Pharmacology,* 84(5), 509–521.

Dietary Patterns of Indian Children: A Bio-Chemical Analysis and Behavioral Management

Rishi Nigam*[1] and Parul Rishi[2]

ABSTRACT

The pace for teens and children is fast and getting faster. Added to the pressures from school and increasing competitiveness, participation in sports and extra activities further changes the nutritional demand and eating patterns of children. Owing to that, it was planned to study the dietary patterns and nutritional status of children using physical and bio-chemical parameters.

A sample of 56 children was selected from the schools of Bhopal city of India. A comprehensive dietary schedule was used by the investigator consisting of Demographic Profile, Physical Profile, Biochemical Profile, Dietary Profile and Cognitive Profile. The total calorie intake of the sample was below or near the normal, however, calories from fat and protein intake were relatively high owing to high junk food diet. Incidence of iron deficiency and serum cholesterol levels above acceptable limits were also found putting them at high risk of developing hypercholesterolemia later. Recommendations for excess fat management, iron deficiency management, total diet management, life style management and dietary behavior management were made.

INTRODUCTION

Modern age is the age of freedom. Freedom may be of thoughts, expression, or action. Diet is no exception to that as far as modern eating patterns of urban life are concerned. In this race for freedom, children are the forerunners, far ahead from the adult generation. Children find themselves amidst a complex society that is undergoing breathtaking changes. Concepts, relationships, lifestyles are meta-morphosised to accommodate the new jet-setting age.

FOOD AND MEDIA

Today's urban child, the architect of new jet era, starts and ends his day with the food of his choice, which is the expression of his independence. His major motivators for

---

* Corresponding author.

[1]DCP Pathology, Barkatullah University, Bhopal, MP, India.
E-mail: nigamrishi@rediffmail.com

[2]Faculty of Personal Management and OB, Indian Institute of Forest Management, Bhopal, MP, India. E-mail: rishiparul@rediffmail.com

eating varieties are TV advertisements, friends, and media. Parental figures and teachers are loosing their power of being the strong motivators for eating patterns and have to compete strongly with powerful media to influence the children. May be, the time has come when parents and teachers will have to refigure their influential strategies to recapture their children from visual media's influence. However, do we think that visual media is behaving in a responsible way as far as eating patterns and nutritional requirements are concerned? Is visual media dependable to decide what a child should eat to protect his health?

The expert panel of American Psychological Association on February 24th, 2004 says that the situation is not so dependable. 'Children under 8 years of age are unable to understand that TV ads are not real and need to be protected from seeing them'. They have estimated that advertisers spend more than $ 12 billion a year in United States, on ads aimed at youth market. The committee also examined the possibilities of putting a ban on children targeted advertising by food and drink companies. Sweden does not permit any TV advertisements directed to children younger than 12 years. Some states in US have imposed 1% additional tax on junk foods to offset junk food advertising.

The whole situation gives the picture that children are to be protected from the overwhelming influence of media on their diet and responsibility lies with parents and teachers in this regard to protect our future architects from any nutritional deficiency as well as health hazards.

FOOD FOR HEALTH

Food is, of course, the prime necessity of life. The food we eat is digested and assimilated in our body to provide us energy and is used for maintenance. Good nutrition is a basic component of health and is of prime importance in the attainment of normal growth, development and maintenance of good health throughout life. The care and promotion of health starts right from childhood. The nutritional and health status of a child greatly influences the future health parameters. Childhood is the growth period from infancy to the beginning of the puberty or adolescence and is marked by many body changes. The school age period has been called the latent time of growth, the rate of growth slows and body changes occur gradually. There is an increased need for all nutrients but the pattern of increased demand varies for different nutrients in selection to their role in growth of specific tissues. Besides health parameters, there is enough evidence to prove that nutrition has a major impact on cognitive development and school performance (Abidoye and Eze, 2000; Bellisele *et al.*, 1998). Therefore, impact of food intake on overall physical, psychological, especially intellectual and cognitive performance of children, can not be disregarded.

URBANIZATION AND NUTRITIONAL DIVIDE

The nutritional divide is increasing between the rich and the poor within and among nations. This increasing dichotomy is particularly alarming in developing countries. The nutritional paradox of South Asia lies in the co-existence of "Grain Mountains and Hungry Millions". This is largely due to inadequate purchasing power arising from lack of sustainable livelihood opportunities.

On the other hand, the urban middle and upper middle class population even without much financial constraints for balanced diet may be presenting a different picture from the general nutritional projections of developing countries. They may not be suffering from nutritional deficiency like Protein Energy Malnutrition (PEM), but may have other nutritional imbalances as a result of changing life styles in urban population. Thus, bridging the nutritional divide is the first requisite for a more equitable and humane world. Improving child nutrition is necessary to safeguard the well-being of future generations.

NUTRITIONAL REQUIREMENTS IN INDIA

In the present endeavour, to find the status of food and nutrition security in India, it is necessary to first examine the 'standards' against which such security is to be judged. At the conceptual plane, it can be stated that a country can be said to have achieved complete food and nutrition security if each and every person in that country is able to consume a minimum quantum and quality of various ingredients, called 'an adequate and balanced diet' on a regular basis. Availability and affordability of such diet, backed by health and educational services in an environmentally sustainable scenario will then enable each member of the society to live a 'good' life; each individual personality getting an opportunity to flower to one's full potential.

It is actually not easy for experts to exactly lay down nutrient requirements and quantities of various ingredients separately for various population and activity groups. Diversity in agro-climatic conditions; food habits; life styles and spiritual/ philosophical inclinations condition the nutritional intakes, apart from the 'measurable physiological needs of the human body.

In India, it is the Indian Council of Medical Research (ICMR) that sets up Nutrition Advisory Committees or Expert Groups and recommend the "Dietary Allowances" in respect of energy (Calories), proteins, fats, minerals, iron, vitamins *etc.* for various age groups within the population and formulated a new set of recommendations with regard to balanced diets for Indians based on the concept of 'least cost'.

ICMR dietary recommendations had specially observed that "RDA (Recommended Dietary Allowance) for Indians are being revised and updated at intervals of about 10 years in view of the changes in our concept of human requirements of several nutrients as a result of studies carried out during the previous decade" (ICMR 1984).

Composition of balanced diet is the end result of the RDAs. The balanced diet is, in a way, the practical prescription for consumption of a basket of food items, which is likely to provide all the required nutrients to the human body.

DIETARY DEMANDS AND NUTRITION OF YOUNG ARCHITECTS

Added to the pressures from school and increasing competitiveness to prepare for college or a job, participation in sports and extra curricular activities further changes the nutritional demand and eating patterns of children. This often means eating on the run. Many factors influence the eating behavior of children. Individual needs and desires, daily moods, social environment, the foods that are available, advertising, *etc*. Children need a lot of nourishing foods to provide them with all of the important nutrients for growth.

Children's tendencies are moving towards sweets, chocolates, and salted snacks and away from vegetables, the important food group, which probably offers the greatest nutritional challenge for parents. Many snacks and treat foods such as potato chips, fast-foods, aerated cold drinks, cheeseburgers, and fries, have high levels of fat, sugar or salt ingredients that are usually best limited to a small portion of diet.

Based on the above background, it was observed that most of the studies, especially Indian studies have targeted the infancy and puberty groups for nutritional studies and that too in the lower to lower middle socio-economic status considering them more prone to nutritional deficiencies. However, the vulnerability of middle and higher socio-economic class who are in major influence of visual media and globalisation cannot be disregarded.

Owing to above probable reasons, it was planned to study the dietary patterns and nutritional status of urban school children of middle to higher socio-economic status using physical growth parameters of height and weight and bio-chemical parameters of haemoglobin, serum iron, blood cholesterol, serum protein and albumin. It also intended to study the relation between dietary patterns and nutritional status, impact of visual media on diet and recommend changes in the responsible adult influential strategies on the diet of children as required.

METHODOLOGY

Sample

A sample of 56 school aged urban middle and upper class physically and mentally healthy children (age ranging from 4 yrs–12 years, M = 7.76 yrs) was selected from the schools of Bhopal city of India using purposive sampling technique. Only those children whose parents consented to participate in the study and allowed the venous blood collection were considered for the sample. In some cases, parents did not co-operate for blood sample collection of their children and in some other cases children were not at all ready for vein puncture. Looking at these problems random selection of sample was not possible.

TOOLS AND TECHNIQUES

A comprehensive dietary schedule was prepared by the investigator, which was divided in five sub-sections.

Demographic Profile—It collected information about personal and family details of the sample and socioeconomic status assessed through family income which may have a marked bearing on the dietary patterns and nutritional status of children.

Physical Profile—Physical profile consisted of actual measurements of standing height in cm and weight in kilograms through standard weighing scale to calculate following indices of nutritional status.

Body Mass Index (BMI) for Age

In children, body mass index is used to assess underweight, overweight, and risk for overweight. Children's body fatness changes over the years as they grow.

Girls and boys also differ in their body fatness as they mature. That is why BMI for children, also referred to as BMI-for-age, is gender and age specific. BMI-for-age is plotted on gender specific growth charts. These charts are used for children and teens 2–20 years of age.

Each of the CDC BMI-for-age gender specific charts contains a series of curved lines indicating specific percentiles. Healthcare professionals use the following established percentile cutoff points to identify underweight and overweight in children. The children having BMI-for-age below 5th percentile can be designated as underweight whereas those having BMI-for-age above 95th percentile can be regarded as overweight. BMI-for-age falling between 85th and 95th percentile indicate the risk of being overweight.

Weight for Age

Weight for age has also been used as an anthropometric method for the evaluation of nutritional status of young children. If a child is healthy, he should reflect appropriate weight and height for his age. This measure, although genetically determined, is strongly influenced by nutrition. If correctly recorded and interpreted, it reflects the pattern of growth and physical state of the individual and indicates how much the individuals deviate from the average at various ages in body size, built and nutritional status.

Biochemical Profile

Biochemical measures involve estimating the level of nutrient in the blood/urine. These measures yield reliable data regarding the nutritional status of the individual with respect to the nutrient estimated.

Serum Protein

Protein forms the major portion of the dissolved substances in blood plasmal forming the basic structural components of the body. They constitute the enzymes present in our body and also act as secondary source of energy.

The measurement of Serum protein reflects the overall picture of protein homeostasis in the body. A number of disorders including the nutritional status affect the Serum total protein and albumin levels. In the present study, serum total protein was estimated by colorimetric method using Biuret reaction. Proteins present in serum or plasma react with copper salt in alkaline medium to form blue colored complex intensity of which is proportional to the protein concentration.

Serum Cholesterol

It is the main lipid found in the blood, bile and brain tissue. Cholesterol is necessary for the formation of cell membrane. It also contributes to the formation of bile salts, adrenal cortical steroids, estrogens and androgens. Increased levels of serum cholesterol are found in various disorders including hyperlipidaemia and hypercholesterolemia, which are closely associated with atherosclerosis and coronary artery disease. Decreased levels are found in malnutrition and malabsorption. Serum cholesterol estimation was done using enzymatic method (CHOD- PAP) which is the standard method.

Haemoglobin

Haemoglobin is most common screening test for diagnosis of Anaemia. Its concentration decreases in different types of anaemia including nutritional anaemia. It is the main intracellular protein of the red blood cell. Its determination is of greatest use in the evaluation of anaemia as the oxygen carrying capacity of the blood is directly related to the haemoglobin level rather than the number of erythrocytes.

Hemoglobin estimation was done by Cyanmethaemoglobin method, which is a standard method, recommended by the International Committee for Standardization of Hematology (ICSH). In this method Drabkin solution on mixing with blood converts haemoglobin to Cyanmethaemoglobin, the color absorbency of which is proportional to the haemoglobin concentration.

Serum Iron

Iron found in the blood is (73%) mainly present in the haemoglobin of the Red blood cells, but iron is carried in plasma bound to the protein transferrin. Decreased serum iron level with increased transferrin level or Total Iron Binding Capacity (TIBC) are found in Iron deficiency anaemia. Decreased iron levels with decreased transferrin levels are seen in anaemia associated with chronic diseases and malnutrition and malabsorption.

Serum iron levels were measured by Ferrozine method in which iron bound to transferring is released in an acidic medium and the ferric ions are reduced to ferrous ions. The ferrous ions react with ferrozine to form a violet colored complex, intensity of which is directly proportional to iron present in the serum.

HEALTH HISTORY

Besides history of chronic and major illnesses and constipation was also taken which is supposed to be quite closely related with dietary patterns and resulting nutritional status. History of any iron supplementation in diet was also taken. Average per day physical activity of the child in the form of outdoor play, games, general P.T at school or cycling was also recorded which may have close relation with the calorie intake of the children.

Dietary Profile—Dietary profile consisted of seeking information about types of foods taken and its approximate quantities in measurable terms. It included reporting of daily dietary schedule of the child in the form of breakfast, school Tiffin, lunch, evening snacks, dinner and any other food taken by the child. Besides, the frequency and quantity of milk intake, milk additives, fat consumption of the family including both saturated and non-saturated, was also asked.

After that, frequency and quantity of specific foods' intake in the diet was tabulated to obtain the concise information. These specific foods were classified as:

- Baked Foods like biscuits, breads, cake, pastries etc.
- Confectioneries like toffees, chocolates, and non-milk based sweets etc.
- Milk Products like cheese, curd, ice cream, milk based sweets etc.
- Healthy foods like fruits, salad, sprouts, dry fruits etc.
- Non-vegetarian foods like egg, fish, chicken, meat etc.
- Fast foods like pizza, burgers, noodles, fried packaged snacks like chips, wafers, etc.
- Cold drinks including only aerated soft drinks.

Based on the above information, total calorie intake, daily protein and fat intake was calculated using standardized tables of approximate nutritive values' of common Indian foods.

Besides, choice of fruits, frequency of eating out, child's demand for media advertised products and frequency of the fulfillment of such demands by parents were also recorded.

Cognitive Profile—Cognitive profile included parental cognitions about the child's diet, its nutritional value for healthy growth, feeding pattern, dietary habits and demands of the child and impact of media on diet. Besides, eating out frequency of the family was also recorded to find out if it is directly or indirectly related with the general nutritional status of the child.

PROCEDURE

After the sample selection, the investigator approached parents of selected children who had already given their consent for the study. They were further explained the importance of this study for managing the dietary behavior of their children. Afterwards the measurement of height and weight was done. Blood sample collection was made for the estimation of biochemical parameters mentioned above. After the blood sample collection, any of the parents was asked to fill the demographic profile of the child as detailed above. They were also asked to report the health history in the schedule.

Dietary profile was taken from the parents, preferably mother, looking at the local culture where mother plays a predominant role in the child's dietary patterns and nutrition. Dietary information as tabulated in the dietary schedule was taken using 24 hours dietary recall and diet history method and was recorded in its respective columns.

ANALYSIS OF RESULTS

Demographic Profile

Demographic profile included the data related to age, sex, socio-economic status, parental qualifications, mother's occupation and family types. All the children of the sample belonged to middle and higher income group families with the income ranging from Rupees, 8,500–40,000/- per month.

Among the children the sex distribution was almost equal with 52% of boys and 48% of girls. Their age ranged from 4 years to 12 years with the mean age of 7.76 years. All the children being from the middle and higher-class families had parents with the educational qualifications ranging from intermediate to Ph.D. including parents with professional qualifications.

Regarding family type, the distribution was quite equal with 48% of children from joint families and 52% of children from nuclear families. In regard to mother's occupation, 45% of mothers were working while 55% mothers of the sampled children were non-working (house wives). Only 10% of the sample had siblings more than one. All the children were studying in the schools in the classes ranging from kindergarten to class seventh.

Physical Profile

Regarding health profile, very few cases reported the history of any chronic or major illness and they were excluded from the sample. About 15% of cases were reported to be suffering from constipation frequently.

Regarding physical profile, the parameters of height and weight were taken through standard measures. The mean height of 122.9 cms was found in the sample. Age wise distribution indicates that mean height of 4–6 yrs was 108.5 cms, while of 7–12 years was 129.45 cms. Regarding weight for age on an average all the children were with in normal weight range however, some cases of overweight or underweight were found. The mean weight for age was 99.7 percentage of the normal.

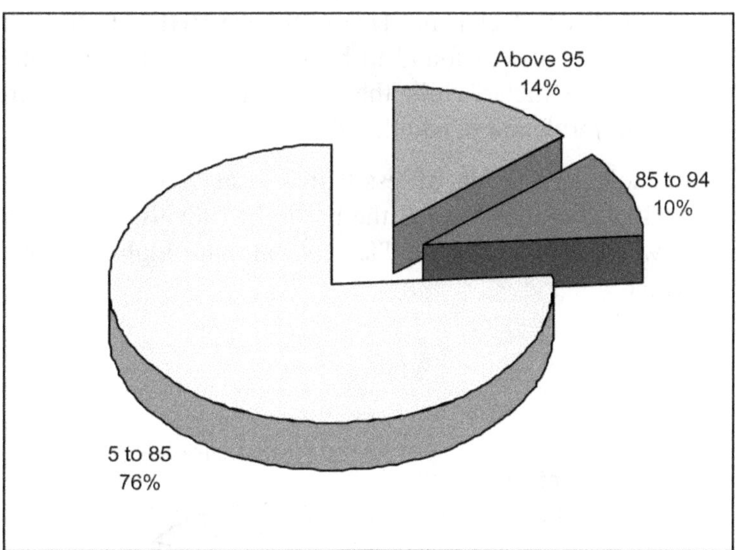

Figure 1: Distribution of BMI for Age in Percentile

B.M.I was calculated based on the obtained heights and weights using the formula:

B.M.I = Weight (Kg) ÷ Height (m) ^{2} and then plotted on gender specific CDC charts.

13.8% of the sample was above 95th percentile indicating the over weight condition while 10.3% of the sample was between 85th–95th percentile of BMI for age indicating the children at risk of being over weight. Rest of the sample was between 5th–85th percentile indicating with in the normal weight range.

BIOCHEMICAL PROFILE

Estimation of various bio chemical parameters like Haemoglobin, Serum Iron, Total Serum Proteins, and total Serum Cholesterol levels were done.

Total mean haemoglobin was found to be 10.51 gms% in the sample. The normal value of haemoglobin in children is 11.0–16.0 gms%. Hb levels of 24% children were above 11 gm% and 73% of the sample suffers from mild anaemia having low Hb levels (9–10.9 gm%). Moderately low levels of Hb (< 9%) were found in only in 3% of the sample.

Mean Serum iron level was found to be 34.3 µg/100 ml. The normal value of serum iron in children is 40–200 ų g/100 ml.

Total Serum protein levels provide an overall picture of protein homeostasis. The mean Serum protein level was found to be 6.1 gm% in the sample. The normal value ranges between 6.0 to 8.0 gm%.

Serum Cholesterol level is one of the important lipid associated with atherosclerosis which is closely related with Ischaemic Heart Disease (IHD). In the present sample mean total serum cholesterol was found to be 170.8 mg%. The acceptable level for children is less than 170 mg% while the levels above 200 mg% are at risk of developing hypercholesterolemia in adulthood.

Acceptable serum cholesterol levels of less than 170 mg% were found in 44% of the sample. However, 38% children were at the borderline levels, *i.e.*, between 170–199 mg% and 18% were above 200 mg%, *i.e.*, at the high risk of developing hypercholesterolemia.

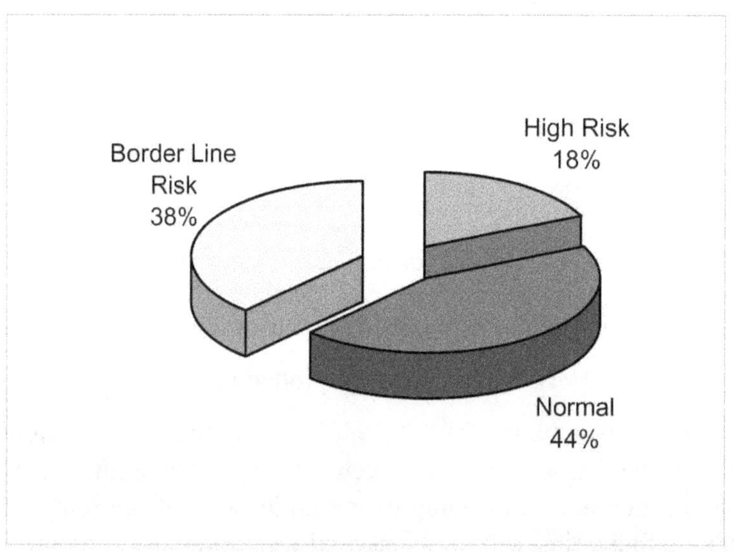

Figure 2: Percentage Distribution of Cholesterol Values

DIETARY PROFILE

It analyzed the type of diet *i.e.,* vegetarian (lacto vegetarian), non-vegetarian or eggetarian, total calorie intake per day, calorie deficiency from RDA, analysis of major food components like protein, fat intake, incidence of Junk food and relation of dietary patterns with different physical, biochemical parameters among the sample population.

Regarding the type of diet, 44.8% of the sample was vegetarian, 31% was eggetarian and 24.2% was non-vegetarian.

On the basis of the dietary history, total calorie intake per day of the sample was calculated. It was found that the mean total calorie intake was deficient among both the groups when compared with Recommended Dietary Allowance (RDA) by Indian Council of Medical Research, 1990 (ICMR). The total deficiency of 7.7% from RDA was found in the present sample.

Age wise comparison of mean values indicated only 2.28% deficiency in the younger age group of 4–6 years and 10.17% deficiency in 7–12 years' age group. When compared, the incidence of deficiency in the sample, it was found that 55.5% of the younger age group had normal calorie intake while 11.2% have 1–5% deficient intake and 33.3% have deficiency in the range of 6–10%.

Regarding the age group of 7–12 years, only 5% of the sample had normal total calorie intake. Rest of the sample had deficiencies ranging from 1–5% in 20% of sample, 6–10% deficiency in 35% of cases and 11–25% deficiency in 40% of cases.

Major Food Components

Major food components are Protein, Fat and Carbohydrates. In the present study, total protein and fat intake was calculated along with the total calorie intake, which was later compared with RDA for respective age groups as per ICMR tabulations of 1990. Apart from calories coming from proteins and fat, rest of the calories were presumed to be coming from carbohydrates.

Protein

In the age group of 4–6 years, RDA has recommended 30 gm protein per day and the mean intake of sample population is 39 gm per day with the range of 28 gm to 44 gm, normal to slightly higher than required. However, in the senior age group, the mean RDA of 7–12 years age group is 50.6 gm while the sample population is taking only 43 gm per day, *i.e.,* the mean protein deficit of 8 grams per day.

Fat

In the age group of 4–6 years, RDA has recommended 25 gm fat per day and the mean intake of sample population is 38.4 gm per day with the range of 30 gm to 48 gm and a mean excess of 13.4 grams. However, in the senior age group, the mean RDA is 23.0 gm while the sample population is taking 35.6 gm per day, *i.e.,* the mean fat excess of 12.6 grams per day.

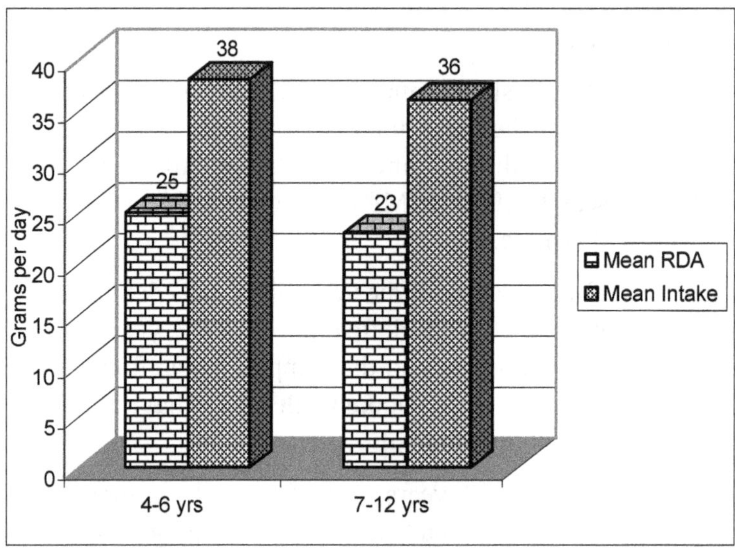

Figure 3: Mean Fat Intake as Compared to RDA across Age Groups

Junk Food—Under dietary patterns, frequency of Junk food intake was also recorded, which primarily included Noodles, especially the Maggi brand, chocolates, branded chips, wafers, cream biscuits, and aerated soft drinks *etc.* Children especially demanded products, which had some plaything as a free gift.

Children, who were consuming junk food at the rate of more than 20% of their calories intake, were found to be 52% in the present sample. Out of these cases, 40% have the cholesterol levels above acceptable limit of 170 mg% and 27% have the levels above 200 mg %, *i.e.,* at the higher risk of developing hypercholesterolemia in adult life. Besides, 26% of the junk food eaters were also found to be having BMI above 85th percentile, which indicates the risk of being over weight.

It was also found that 87% of such children demanded junk food based on media advertising and free gifts of different nature. However, in rest of the cases, parents willingly provided such food without any specific demand. Another finding was that 67% of Junk Food eaters were also reported to be fussy eaters by their parents and among them, 53% parents admitted that their children are not taking nutritive diet.

Relation of Dietary Patterns with Physical and Biochemical Parameters—Inter co-relations were calculated to see the relationship between different bio-chemical parameters and anthropometrical indicators of nutritional status.

BMI is an acceptable anthropometric measure for nutritional assessment, especially to classify obesity in adults. However, recently it is also being used to assess under weight and over weight in children in western countries with a slight modification in the form of BMI for age depicted in percentile.

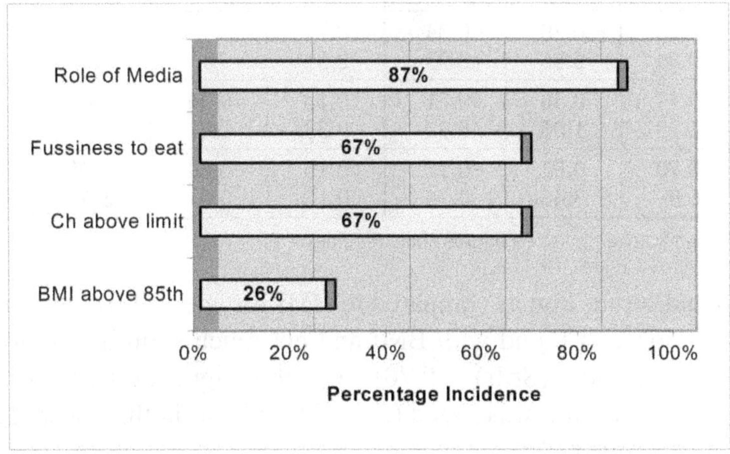

Figure 4: Incidence of different Features in Junk Food Eaters

To cross check the validity of this measure, the inter co-relation between weight for age, the acceptable parameter for children in India and BMI for age was calculated and a moderately high coefficient of co-relation was found ($r = 0.64$) which was significant at .01 level ($F = 4.7$). It indicates that BMI for age can be taken as an acceptable measure for nutritional assessment of Indian children and there is a need to plot gender specific B.M.I. for age percentile curves, specifically for Indian children.

When compared with calorie deviation from RDA, it was found that most of the children were taking deficient calories and as the calorie deficiency increased, both BMI for age and Weight for age decreased (r (BMIa) = –0.69, r(WFA) = –0.69). Significant values of F(6.28 and 6.4) also confirm the above findings.

Serum Protein was also found to be negatively co-related with calorie deviation from RDA($r = -0.71$). Children with deficient calories intake were also low in serum protein levels. However, children with higher serum protein had relatively higher WFA($r = 0.44$).

Table 1: Inter Correlations among Physical and Bio-Chemical Parameters

	WFA	*BMIa*	*Cal.D*	*Hb*	*S.Ir*	*S.Pr*	*Chol*
WFA	–						
BMIa	r = 0.64 F = 4.7	–					
Cal.D	–0.69 6.4	–0.69 6.28	–				
Hb	0.16 0.19	0.53 2.75	–0.22 0.36	–			
S.Ir	0.33 0.84	0.70 6.56	–0.34 0.93	0.74 8.31	–		
S.Pr	0.44 1.73	0.36 1.06	–0.71 6.92	0.13 0.33	0.34 0.91	–	
Chol	0.70 6.8	0.52 3.46	0.11 0.24	0.15 0.16	0.04 0.01	0.71 6.9	–

Bold Indicates Significance. Coloured figures show F Values.

Regarding Hb and serum iron as compared to BMI for age and weight for age, a good moderate co-relation was found with BMI and not much significant co-relation with WFA (r (hb) = 0.53 and r (Sr.Ir) = 0.70). A highly significant correlation between haemoglobin and serum iron was found (r = 0.74) indicating that most of the anaemia in children is mainly due to iron deficiency.

In regard to cholesterol levels, a high co-relation was found with WFA and serum cholesterol (r = 0.70) and a good co-relation with BMI for age (r = 0.52). As most of the children have high fat intake and its large portion is in the form of saturated fat which is biochemically depicted in the form of higher levels of serum cholesterol. Most of such children have relatively higher WFA too. Regarding serum protein too, the high correlation with cholesterol (r = 0.71) can be interpreted in terms of larger proportion of protein and fat both in combination in the diet of middle and above socio economic group.

Cognitive Profile

Parental awareness about the nutritive status of diet taken by their children, their satisfaction with the diet intake and other cognitive issues were analyzed under this section. It was found that 51.7% of parents considered their child's diet nutritive enough for their growth and were satisfied to some extent. However, rests of the parents were either dissatisfied or uncertain about the nutritive status of their children's diet. Parents of 58.6% children of the sample reported them as fussy eaters and interestingly, most of this percentage was among high junk food eating children.

DISCUSSION

The study has certain special features like it catered children from middle and above socio-economic status, the group which is generally regarded as a privileged group as far as food availability is concerned. This group also had relatively greater exposure to mass media and associated advertising, which might be substantially associated with food demand and food choices of such children. Besides, being from the urban elite class, parental cognition about the diet and nutrition of children was also considered to be quite high.

Owing to the above reasons, various dietary patterns of the sample group were analyzed. The sample distribution was quite equal as far as demographic variables of sex, family type, and mothers' working/non-working status were concerned.

As far as the physical parameters of height and weight are concerned, it was found that the mean height of the junior group of the sample was relatively at the higher level of the mean height for this age group. Regarding senior group (7–12 years), the mean height of 129.45 cms was also in the normal range (Swaminathan, 1989). Besides, weight for age measure also confirmed that all the children were in the normal and above normal range as per IAP classification.

When BMI for age was calculated on gender specific percentile curves (CDC Growth Charts, 2000), it was found that 76% of children were in the normal range, but the remaining percentage (24%) was either over weight or at risk of being over weight. Another special feature of BMI for age was, that this 'at risk' condition was more among 4–6 years age group as compared to the senior age group. However even with normal to mildly deficient calories intake, its combination with reduced physical activities of children may be responsible for normal to high BMI in this population. Their protein intake was also above recommended level and correspondingly, their serum protein levels were also in the normal range. However, they were relatively low in Hb and serum iron levels indicating the high prevalence of iron deficiency anaemia. Its one reason might be that their diet may be lacking in protecting food groups like green leafy vegetables and fruits. Another reason may be relatively poor absorption of iron from the diet or less bio-availability of iron. The non-vegetarian foods have iron (haem) with very high bio-availability and the absorption of this is not affected by any other factor in the lumen including various food ingredients, whereas the diet of vegetarian or non-vegetarian children the main part was from the vegetarian group which had poor iron bio-availability. Absorption of iron from vegetarian sources was affected by various factors. Besides, more prevalence of parasitic infestations in this age group can also be an additional significant cause.

Iron deficiency anemia is a common childhood nutritional problem in developing countries, no matter what the diet. The nutritional anemia has major consequences not only on the morbidity and mortality in children but also affects growth and intellectual development of these children. Good iron sources include whole or enriched grains and grain products, iron-fortified cereals, legumes, green leafy vegetables and dried fruits. Vitamin C helps the body to absorb iron, so citrus fruits with iron-rich foods are a good combination.

At the senior age group, total calorie intake was relatively lower at their age and deficiencies were up to 25% from recommended intake of their age. A significant observation was that their total dietary intake was not increasing with age and increased requirements for growth and body building as it should. Besides, their Hb was also below the low normal range, again indicating the prevalence of anaemia which might be with the reasons common to the junior age group which were continuing at this stage too along with the increased body requirement of iron with increased blood volume.

Energy needs of children at different ages and under various conditions vary greatly. The approximate average expenditure of energy by the child of 6–12 yr of age are basal metabolism 50%, growth 12%, physical activity 25%, fecal loss about 8%, mainly as unabsorbed fat and thermic of food 5% of the remainder (Behrman, Kliegman and Jenson, 2000).

A child will meet protein needs if a variety of plant foods are eaten and calorie intake is adequate. It is unnecessary to precisely plan and complement amino acids within each meal as was once thought, as long as children eat several meals and snacks a day. Children who are most likely to be at risk for inadequate protein intake are those who have multiple food allergies or those who have limited food selections because of fat diets, behavioral problems or limited access to food. Variety is the key to a healthy diet. Sources of protein include pulses, grains, soya products, beans, meat analogs, nuts, egg and milk products, which should be added to the diet to meet the required protein, need as per age.

As children are growing and developing bones, teeth, muscles *etc*, they need more nutritious food that is proportionate to their weight. Food consumed by children should contain proper level of calcium, iron, zinc, vitamin B, C and vitamin A. The energy needs of a child are determined on the basis of basal metabolism, rate of growth, and activity. Dietary energy must be sufficient to ensure growth and spare protein from being used for energy, without being excessive that it results in obesity. Energy intakes of healthy, growing children of the same age and sex vary depending mainly on their activity level.

A major finding of this study revolves around high fat intake in general, in both the age groups and its possible short term and long term consequences. The dietary fat per day was found to be in the excess of 12–13 gms which was also being depicted in the biochemical parameter of serum cholesterol levels of these children. Around 56% of the sample had border line to high risk levels of serum cholesterol (< 170 mg%). A high intake of fat, especially the high percentage of saturated fat in the diet of children may be one of the reasons for elevated cholesterol levels.

Secondly, children and adolescents with elevated serum cholesterol levels, particularly LDL-cholesterol levels, often come from families in which there is a high incidence of coronary heart disease in the adult relatives. (AAP, 1998). A strong familial aggregation of total, LDL-, and HDL-cholesterol levels exists in children and parents. Familial aggregation of blood cholesterol levels results because of shared environments and genetic factors. The monogenetic factors that cause high cholesterol levels include familial hypercholesterolemia and familial-combined hypercholesterolemia. Polygenic disorders that result from the expression of a number of genes, each with a small but additional effect, combined with environmental contributions such as a diet high in saturated fat and cholesterol are likely the most frequent causes of high cholesterol levels during childhood.

Nelson (2000) stated that there is an association between fat intake and cholesterol levels in adult Coronary Heart Disease (CHD). Adult Cardiovascular disease has its roots in childhood. The strongest data linking factors in childhood with adult CHD come from the Bogalusa heart study. The survey has found significant correlations between early atherosclerotic changes identified at autopsy of children and both total and LDL cholesterol levels. For a child, the following pattern of nutrient intake is recommended: 1) saturated fatty acids < 10% of total calories; 2) total fat over several days of ≤ 30% of total calories and no less than 20% of total calories; and 3) dietary cholesterol < 300 mg per day.

Thirdly, the combination of excess dietary fat with continuously reducing physical activity levels in urban children makes the situation grimmer. Today's urban child spends most of its free time in watching TV, playing video games or sitting on computer apart from highly competitive studies, which take most of the time. The out door activities and sports either during schools hour or in the evening has been drastically curtailed. This has reduced the calorie demands for children as per their age. Overall, children spent an average of 20 to 25 minutes a day being physically active, compared with the recommended minimum of 60 minutes. Fewer children playing sport and parents' fears about security, which have kept children indoors, cause the declining level of physical activity among children, which has been noted for years. Fewer children walk or cycle to school than in past generations and more are driven to school.

The impact of visual media, especially the TV advertisements of junk foods and aerated drinks aimed at children, further promote the consumption of these products, which are high in free calories, and contain saturated fat in high proportion. In this study it is found that 52% of the children had higher frequency of junk food consumption either daily or at least three to four times a week which is associated with a high impact of media advertising and associated free games. Children who become habitual to junk foods consequently become more fussy eaters and deny or resist conventional healthy foods. This situation is further worsened if parents satisfy such demands frequently without showing much resistance and children start considering it as an acceptable eating behavior.

Not surprisingly, junk food not only has physiological repercussions, but also psychological ones, far-reaching ones that affect the child's intellect and personalities. Coping intelligently with their dietary needs increases their self-esteem, and encourages further discovery. School days are full of educational challenges that require long attention spans and stamina. Poor nutritional habits can undermine these pre-requisites of learning, as well as sap the strength that children need for making friends, interacting with family, participating in sports and games or simply feeling god about themselves.

Junk foods are often eaten in instead of regular food, an essential Indian diet that consists of wholesome chapatis and vegetables or snacks like upmas and idlis. Not surprisingly eating junk food leads to a sense of starvation both physically and mentally, as the feeling of satiation and contentment that comes after a wholesome meal is absent. On the other hand, parental perception for good nutrition for children starts with fat rich diet only disregarding the essential micronutrients and vitamins present in the protective food groups which make the diet balanced. Combination of all these factors might contribute to increased incidence of childhood obesity. Childhood obesity is a growing problem in India. Since obesity is a known risk factor for many adult diseases, curtailing childhood obesity is vital to ensuring children grow up to be healthy adults.

A study published in the Archives of Pediatrics and Adolescent Medicine (2003) was conducted among about 320 sixth- and seventh-grade students in three schools. All were measured for height and weight, and BMI was calculated. The children also completed a questionnaire aimed at gauging television viewing habits and consumption of soft drinks.

Results showed about a third of the children had a BMI at or above the 85th percentile. Children who watched TV for two or more hours per night had higher BMIs than those who watched for less than two hours, and those who drank three or more sodas per day had higher BMIs than those who drank less than that amount.

Its possible reasons may be more access to media advertised fast foods and packaged foods, more exposure to junk foods with peer group influence, lack of parental quality time for taking care of children's nutritional requirements, increasing fussiness of children because of growing nuclear families and single child families, reducing physical activity levels due to computers, television, video games *etc.* providing convenient entertainment on one hand and increasing study loads, reducing total free time for games, entertainment or social activities on the other.

Dietary Behavior Management

Dietary behavior management was recommended as follows:

Excess Fat Management—There is a need to repeat Serum Cholesterol levels of children whose current levels are above 170 mg% after a month and a watch should be on their levels further. Complete lipid profile is also recommended for children with levels above 200 mg%. To make the diet of children more balanced, taking fewer amounts of food rich in saturated fats, should reduce intake of the fat in their diet. Especially the junk foods like chocolates, wafers, cream biscuits and sweets. As they begin to consume fewer calories from fat, children should replace these calories by eating more grain products, fruits, vegetables, low-fat milk products or other calcium-rich foods, beans, lean meat, poultry, fish, or other protein-rich foods. These recommendations are for average intakes over several days, so that if foods high in total fat, saturated fat, and cholesterol are eaten, eating less of these nutrients at other times can compensate them for.

Iron Deficiency Management—To combat the high prevalence of iron deficiency anaemia, foods high in iron contents like green leafy vegetables and fruits should be increased in diets of vegetarians, and they should be combined with fruits containing ascorbic acid (Vit. C), which enhances the absorption of iron from vegetarian source. Intake of tea and coffee containing phytates should be discouraged. Children who are non-vegetarian, intake of read meat and liver should be encouraged. Cooking of vegetables in iron utensils along with addition of *khatai* (acidic sour substances) increases the absorbable iron content.

Fortification of common salt, biscuits, cornflakes, chocolates, toffees and other food items commonly consumed by the children can be a good option to tackle iron deficiency. In cases of severe iron deficiency iron supplementation under medical supervision is recommended.

Total Diet Management—Because no single food item provides all the essential nutrients in the amounts needed, choosing a wide variety of food from all the food groups will ensure an adequate diet. Nutritional adequacy should be achieved by eating a wide variety of foods and caloric intake should be adequate to support growth and development and to reach or maintain desirable body weight.

Regular meals and healthy snacks that include carbohydrate-rich foods, fruits and vegetables, dairy products, eggs, legumes and nuts should contribute to proper growth and development without supplying excessive energy to the diet. Children need to drink plenty of fluids, especially if it is hot or they are physically active. Water is obviously a good source of liquid and supplies fluid without calories. Variety is important in children's diets and other sources of fluid such as milk and milk drinks, fruit juices and soft drinks can also be chosen to provide needed fluids.

Life Style Management—Looking at the emerging trend of sedentary life style of school aged children, there is a strong need to increase the physical activities of the children both at schools and thereafter at home. Outdoor games, sports and general physical training at school should be not only encouraged but should be made compulsory with due monitoring. Parents should also encourage their children to play out door games to burn their calories. An increasing competition in study, associated hobby classes and high-tech entertainment in the form of TV viewing, computer/video games should not compensate the outdoor games and cycling, the conventional modes of entertainments which were also having dietary blessings in disguise.

Dietary Behavior Management—Children, often tend to eat less than most parents think they should. This is generally due to a developing sense of independence and a slow down in growth. All parents should schedule regular check-ups with their child's pediatrician, in order to monitor growth, development, and health. All parents need to make sure what their child eat gives the child the nutrients he or she needs. The preschool years are an important time for developing healthy eating patterns, which can set the stage for a healthful adult diet. Parents should make the children regularly aware about the impact of type of diet on health and encourage them for healthy eating. They should themselves present the model of Food for Health before them.

CONCLUSIONS

Owing to the impact of media and modern social environment of schools and neighborhood, convincing children for consuming nutritive diet is a big challenge for today. To tackle that, healthy dietary habits should be made a part of curriculum and should be encouraged at schools, so that its wider impact can be made on the psyche and cognitions of children right from early childhood. However, healthy eating does not mean tasteless food. Parents must bring variety to the taste and appearance of food by making it attractive and desirable along with nutritious to best manage the dietary behavior of today's fussy children addicted to junks.

Finally, there is simply no substitute for the feeling that descends, when you wake up and find that you are ready to take on the world and this primarily stems from Good Health! There is no better time than now to build a supportive environment for nurturing our children and endowing them with a legacy of good health.

Extensive study on a larger sample is required to study the incidence of cholesterol in Indian children with a special emphasis on more in depth lipid levels like LDL, HDL and triglycerides in relation to the familial history. Besides, physical and psychological correlates of junk food intake by children and appropriateness of role of media in this regard is also to be investigated further. There is also a need to develop BMI for age percentile curves for Indian children and adolescent population looking at its role in diagnosing the over-weight risk as the childhood obesity problem is on the rise in India too.

REFERENCES

Abidoye, R.O. and Eze, D.I. (2000). *Comparative School Performance through Better Health and Nutrition in Nsukka,Enugu, Nigeria,* 20(5), 609–620.

American Academy of Pediatrics (1998). "Cholesterol in Childhood." *Pediatrics,* 101, 1, 141–147.

Archives of Pediatrics and Adolescent Medicine (2003). 157, 882–886.

Behrman, Kliegman and Jenson (2000). *Nelson Textbook of Pediatrics.* Saunders: Philidelphia.

Bellisele, F., Blundell, J.E., Dye, L. Fantino, M. *et al.* (1998). *Functional Food Science and Behavior and Psychological Functions.* London: CAB International.

Dorbuschs, M. (1991). "Standardized Percentile Curves of Body Mass Index for Children and Adolescents." *Amercian Journal of Diseases of Child,* 145, 259–265.

Gulati, S. and Saxena, A. (2003). "Study of Lipid Profile in Children of Patients with Premature Coronary Artery Disease." *Indian Pediatrics,* 40, 556–560.

Haddad, L.J.R. and Gillespie, S. (2003). "India has Enormous under Nutrition and Over Nutrition Problem." *Express Pharma Pulse,* March 27, 2003.

ICMR (1984). *Dietary Recommendations.*

ICMR (1990). *Nutrient Requirement and RDIs for Indian Children.*

Klish, W.J. (1998). "Cholesterol in Childhood", *Pediatrics*, 101(1), 141–147.

Nelson (2002). *Nelson Textbook of Paediatrics,* Saunders: Philidelphia.

Swaminathan, M.S. (2002). "Nutrition in the Third Millennium" in *Countries in Transition, 17th International Congress of Nutrition*, Vienna.

Clinical Profile of Psychosomatic Symptoms in Children in a Tertiary Level Hospital of North India

Bindu Dhingra*[1] and Anjoo Bhatnagar[2]

ABSTRACT

A retrospective study was undertaken in the Department of Pediatrics of a tertiary level hospital to describe the clinical profile of psychosomatic symptoms in children and adolescents upto 18 years of age between 2004 and 2007. A total of 349 cases were identified as having psychosomatic symptoms, of which 51.3% were females and 48.7% were males. Mean age was 11.1 years. The findings showed that the most common presenting symptom was multiple symptoms (31.2%) followed by hyperventilation (18.6%), headache (15.1%) and fainting (12.3%). Other symptoms like pain in abdomen (8.8%), pseudo seizures (4.5%), chest pain (2.8%), cough (2.8%) and vomiting (2.2%) were also present along with other minor symptoms like hiccups, excessive urination and dizziness (1.7%). Majority of the cases (61%) presented to the out-patient department while 39% were emergency indoor admissions. 1.7% of the cases even required admission to the Intensive Care Unit due to the severity of physical symptoms. Stress factors which resulted in the psychosomatic symptomatology were predominantly scholastic problems.

INTRODUCTION

The influence of mind and emotions over physical functions has been well recognized in medicine. Psychosocial concerns are becoming increasingly prominent in pediatric practice. Behavioral, developmental and psychosocial problems were first identified as the new morbidity of pediatrics more than 30 years ago (Hack, S. and Jellinek, M.S., 1998). With more persistent symptomatology such as chronic abdominal pain or persistent headaches, the medical practitioner often recognizes the flavour of a psychosomatic presentation and needs to differentiate such symptoms from those of underlying organic pathology (Brill, S.R. *et al.,* 2001).

Psychosomatic symptoms are by definition clinical symptoms with no underlying organic pathology (Brill, S.R. *et al.,* 2001). These symptoms are related to children's psychological functioning and cause significant distress and functional impairment thus interfering with their quality of life during a sensitive developmental period.

High rates of psychopathology "hidden" at presentation have been identified amongst children and adolescents attending general practice and pediatric services ostensibly for physical symptoms. About one in ten children in the general population complain

---

*Corresponding author.

[1, 2]Department of Pediatrics, Fortis Escorts Hospital and Research Center, Faridabad, Haryana, India.

of recurrent physical symptoms, the majority medically unexplained (Garralda, M.E., 2004). Existing evidence suggests that these symptoms are theorized to be a normal response to excessive stress or a heightened response to normal amounts of stress especially school related (Brill, S.R. *et al.,* 2001; Garralda, M.E., 2004; Cederquist, A.V., 2006).

The prevalence rate for psychosomatic complaints in children and adolescents has been reported to be between 10 and 25% (Brill, S.R. *et al.,* 2001; Garralda, M.E., 2004). The prevalence and nature of these symptoms may vary by age, gender, culture and developmental stage of the child. The most commonly reported symptoms are abdominal pain, headache, musculo-skeletal pain and chest pain (Brill, S.R. *et al.,* 2001). Other common symptoms are fatigue, weakness, nausea, hyperventilation (over breathing), difficulty in breathing, back pain, pseudo seizures (psychogenic non-epileptic seizures) dizziness and fainting (Brill, S.R. *et al.,* 2007). Many children are found to suffer from multiple pains, most commonly from the combination of headache and abdominal pain (Santalahti, P.S. *et al.,* 2005; Bentsen, L.T. *et al.,* 2001; Ostberg, V. *et al.,* 2006).

AIM

The aim of the present study was to describe the clinical profile of psychosomatic symptoms in children upto 18 years of age presented to the Department of Pediatrics from April 2004 to March 2007.

SETTING

Department of Pediatrics, Tertiary Level Hospital, North India.

SUBJECTS AND METHODS

Inclusion Criteria: Children upto 18 years of age presenting to Department of Pediatrics between April 2004 to March 2007 with psychosomatic symptoms as diagnosed by a team of pediatricians and a child psychologist.

Exclusion Criteria: Children with organic disorders as shown by physical examination, laboratory and other investigations.

Retrospective study of the case records of pediatric patients referred to child psychologist was done to identify the type of psychosomatic symptoms, age, sex, presentation to Out-Patient Department (OPD), In-Patient Department (IPD) and the stress factors causing the symptomatology. The data was tabulated and analysed. Statistical analysis was done with the help of probability estimation.

Study Design

The study was a retrospective, institutional, non-randomized, clinical case series.

Results

Total of 349 cases were identified as having psychosomatic symptoms of which 179 cases (51.3%) were females and 170 cases (48.7%) were males. The male:female ratio was approximately equal. The age range of the subjects was 2.5 years to 18 years and the mean age was 11.1 years.

The distribution profile of children presenting with psychosomatic symptoms is shown in Table 1. Most common presentation was multiple symptoms (31.2%, P = 0.312) followed by hyperventilation (18.6%, P = 0.186), headache (15.1%, P = 0.152) and fainting (12.3%, P = 0.123). Other symptoms like pain in abdomen (8.8%) pseudo seizures (4.5%) and vomitting (2.2%) were also present. Pain in chest and cough were present in 2.8% of cases respectively while other symptoms like hiccups and excessive urination were present in only 0.6% cases each. Dizziness was present in only 2 cases (0.5%). Though overall sex ratio is equal but headache and abdominal pain were reported more by girls.

Table 1: Distribution Profile of Children Presenting with Psychosomatic Symptoms (percentages)

Symptoms	*Total* (n = 349)	*OPD* (n = 213)	*IPD* (n = 136)	*p*
Multiple Symptoms	31.2	70.6	29.4	0.312
Hyperventilation	18.6	67.7	32.3	0.186
Headache	15.1	71.7	28.3	0.152
Fainting	12.3	32.6	67.4	0.123
Abdominal Pain	8.8	38.7	61.3	0.08
Pseudo seizures	4.5	56.3	43.7	0.046
Chest Pain	2.8	90.0	10.0	0.029
Cough	2.8	60.0	40.0	0.029
Vomiting	2.2	12.5	87.5	0.023
Hiccups	0.6	100	0	0.003
Excessive Urination	0.6	100	0	0.003
Dizziness	0.5	50	50	0.006

Majority of the cases (61%) presented to the OPD while 39% presented to casualty requiring indoor admission. A few patients (1.7%) even required admission to Intensive Care Unit (ICU) due to the severity of physical symptoms but turned out to be psychosomatic.

The stress factors causing the somatization response were varied. Predominant among them were school related problems *viz.* academic workload, academic performance, examination anxiety, punishment by teachers, phobia of Mathematics, inability to cope with English language, high expectations of parents regarding marks, adjustment to new school *etc.*

DISCUSSION

It is well documented that stress causes various physical symptoms mediated through the autonomic nervous system. The present study showed that cluster of physical symptoms was the most common presentation in both sexes. In a study on pain among children, one half of the children who had experienced pain reported having multiple pains. This shows that psychosomatic symptoms often cluster with each other (Brill, S.R. *et al.,* 2001; Santalahti, P.S. *et al.,* 2005). Other studies (Santalahti, P.S. *et al.,* 2005; Bentsen, L.T. *et al.,* 2001; Ostberg, V. *et al.,* 2006) have found headache and abdominal pain to be most common with prevalence higher in girls than in boys. In a small pediatric sample from rural India (Ghosh, J.K. *et al.,* 2007) found that the most common presenting symptom was psychogenic seizures with precipitating factors being predominantly scholastic problems. Another study of Norwegian adolescents (Brill, S.R. *et al.,* 2001) also found increased school distress to be associated with several psychosomatic symptoms, while social support *via* teachers or other students reduced the risk of symptoms. In the present study also school related problems were predominant.

Hyperventilation, often concurrent with anxiety states, is a common psychosomatic symptom in adolescents. Associated symptoms may include dizziness, fainting or palpitations. This was the second most common presentation in the present study (18.6%). In one study, thirteen out of twenty-three patients with hyperventilation referred for psychiatric evaluation were diagnosed with anxiety disorder and three met criteria for depression (Brill, S.R. *et al.,* 2001).

Headaches in adolescents are common and are generally presumed to be stress related, tension headaches. They are often coupled with other somatic symptoms, and, like abdominal pain, can comprise a "pain syndrome" (Brill, S.R. *et al.*, 2001). In the present study 15.1% of the subjects reported headaches. Prevalence figures of headache in adolescents are not known as the majority of teens do not seek medical care for headaches as they are often ameliorated with common analgesics and are perceived as benign. Thus the adolescent presenting with a complaint of recurrent headaches may represent a more select population.

Although not as common as headaches and abdominal pain, chest pain is also a frequent presentation in pediatric emergency departments and majority of cases (up to

85%) have no clear medical etiology. Lipsitz, J.D. *et al.* (2005) found 59% of pediatric patients reporting with chest pain to be psychosomatic. In the present study, only 2.8% of the subjects presented with psychosomatic chest pain.

Studies have found significant age differences in the incidence of symptoms. Tanaka, H. *et al.* (2000) found that older children (aged 10–12 years) had higher psychosomatic complaints than younger children (aged 7–9 years). This was also seen in our study as the mean age of our sample was 11.1 years.

The degree of impairment from psychosomatic symptoms can range from minor to major who may even require pharmacologic treatment or hospitalization (Hack, S. *et al.,* 1998; Garralda, M.E., 2004). In the present study, majority of the cases (61%) were seen in OPD and 39% needed hospitalization.

This was an uncontrolled study. The patient population was predominantly of middle to upper socio-economic status, which limits generalizability of the findings. More studies over a longer time period are needed to investigate the associations between psychological problems and psychosomatic symptoms in children.

Treatment requires a paradigm shift in the approach to patient care from the traditional biomedical model, which presumes organic pathology and psychological disturbance to be separate entities, to the biopsychosocial model. The present study highlights school related stress and the importance of mental health consultation in pediatric population for treatment of psychosomatic symptoms in our country.

CONCLUSION

1. Psychosomatic symptoms in children are often encountered in pediatric practice in both sexes.
2. It mostly presents as multiple symptoms.
3. Hyperventilation, headache, fainting, abdominal pain, pseudo seizures, chest pain, cough and vomiting were other psychosomatic presentations.
4. Symptoms may be so severe to require indoor and ICU admission but turned out to be psychosomatic.

REFERENCES

Bentsen, L.T., Kohler, L., Gustafsson, J.E. (2001). "Psychosomatic Complaints in School Children: A Nordic Comparison." *Scand J. Public Health,* 29, 44–54.

Brill, S.R., Patel, D.R. and MacDonald, E. (2001). "Psychosomatic Disorders in Pediatrics." *Indian Journal of Pediatrics,* 68(7), 597–603.

Cederquist, A.V. (2006). "Psychiatric and Psychosomatic Symptoms are Increasing Problems among Swedish School Children: A Commentary." *Acta Pediatrica,* 95, 901–903.

Garralda, M.E. (2004). "The Interface between Physical and Mental Health Problems and Medical Help Seeking in Children and Adolescents: A Research Perspective." *Child and Adolescent Mental Health,* 9(4), 146–155.

Ghosh, J.K., Majumdar, P., Pant, P., Dutta, R. and Bhatia, B.D. (2007). "Clinical Profile and Outcome of Conversion Disorder in Children in a Tertiary Hospital of North India." *Journal of Tropical Pediatrics,* 53, 213–214.

Hack, S. and Jellinek, M.S. (1998). "Historical Clues to the Diagnosis of the Dysfunctional Child and Other Psychiatric Disorders in Children." *Pediatric Clinics of North America,* 45(1), 25–48.

Jellesma, F.C., Rieffe, C. and Terwogt, M.M. (2007). "Evaluation of Somatic Complaint List in Children." *Journal of Psychosomatic Research,* 63(4), 399–401.

Lipsitz, J.D., Maria, C., Apfel, H., Marans, Z., Gua, M., Duent, H. and Ftyer, A.J. (2005). "Non-cardiac Chest Pain and Psychopathology in Children and Adolescents." *Journal of Psychosomatic Research,* 59(3), 185–188.

Ostberg, V., Gosta, A. and Hjern, A. (2006). "Living Conditions and Psychosomatic Complaints in Swedish School Children." *Acta Pediatrica,* 95, 929–934.

Santalahti, P.S., Aromaa, M., Sourander, A., Helenius, H. and Piha, J. (2005). "Have There been Changes in Children's Psychosomatic Symptoms? A 10 Year Comparison from Finland". *Pediatrics,*115(4), 434–442.

Tanaka, H., Tamai, H., Terashima, S., Takenaka, Y. and Tanaka, T. (2000). "Psychosocial Factors Affecting Psychosomatic Symptoms in Japanese School Children." *Pediatrics International,* 42, 354–358.

Psychology of TB Patients Under Dots: An Investigation in Agra (UP)

R. Bhatnagar[1], G.P. Mathur[2] and S. Bhatnagar*[3]

ABSTRACT

The World Health Organization declared Tuberculosis (TB) a global health emergency in 1993. Four fifth of the new TB cases are reported from 22 high-burden countries in the world. India being the highest burdened country contributes 20% of TB patients in the world. Realising its responsibility, the Government of India started the Revised National TB Control Programme (RNTCP) using the Directly Observed Treatment, Short-course chemotherapy (DOTS) strategy in 1997. Out of the two objectives of RNTCP, the second one about the detection of 70% of New Sputum Smear Positive (NSP) patients is not achieved in a few districts, for example Agra (UP). An investigation has been attempted to know the reasons for not achieving the same in the present article. Lack of knowledge was observed as the patients were neither aware of the natural course of the disease nor about the facility of DOTS. Stigma of the disease was observed in some of the patients. A few patients had stress and anxiety. Poor physical and mental health was conritbuting to each other. It was observed that more interaction with patients, family members and neighbours should be done. Extensive community meetings and patient- DOT provider meetings leading to good interpersonal relationship are not only essential but mandatory for the continued success of the programme.

INTRODUCTION

Tuberculosis is a common and deadly infectious disease caused by *mycobacteria*, affecting most commonly the lungs. Progression from TB infection to TB disease occurs when the TB bacilli overcome the immune system defences and begin to multiply. TB is spread by aerosol droplets expelled by people with the active disease of the lungs when they cough, sneeze, speak or spit. A person with untreated, active tuberculosis can infect 10–15 other people per year. The chain of transmission can therefore be broken by starting effective anti-tuberculous therapy. After two weeks of such treatment, people with non-resistant active TB generally cease to be contagious. The treatment under DOTS is free and long (6–8 months usually) comprising of Intensive and Continuation phases. It must be regular and complete to achieve the cure and prevent the multi drug resistance. This knowledge should be imparted to the

* Corresponding author.

[1] ACME Iinstitute of Management and Technology, Sikandara, Agra, UP, India.

[2] I.G. Government Girls' Degree College, RaeBareli, UP, India.

[3] State TB Training and Demonstration Centre, Agra, UP, India.

E-mail: drshailendrabhatnagar@yahoo.com

patients and their family members by continued interactions. A healthy individual maintains good adjustment with social situations, and is engaged in some or other good project intended to benefit the society directly or indirectly. The stress and anxiety in TB patients should be addressed by the health providers during motivation sessions. Social relationships are a part of everyone's life. Family of the patient has the greatest importance in maintaining a condition of mental health. The initial counselling of the family by the health personnel is therefore very important. The patients should be told how to prevent the next generation from the disease. Thus during the long treatment of TB patients, their psychological aspects should also be kept in mind for the complete success of DOTS.

REVIEW OF LITERATURE

The objectives of RNTCP are to achieve and maintain:

- A cure rate of at least 85% among newly detected infectious (new sputum smear positive) cases.
- Detection of at least 70% of such cases in the population.

A new TB patient is one who has never had treatment for tuberculosis or has taken anti-tuberculosis drugs for less than one month.

A Treatment-After-Default (TAD) is a TB patient who received anti-tuberculosis treatment for one month or more from any source and returns to treatment after having defaulted, *i.e.,* not taken anti-TB drugs consecutively for two months or more, and is found to be sputum smear positive.

DOT provider is a person trained in RNTCP for providing the anti-TB drugs to the patient at a place called DOT centre.

In the world, 3.9 million NSP pulmonary TB cases were reported in 2004.

In India, about 400 million people are estimated to be infected by *T. bacilli.* More than 70% of TB cases are seen in economically productive age group (15–54 years). 75 NSP PTB cases/1 lakh population per year are expected. 2 patients die due to TB every 3 minutes.

Effect on Human Health in India	*Estimated Burden Per Year*
Indirect costs to society	$3 billion
Direct costs to society	$300 million
Productive work days lost due to TB illness	$100 million
Productive work days lost due to TB deaths	$1.3 billion
School drop outs due to parental TB	$0.3 million
Women rejected by families due to TB	$0.1 million

Directly Observed Treatment Short-Course (DOTS)

DOTS Strategy, 1994 is a major plank in the *WHO* global TB control programme:

1. Government commitment to TB control.
2. Diagnosis by smear microscopy mostly on self reporting symptomatic patients.
3. Standardized short course chemotherapy (SCC) with direct observation of treatment (DOT).
4. Efficient system of drug supply.
5. Efficient recording and reporting system with assessment of treatment results.

According to DOTS, all TB patients should have at least the first two/three months of their therapy observed. Standardized Treatment Regimens are one of the pillars of the DOTS strategy.

DOTS had been implemented in 183 countries by 2004.

Stop TB Partnership proposed a "Global Plan to Stop TB", which aims to save 14 million lives between 2006 and 2015.

Stop TB Strategy, 2006 has a vision of a world free of TB, dramatically reducing the global burden of TB by 2015.

The result of above strategies would be a TB free environment, necessary for sustained development of our society.

Global Situation of DOTS

Since 1995, more than 21 million patients have been diagnosed and treated in DOTS programme. Of 1.7 million NSP patients registered in 2003, 82% were successfully treated under DOTS.

Indian Situation of DOTS

The Revised National Tuberculosis Control Programme (RNTCP) implementing in a phased manner, covered the entire country by March 2006. 6.7 million patients have been initiated on DOTS, preventing 1.2 million deaths.

Physical and mental health are complementary to each other especially in TB patients due to their long treatment. They need not only the drugs but emotional and social support by family members and the health providers.

MATERIAL AND METHOD

RNTCP using the DOTS strategy was started in District Agra in the state of Uttar Pradesh on 31st May, 2003. Out of about 600 TAD patients on treatment in 4Q07, 107 were interviewed using a self made format of statements in the study in some of the

Designated Microscopy Centres of district Agra. It was tried to elicit the knowledge of patients about TB, their treatment seeking behavior, their physical and mental health, their level of satisfaction about the present treatment and the reasons of earlier drop outs.

OBSERVATIONS

Almost all the patients were from the low socioeconomic group with low literacy level.

Knowledge of Patients

- About 50% of patients felt that their condition improved with DOTS.
- About 60% of patients knew their diagnosis (TB).
- Minority (about 20%) were aware of the natural course of TB and its prevention.
- About 50% of patients were aware of the duration of the treatment.
- Majority (about 90%) were not aware about the existing facility of DOTS earlier.
- About 60% of patients were not aware about the mode of spread of the disease.

Treatment Seeking Behavior by the Patients

- Majority (about 90%) consulted qualified private practitioners before taking DOTS.
- Almost all patients wanted to discuss about their illness in detail.
- All patients resided permanently in district Agra.
- They came to know about DOTS by various sources: DOT provider, OPD, Health Care Worker (HCW), cured patient, private practitioner and friend.
- About 30% of patients did not want to disclose the diagnosis to others.
- The earlier treatment was interrupted due to lack of money (about 60%)/ alcoholism/work/associated illness.

Mental and Physical Health of the Patients

- About 20% of patients had stress and anxiety related to their illness.
- Associated illness (about 10%) frustrated the patient without taking proper remedy leading to apathy towards DOTS.
- About 20% of patients were unable to earn their livelihood.
- About 10% paediatric patients dropped out of school.
- About 10% women patients were rejected by their families.

Technical and Administrative

- Majority (about 80%) had 3 samples of sputum examined at the time of diagnosis.
- Almost all patients had no difficulty in sputum examination.

- Almost all patients were fully satisfied with the DOT provider and personnel at the Designated Microscopy Centre (DMC).

DISCUSSION

Annualised total case detection rate is more in district Agra than optimum, with 163 (Agra), 118 (UP) and 124 (India) cases per lakh population for 1Q07 (Figure 1).

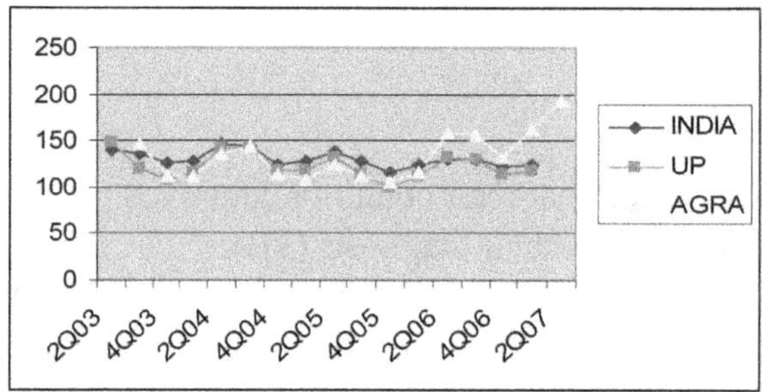

Figure 1: Annualized Total Case Detection Rate

The first objective of RNTCP, the cure rate among NSP patients has been achieved and maintained at all levels (Figure 2). Cure rate of NSP patients is almost at par with national and state level with 83% (Agra), 83% (UP) and 84% (India) in 1Q07.

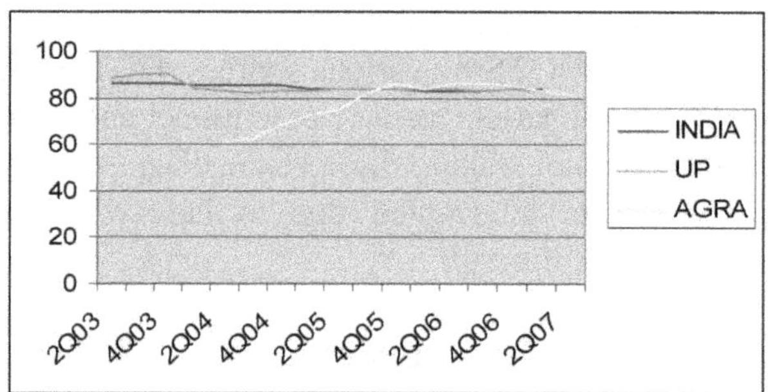

Figure 2: Cure Rate of New Smear Positive Patients

The second objective of RNTCP, the detection of new sputum smear positive (NSP) patients (57% in 2Q07) is less than optimum in district Agra (Figure 3).

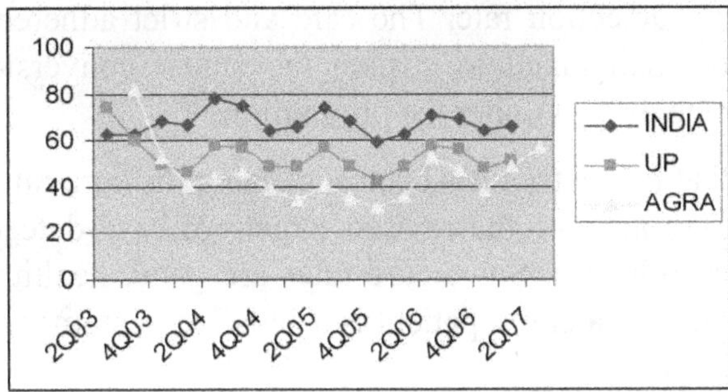

Figure 3: Annualized NSP Case Detection Rate (%)

DOTS is the sure treatment for cure of TB. This is the simplest method to prevent the next generation from this menace. The positivity rate in the TB suspects in the district is optimum. All the smear positive results are recorded in the TB register in general.

Inferences of the study are

1. The community meetings should be done frequently, effectively and at right time in the presence of at least a Medical Officer.
2. Patient-provider interaction meetings should be done sincerely in the presence of at least Supervisors.
3. Review of slides read as negative particularly if placed on DOTS should be intensified by Senior TB Laboratory Supervisor (STLS).
4. Training status of the lab technicians should be assessed periodically.

The counselling by a Psychologist can be sought in inference 1 and 2.

The total case detection rate has been consistently increasing due to participation of SN Medical College (especially deptt. of TB and Chest, Paediatrics); Medical Care Unit; K.B. Patel Hospital, Saran Ashram Hospital, Mina Charitable Hospital (NGOs); Air Force Hospital and Cantonment Board Hospital *etc*. The number of NSP cases is improving but needs to accelerate. Efforts are being made at all levels with spreading the information about DOTS in the community using more and more IEC methods.

NSP case notification rate indicates the extent to which patients with new smear positive TB is being treated by the public health system. From the Figure 3 it can be seen that Distt. Agra has achieved the detection of 45% of NSPs in the community for most of the quarters. More efforts are expected when compared to All India performance.

Agra has witnessed beautiful example of Public Private Mix with plenty of NGOs, private practitioners, hospitals of other sectors and community DOT providers contributing in the programme. The district could also intensify the IEC activities, including building and strengthening partnerships with all major health providers to improve its NSP case detection rate. The care and strict adherence to the RNTCP guidelines should be maintained to sustain the smear conversion and cure rates already achieved by the district under the programme.

The sliver lining is that the district has been sustaining the cure rate of around 85%. It is therefore possible to achieve the revised targets of case detection with strategic advances in public health care. Since cure rates are good, health facilities will start attracting more patients, as a cured patient is a satisfied customer and would serve as a pamphlet for the programme.

Regular motivation of the patient is very vital. Knowledge of patients should be increased. They should be explained about the diagnosis, natural course of the disease and its prevention, duration of treatment and the mode of its spread. Regular workshops for the involvement and follow up of more and more of private practitioners and hospitals should be undertaken in each DMC. Agra is one of the few districts to have an Urban TB Coordinator for this task.

The Programme Officers, initiating doctors, technicians, field supervisors should devote more effective time with the patient resolving all the queries in his/her mind about TB. Frequent and regular community meetings should be organized with more higher officials attending them. The DOT providers, Medical Officer and HCWs of the DMC, cured patients, private practitioners and community in general should be involved in the community meetings. Patient-provider meetings can remove the ignorance of the patients and community at large about TB. More and more publicity should be done about free sputum diagnosis and International standard of treatment of TB.

The behavior of all the health providers must be sympathetic towards the patients. If necessary, psychological help or anti anxiety drugs (as advised by a qualified doctor) can be used. Children dropped out of school should be sent back to the school at the earliest. Family members who rejected the woman patient should be counselled. Associated illness should be dealt at the time of treatment. All the technicians should be asked to take three samples at the time of diagnosis. The DMC personnel and DOT providers should continue to work with devotion.

The patients should be told about the harm of excessive crowding in unhealthy small houses. Cooperative effort on the part of the government, teachers, social and religious leaders should be sought regularly. Inter Personal Communication skills should be practiced regularly with sincerity at all levels by the health providers.

The greater the balance of the social relationships and the greater their simplicity, the better would be the mental and physical health of the TB patients. Hence proper behavior and sympathetic attitude by the health providers are essential towards the

TB patients during their frequent visits to the DOT centres for taking DOT. It is our responsibility to help TB patients come out of the clutches of the vicious cycle of poor physical and mental health.

> "The successive reports from India on the progress of the national DOTS programmes for TB have astonished and delighted me. All concerned deserve the greatest credit for facing up to this enormous challenge with such speed and such success. India is an example to the world."
>
> —*Sir John Crofton, Eminent Pulmonologist*

REFERENCES

Central TB Division, Directorate General of Health Services (2005). "Managing Revised National Tuberculosis Control Programme in Your Area", *A Training Course Module 1.*

Central TB Division, Directorate General of Health Services (2007). New Delhi: *RNTCP Performance report—First quarter.*

Gopi, P. *et al.* (2005). (TRC), IJMR.

Shailendra Bhatnagar (2007). "DOTS as Community Health Care Initiative as Seen in Agra (UP)", *International Conference on Environmental Parasitology and Community Health Care Initiatives*, Dayalbagh Educational Institute Agra, Proceedings, 74–78.

TB India (2007). *RNTCP Status Report.* Central TB Division, Directorate General of Health Services.

Technical and Operational Guidelines for Tuberculosis Control (2005), 16–18.

TRC (1999). Socio-Economic Impact of TB on Patients and Family in India, *Int J Tub Lung Dis,* 3, 869–877.

WHO (2006). *Global Tuberculosis Control; Surveillance, Planning and Financing.* WHO: Geneva.

Intellectual Angst and Mental Despair: Virginia Woolf's *Mrs Dalloway*

Prem Kumari Srivastava*

ABSTRACT

Encapsulated in the general landscape of English literature and psychology, within the rubric of the academia, is a marriage and a mating. They converge and impinge upon each other at several junctures, thereby establishing themselves as mutually inclusive domains. This paper captures an important intersection of modernism's isolationist agenda and a defining moment in early twentieth century feminism. Here, stands the British novelist, Virginia Woolf and her poignant study of insanity and suicide in her novel, *Mrs. Dalloway* (1925). The novel traces the lifespan of a pre-menopausal woman, Clarissa Dalloway and her shifting loyalties between a lost past with Peter, her poor friend-lover and a present with the successful, rich husband, Richard. Set in the tumultuous and depressed post World War I period of Victorian England, the novel also foregrounds the transgressions of the displaced psyche of the soldier, Septimus Warren Smith, who doubles up as Clarissa's alternate self, representing two halves—the living and the dying—of the same soul. Here, woman is the primary signifier and her mental health in terms of the use of past and memory as a means to respond to contemporary reality is at the centre. Tackling anxieties that plague women's health and psyche, the paper explores the intellectual angst and psychological despair of a woman writer/ protagonist, bordering on schizophrenia, relapsing into madness on numerous occasions, leading to her eventual suicide.

INTRODUCTION

One of the most 'read' writers of Victorian feminism as also extensively researched; what legitimizes Virginia Woolf's relevance as well as inclusion in detailed studies and researches on mental health and psychology even today is the unique relationship between madness and creativity in her works. In the present war-ridden, divisive world, her signature statement on insanity and suicide continue to engage scholars the world over for its contemporariness. Though, the novel is by no way a self portrait, but many of the concerns that Woolf voices in her diary entries[1]: the passage of

---

*Institute of Lifelong Learning, University of Delhi, India (on deputation from Maharaja Agrasen College, University of Delhi, India). E-mail: premksri@gmail.com

[1]According to Lyndall Gordon, one of Woolf's best-known literary biographers," Virginia Woolf shaped and defended the modern novel and left nearly 4,000 letters and thirty volumes of a diary. No writer's life can be so fully documented" Gordon, Lyndall. *Virginia Woolf: A Writer's Life.* Oxford: Oxford University Press, 1986, 5.

time;[2] wanting to prove even to oneself; coping with failures, death, childlessness; growing old; and nihilistic despair;[3] slip smoothly and tenderly into each other, building a complex matrix of human fallibilities in the novel. Interestingly, the novel is also read as "a celebration of the ecstasy of living and an elegy for the swift passage of that ecstasy"[4].

I

"The most schizophrenic of English novels"[5]

Born on 25 January 1882 to Leslie and Julia (Duckworth) Stephen at Hyde Park Gate, Kensington, Virginia Woolf battled poor health all her life compounded with bouts of mental illness. Her location in the war-ridden England impacted her intellectual make-up. Her personal traumas (death of mother in 1895, half-sister Stella Duckworth, two years later, father in 1904, brother, Thoby in 1907 and her friend Kitty Maxse in 1922) as also her domestic life led to five debilitating rounds of mental breakdowns as well as minor disturbances between 1897 and 1915. In 1898 Virginia met Kitty Maxse, who later became the model for Mrs. Dalloway. In 1904, upon the death of her father Sir Leslie Stephen, Virginia suffered her second and far more serious breakdown, during which she attempted suicide. The same year, the Stephen siblings moved to Bloomsbury; soon, Thoby started 'Thursday Evenings' at their 46 Gordon Square residence hosting his university friends, which marked the beginnings of the famous 'Bloomsbury Group'. In August 1912 she married Leonard Woolf, after an attack of mental illness earlier that year; the following year she was again seriously ill and attempted suicide by overdose. However, she began to recover after the publication of the *The Voyage Out* in 1915, and in 1917 the Woolfs started The Hogarth Press at home. Woolf continued to write and publish fiction and prose—*Night and Day* (1919), *Monday or Tuesday* (1921) and their publishing venture began to flourish amongst intellectuals. 1922 was an eventful year in Woolf's life: she published *Jacob's Room*, her friend Kitty Maxse died, and she met Vita Sackville-West, with whom she was to have a long and rich love affair, both emotional and physical.

From there on, the years were astonishingly busy and fruitful for Woolf. Both *The Common Reader* and *Mrs. Dalloway* were published in 1925, and *To the Lighthouse*

---

[2]Virginia Woolf. "*I think too much of whys and wherefores: too much of myself. I don't like time to flap around me....*". From *The Diary of Virginia Woolf,* Vol. 2 1920–24. Ed. Anne Olivier Bell. London: Penguin, 1981, 72.

[3]Poole, Roger. *The Unknown Virginia Woolf.* Cambridge: Cambridge University Press, 1995 (1st pub. 1978).

[4]Rose, Phyllis. *Woman of Letters: A life of Virginia Woolf.* London: Routledge & Kegan Paul 1978, 125.

[5]Ibid, 125.

in 1927. While her relationship with Vita blossomed, she began to write *Orlando*, which was published in 1928. The same year, she delivered lectures at Cambridge that later became *A Room of One's Own* (1929). *The Waves* appeared in 1931. By the mid-30s, however, the strains of her emotional and intellectual struggles were beginning to overtake her. She labored over *The Years* through 1935–36, and published *Three Guineas*, her most political tract besides *A Room of One's Own*, in 1938. In February 1941 she managed to finish writing *Between the Acts*, but the curtain was about to descend on her own tumultuous life: her mental health deteriorated rapidly, and on 29 March she drowned herself in the River Ouse. It is almost impossible, in fact, to talk about Woolf's literary achievements without considering the vital connection between identity (female), writing (memory and experience) and social reality (the times) that she embodies; it is for this reason that her non-fictional writings are so crucial to the understanding of her fiction. The richest source of this material certainly lies in the wealth of Woolf's own writings—her letters, diary, essays, short stories, novels and the remarkable characters she created. *Mrs Dalloway* is a wonderfully representative modernist text, not simply because Woolf practices in it her famous 'Stream of Consciousness' narrative technique, but also because it captures so brilliantly the fragmented consciousness that is symptomatic of life in the twentieth century.

The narrative of *Mrs. Dalloway* runs on parallel courses between the worlds of Clarissa Dalloway and Septimus Warren Smith on a single given day (June the 13th) in London in 1923.[6] It traces the lifespan of pre-menopausal, wife, mother and gracious hostess, Clarissa Dalloway's shifting loyalties between a lost past with her one time suitor Peter (who still enchants her) and her childhood friend/lover Sally Seton; and a present with the successful, rich husband Richard and her seventeen-year-old grown up daughter Elizabeth. Set in the tumultuous and depressed post World War I period against the backdrop of Victorian England, the novel also foregrounds the transgressions of the displaced psyche of Clarissa and the soldier, Septimus Warren Smith, who doubles up as Clarrisa's alternate self, representing two halves—the living and the dying—of the same soul. Peter's return, back from his imperialistic adventures in India to torment her with the flicking of his penknife (a weirdly phallic symbol) and memories of her youthful passion for the "amazing" Sally Seton, add to her emotional turmoil. Septimus Warren Smith, back from the War and emotionally ravaged by it, struggles to cling to the promise of a normal sane existence as he sees it embodied in his young wife Lucrezia, but finds himself slipping away into the dark and blessed oblivion he desperately craves. If there is any confusion about the disjunction between the two worlds—for Clarissa and Septimus are never acquainted—it is cleared with the realization that by the working of some

[6]We have James Joyce's *Ulysses* (1922) tracing a mythic passage of a single day in the city of Dublin.

strange logic of fiction, Septimus emerges as Clarissa's double at the end of the novel, her death-wish fulfilled in his leap from the window.[7] Septimus, in killing himself at the end of the novel, proves himself to be Clarrisa's soul twin who dies so that she can survive. And yet they have never really met in the novel. The classical unities of time (one summer's day) and place (the city of London) are, after all, easily maintained; the regular chiming of the Big Ben alerts us to the passing of hours as the two worlds—Clarissa's and Septimus's—meet and part, each oblivious of the other until they merge briefly at the end when Peter registers the sound of the ambulance's alarm as the vehicle rushes towards Septimus's now-dead body, and the Bradshaws bring the news of his suicide to Clarissa's party.

Her short story, *'Mrs Dalloway in Bond Street'*, written in August 1922, was the genesis of the novel. Woolf first envisaged the novel as a series of vignettes; her working title in October 1922 was 'At Home' or 'The Party', in which separate stories would connect at the end, perhaps by a climactic event: "There must be some sort of fusion. And all must converge upon the party at the end."[8] Later that month Woolf realized that "*Mrs Dalloway* has branched into a book; and I adumbrate here a study of insanity and suicide: the world seen by the sane and the insane side by side …." (28)[9]

II

"It might be possible, Septimus thought, looking at England from the train window, as they left Newhaven; it might be possible that the world itself is without meaning."

These are, philosophically and humanly, the central lines in the book.[10] Throughout the nineteenth century, the British Empire seemed invincible. It spread into many other countries, such as India, Nigeria, and South Africa, becoming the largest empire the world had ever seen. World War I was a violent reality check. For the first time in nearly a century, the English were vulnerable on its own land. The Allies technically won the war, but the extent of devastation England suffered made it a victory in name only. Entire communities of young men were injured and killed. In 1916, at the Battle of the Somme, England suffered 60,000 casualties—the largest slaughter in

---

[7] Ibid. "Woolf has recorded her earlier intentions to have Clarissa die at the end of *Mrs Dalloway,* before she conceived of the rather more sophisticated—if confusing—inclusion of Septimus Smith as an unknown, and unacknowledged, soul twin, who also doubles up as a curious scapegoat figure in the text", xxxv.

[8] Woolf, Virginia. *Jacob's Room* notebook 3, 6 October 1922, 131, Berg Collection, New York Public Library.

[9] Woolf, Virginia. *Diary,* Vol. II, 14 October 1922, 207.

[10] Poole, Roger. *The Unknown Virginia Woolf.* Cambridge: Cambridge University Press, 1995 (1st pub. 1978).

England's history. Not surprisingly, English citizens lost much of their faith in the empire after the war. No longer could England claim to be invulnerable and all-powerful. Citizens were less inclined to willingly adhere to the rigid constraints imposed by England's class system, which benefited only a small margin of society but which all classes had fought to preserve.

In 1925, when *Mrs. Dalloway* takes place, the old establishment and its oppressive values are nearing their end. English citizens, including Clarissa, Peter, and Septimus, feel the failure of the empire as strongly as they feel their own personal failures. Those citizens who still champion English tradition, such as Aunt Helena and Lady Bruton, are old. *Mrs. Dalloway* takes place after World War I, a time when the English looked desperately for meaning in the old symbols but found the symbols hollow. The prime minister in *Mrs. Dalloway* embodies England's old values and hierarchical social system, which are in decline. The old pyramidal social system that benefited the very rich before the war is now decaying, and the symbols of its greatness have become pathetic.

Throughout *Mrs. Dalloway*, Clarissa, Septimus, Peter, and others struggle to find outlets for communication as well as adequate privacy, and the balance between the two is difficult for all to attain. Clarissa in particular struggles to open the pathway for communication and throws parties in an attempt to draw people together. At the same time, she feels shrouded within her own reflective soul and thinks the ultimate human mystery is how she can exist in one room while the old woman in the house across from hers exists in another. Even as Clarissa celebrates the old woman's independence, she knows it comes with an inevitable loneliness. Peter tries to explain the contradictory human impulses toward privacy and communication by comparing the soul to a fish that swims along in murky water then rises quickly to the surface to frolic on the waves. The war has changed people's ideas of what English society should be, and understanding is difficult between those who support traditional English society and those who hope for continued change. Meaningful connections in this disjointed postwar world are not easy to make, no matter what efforts the characters put forth. Ultimately, Clarissa sees Septimus's death as a desperate, but legitimate, act of communication.

The characters mental states are often reflected through certain symbols associated with the war and weapons in the novel. Peter Walsh's constant opening, closing, and fiddling with the knife suggests his inability to decide what he feels. He doesn't know whether he abhors English tradition and wants to fight it, or whether he accepts English civilization just as it is. The pocketknife reveals Peter's defensiveness. He is armed with the knife, in a sense, when he pays an unexpected visit to Clarissa, while she herself is armed with her sewing scissors. Their weapons make them equal competitors. Knives and weapons are also phallic symbols, hinting at sexuality and power. Peter cannot define his own identity, and his constant fidgeting with the knife suggests how uncomfortable he is with his masculinity. Septimus, psychologically crippled by the literal weapons of war, commits suicide by impaling himself on a metal fence, showing the danger lurking behind man-made boundaries.

Human psyche has been irrevocably bruised. Thoughts of death lurk constantly beneath the surface of everyday life in *Mrs. Dalloway*, especially for Clarissa, Septimus, and Peter, and this awareness makes even mundane events and interactions meaningful at the same time, even threatening. At the very start of her day, when she goes out to buy flowers for her party, Clarissa remembers a moment in her youth when she suspected a terrible event would occur. Big Ben tolls out the hour, and Clarissa repeats a line from Shakespeare's *Cymbeline* over and over as the day goes on: "Fear no more the heat o' the sun/Nor the furious winter's rages." The many appearances of Shakespeare specifically and poetry in general suggest the psychological succour that is often termed-hopefulness, the possibility of finding comfort in art, and the survival of the soul in *Mrs. Dalloway.* Clarissa quotes Shakespeare's plays many times throughout the day. The line is from a funeral song that celebrates death as a comfort after a difficult life. Middle-aged Clarissa has experienced the deaths of her father, mother, and sister and has lived through the calamity of war, and she has grown to believe that living even one day is dangerous. Death is very naturally in her thoughts, and the line from *Cymbeline*, along with Septimus's suicidal embrace of death, ultimately helps her to be at peace with her own mortality. Peter Walsh, so insecure in his identity, grows frantic at the idea of death and follows an anonymous young woman through London to forget about it. Septimus faces death most directly. Though he fears it, he finally chooses it over what seems to him a direr alternative—living another day. Waves and water regularly wash over events and thoughts in *Mrs. Dalloway* and nearly always suggest the possibility of extinction or death. Time sometimes takes on water-like qualities for Clarissa, such as when the chime from Big Ben "flood[s]" her room, marking another passing hour. Traditional English society itself is a kind of tide, pulling under those people not strong enough to stand on their own. Lady Bradshaw, for example, eventually succumbs to Sir William's bullying, overbearing presence.

Oppression is a constant threat for Clarissa and Septimus in *Mrs. Dalloway*, and Septimus dies in order to escape what he perceives to be an oppressive social pressure to conform. It comes in many guises, including religion, science, or social convention. Miss Kilman and Sir William Bradshaw are two of the major oppressors in the novel: Miss Kilman dreams of felling Clarissa in the name of religion and Sir William would like to subdue all those who challenge his conception of the world. Both wish to convert the world to their belief systems in order to gain power and dominate others, and their rigidity oppresses all who come into contact with them. More subtle oppressors, even those who do not intend to, do harm by supporting the repressive English social system. Though Clarissa herself lives under the weight of that system and often feels oppressed by it, her acceptance of patriarchal English society makes her, in part, responsible for Septimus's death. Thus she too is an oppressor of sorts. At the end of the novel, she reflects on his suicide: "Somehow it was her disaster—her disgrace." She accepts responsibility, though other characters are equally or more fully to blame, which suggests that everyone is in some way complicit in the oppression of others.

Tree and flower images have close connection with health, well being and goodness as also life, death and decay. They also symbolically represent mental states in *Mrs. Dalloway*. The color, variety, and beauty of flowers suggest feeling and emotion, and those characters who are comfortable with flowers, such as Clarissa, have distinctly different personalities than those characters who are not, such as Richard and Lady Bruton. The first time we see Clarissa, a deep thinker, she is on her way to the flower shop, where she will revel in the flowers she sees. Richard and Hugh, more emotionally repressed representatives of the English establishment, offer traditional roses and carnations to Clarissa and Lady Bruton, respectively. Richard handles the bouquet of roses awkwardly, like a weapon. Lady Bruton accepts the flowers with a "grim smile" and lays them stiffly by her plate, also unsure of how to handle them. When she eventually stuffs them into her dress, the femininity and grace of the gesture are rare and unexpected.

The old woman in the window across from Clarissa's house represents the privacy of the soul and the loneliness that goes with it. Clarissa sees the future in the old woman: She herself will grow old and become more and more alone, since that is the nature of life. As Clarissa grows older, she reflects more but communicates less. Roger Poole along with several other scholars, points out that her failures find a symbolic reference to Greek scattered profusely in novels, in essays, in letters and diaries. For Virginia Woolf, Greek was a symbol for everything that she personally would never be able to attain to Greek was an ideal, a touchstone, an abstraction of pure intellection. It was a symbol for her own failure, her own impracticality, her own shifting nature, her irrepressible unlearnedness, so she thought.

III

"The autobiographical element both constructs as well as deconstructs the text."

It would be worthwhile to open certain pages of Virginia Woolf's diaries and letters that outline her health issues while looking at *Mrs Dalloway*. Lyndall Gordon's (1986) pioneering work is of great importance here.[11] In Virginia's case, the line

[11] Gordon, Lyndall. "The Question of Madness" in *Virginia Woolf: A Writer's Life*. Oxford: Oxford University Press, 1986.

between madness[12] and creativity are harder to draw. Her worst episodes—in 1904, in 1915, and finally in 1941—were invariably heralded by voices which spoke to her alone. The text can be read wholly as fiction and as one inspired and engendered with social reality. In September 1897, Virginia Stephen first fought a wish to die. 'This diary is lengthening indeed', she wrote, 'but death would be shorter and less painful.' And 'Life is a hard business', she scribbled into the void, 'one needs a rhinoceros skin—and that one has not got!' She told her sister that to escape, 'I shall soon have to jump out of a window.' And Septimus did!

In inventing the character of Septimus Warren Smith, Virginia found an extremely subtle and cogent symbol, a perfect 'objective correlative' for her own state of mind in 1912–13. For Septimus Smith's root problem is that 'he could not feel'. Septimus Smith is presented as a young man who goes to the war, makes friends with his officer, Evans, sees Evans killed, and prides himself on being able to take this in his stride without faltering. His career is given in a very few words:

> "Septimus was one of the first to volunteer. He went to France to save an England, which consisted almost entirely of Shakespeare's plays, and Miss Isabel Pole in a green dress walking in a square. There in the trenches the change which Mr. Brewer desired when he advised football was produced instantly; he developed manliness; he was promoted; he drew the attention, indeed the affection of his officer, Evans by name.... when Evans was killed, just before the Armistice, in Italy, Septimus, far from showing any emotion or recognizing that here was the end of a friendship, congratulated himself upon feeling very little and very reasonably. The War had taught him. It was sublime."

In her own case, she was treated in an entirely external and 'behavioral' way, which took no account of her inner dilemma. In Septimus Smith, and the 'treatment' he receives, Virginia has the symbol she needs.

> "The War had taught him. It was sublime.... He became engaged one evening when the panic was on him—that he could not feel.... Even taste... had no relish to him.... his brain was perfect; it must be the fault of the world then."

Having established, in symbolic form, that extreme shock can anaesthetize the feelings, Virginia goes on to show that such a shock can lead *directly* to the conviction that the world itself is entirely without meaning. Since doctors are the official prescribers of normality, Virginia Woolf examines how, precisely, they define mental illness. The specialist, Sir William, takes the opposite position on

[12] Gordon points out, "'Madness' or 'sanity', like all such defining terms, are absurd simplifications. The most subversive element in Virginia Woolf's work—more so than her challenge of notions of madness and sanity—is her challenge of the category *per se*.... She told a friend that in 'the lava of madness' she found her subjects...".

mental illness, but his notion is equally thin. He regards abnormality primarily as a form of radicalism, a social danger to wipe out. When Smith repeats the word 'war' interrogatively, the doctor notes a serious symptom in his 'attaching meanings to words of a symbolical kind'. Like Virginia's specialists, Sir William insists that Smith is dangerously ill and must be shut up in sanatorium where there are to be no ideas and no contacts until the patient comes to heel:

> "Sir William not only prospered himself but made England prosper, secluded her lunatics, forbade childbirth, penalised despair, made it impossible for the unfit to propagate their views until they, too, shared his sense of proportion—his if they were men, Lady Bradshaw's if they were women.".

When Septimus kills himself he waits until the last possible moment. He does not want to die but Holmes, Bradshaw's agent, is coming to take him away. Septimus knows that suicide is tiresomely melodramatic. It is not his idea of tragedy, merely the only means of escape from the indignity of brutes.

The relation between Clarissa Dalloway and her husband Richard is in all points identical to the relation between Virginia and Leonard: one passage from the novel sums it all up, her husband's divine simplicity', the doctor's eternal regime:

> "And there is a dignity in people, a solitude; even between husband and wife a gulf; and that one must respect, thought Clarissa.... He returned with a pillow and a quilt. 'An hour's complete rest after luncheon,' he said. And he went. How like him! He would go on saying 'An hour's complete rest after luncheon' to the end of time, because a doctor had ordered it once. It was like him to take what doctors said literally; part of his adorable divine simplicity, which no one had to the same extent"

Poole (1995) says that, "It seems to me clear that this is how Virginia regarded Leonard—a good, naïve, trusting soul, literal, loving and essentially 'other': someone she hardly knew, and who hardly knew her."[13]

Thus, Woolf uses her inadequate marriage, as well as her brushes with insanity, in *Mrs Dalloway*, by dividing up the experiences between her dual protagonists, Clarissa and Septimus. She further complicates the story of madness by merging it with the experience of war. Septimus is important to the text for two reasons: first, for bearing the weight of Woolf's response to war, and second, for providing her with the scope to explore the phenomenon of psychosis/neurosis that plagued her particularly through the war years 1914–18.

---

[13] Poole, Roger. *The Unknown Virginia Woolf.* Cambridge: Cambridge University Press, 1995, (1st pub.1978).

IV

"Forbade childbirth, penalized despair"

Woolf's intellectual angst was reflected rather seriously in her concerns about the position as well as condition of women in an overtly masculinist society. In a letter to her friend Ethel Smythe written on Christmas Eve, 1940, three months before committing suicide, Woolf declared rather curiously:

> "There has never been a woman's autobiography", going on to muse, "Chastity and modesty I suppose have been the reason. Now, why shouldn't you be, not only the first woman to write an opera, but equally the first to tell the truths about herself? .... More introspection. More intimacy."[14]

As an artist who was a responsible social and political being, she believed a woman had as much right to know about, and participate in, public life; as a woman writer should find the freedom to write whatever she willed. In her charter for women writers' rights—*A Room of One's Own* (1929), where she demanded a private space (both actual and metaphorical) for the female artist—Woolf indicated that the future of fiction was inextricably bound to changing attitudes to men, to themselves and to other women. She recognized the difficulty of reforming a male-centric world, but also reminded her female audience that the responsibility for such a task lay with them. Her significant pronouncement is encapsulated in these lines: "Women have served all these centuries as looking-glasses possessing the magic and delicious power of reflecting the figure of man at twice its natural size. Whatever may be their use in civilized societies, mirrors are essential to all violent and heroic action. That serves to explain in part the necessity that women are often to men. And it serves to explain in part how restless they are under her criticism. For if she begins to tell the truth, the figure in the looking-glass shrinks; his fitness for life is diminished.[15]

The turn of the century was a period of gender crisis. *Mrs Dalloway* addresses it *absolutely* ably. (Emphasis mine) Septimus's homoerotic romance with his officer Evans ends in a partnership with death. The resultant madness represents, according to Kristeva, the fragility of the patriarchal enterprise.[16] The madness parodies and subverts the central tenets of heroes and hero worship. Other same-sex relations (Sally Seton and Clarissa, Doris Kilman and Elizabeth) are not redemptive either. The most crucial relationship emerges thus, is between two people who never met.

Woolf developed a consistent analogy between the (passing of) hours and the female life cycle, or more aptly for this purpose, the biological clock. She introduced the

---

[14] Woolf, Virginia. *The Letters,* Vol. VI. Ed Nigel Nicholson. London: Hogarth Press, 1980, 453.

[15] Woolf, Virginia. *A Room of One's Own.* London: Grafton, 1929, 35–6.

[16] Bose, Brinda (Ed). *Mrs Dalloway.* New Delhi: Worldview Publications, 2001.

striking of the Big Ben to act as a temporal grid to organize the narrative simply because the passing of time is central to this novel. Her working title initially was 'The Hours', and she drew up an elaborate plan for the passage of hours during the one day that her parallel narratives were to span. The city of London grew to be a living protagonist in the novel. But ultimately, Woolf recognized that the focus of the novel was Clarissa herself. According to Elaine Showalter (1922), "Woolf gives us a full range of portraits spanning the seven ages of woman. Elizabeth Dalloway is almost eighteen, just beginning her adult life. Lucrezia Smith is in her twenties. Milly Brush and Doris Killman are in their forties. Clarissa and Sally Seton are in their fifties. Millicent Bruton is sixty-two… Miss Helena Parry, past eighty…Finally, there is the nameless old woman Clarissa sees from her window, alone, putting out her light and going to bed…."[17] This way the passage of time got irrevocably linked with the several women's stories in the novel.

Closely linked to this study of sane insane was her portrayal of Clarissa's experience of menopause, a condition that is even at this turn of the century implicitly linked with illness. Woolf was only in her early forties when she wrote *Mrs Dalloway*, but because she had been forbidden—in a joint decision taken by her psychiatrist (caricatured in Sir William Bradshaw in the novel) and her husband—to have children, she morbidly awaited menopause as the final symbol of the end of her childbearing years. According to Showalter (1922), "The novel is preoccupied with these questions on many levels—in Septimus's mad horror of the body and reproduction, in Rezia's longing for a baby and in Clarissa's coming to terms with the finality of a central aspect of her personality. Moreover, according to the medical opinion of Woolf's day, menopause was a condition to be dreaded and feared as much as insanity, and indeed closely allied with it."[18]

The novel is essentially a description of a man and a woman living together in a marriage which has long since resigned itself to having no physical base. Although *Mrs Dalloway* does have a daughter, this event is so long in the past that it is almost a mythical remembrance. Her daughter is grown up, and leading her own life, partly under the malign tutelage of Miss Kilman. Apart from a certain pride in her daughter, *Mrs Dalloway* seems to have no relation to her. She lives a nun-like, chaste existence, sleeping alone in her bedroom, and resting during the afternoons while her husband is away on committee work. There is no suggestion that there has been any physical contact for decades. The sense of childlessness is engendered partly by the awareness in the reader of this fact, and partly by the extreme distance, which exists between *Mrs Dalloway* and her daughter. At one juncture in the novel even Peter felt, "There

[17] Showalter, Elaine. 'Introduction' to *Mrs Dalloway*. London: Penguin Twentieth Century Classics, 1922, xxx–xxxi.

[18] Showalter, xxx–xxxi.

is some emptiness in her" For her, "The sheet was stretched and the bed narrow". Mrs. Dalloway, in the novel, is not childless, yet the novel aches with a sense of childlessness. Despair has indeed been penalised through the forbidding of childbirth. But childbearing, the continuance of life, is refused because according to certain propagandists of that time, those who despair are unfit to propagate.

V

"For there she was"

Towards the end, we see that these problems lead to a state of nihilistic despair, and the conviction that the world is really meaningless and hostile. And it is in this state, and unable to utter a word, that Virginia is seen by Henry Head on 9 September 1913, and Septimus Smith is seen by Sir William Bradshaw in the novel of ten years later. Virginia's subtle use of the psychic cause of Septimus's mental collapse ('the War') allows her to reinforce her symbol twice over. Her fictional suicide through Septimus in *Mrs Dalloway*, suffer from mental isolation. She demonstrates through these characters the most terrifying experience she herself knew, which is to lose communication with the world outside one's mind. Septimus Warren Smith feels like a:

> "'relic straying on the edge of the world, this outcast who gazed back at the inhabited regions, who lay like a drowned sailor, on the shore of the world'. This is what 'breakdown' meant to her, not so much collapse,… but thought so rapid that language, the main route of communication, became incoherent. Here, if anywhere, is the link between Virginia Woolf's madness and creativity."[19]

Septimus acts out instincts suppressed in *Mrs Dalloway*. He withdraws to live in a self-enclosed dream world, which frequently becomes a nightmare. Finally, opts for death while Clarissa continues to connect with people. Septimus without Clarissa is as incomplete a portrait as she without him. They suggest a polarity, the mad fragmented visions of a shell-shocked soldier and the orderly socialite/Westminster hostess. Of the two, "Clarissa is the most complete figure—because of her creative engagement with life."[20] When Clarissa learns of the death of the young man she never knew, she feels a curious empathy:

> "Death was defiance. Death was an attempt to communicate, people feeling the impossibility of reaching the centre which, mystically, evaded them; closeness drew apart, rapture faded; one was alone. There was an embrace in death...She had escaped. But that young man had killed himself. Somehow it was her disaster—her disgrace."

[19] Gordon, Lyndall. "The Question of Madness" in *Virginia Woolf: A Writer's Life.* Oxford: Oxford University Press, 1986.

[20] Rose, 139.

Despite the horrific death of Septimus by suicide right at the end of *Mrs Dalloway*, Woolf is able to close the novel on an affirmative note. This is partly possible because Clarissa's double is dead while she survives (though she is unsure whether it is an "escape" or a "disaster"/"disgrace"). Clarissa's party itself also strikes the positive note at the end, and there are two relationships that Woolf appears to endorse as signifiers for the emotional survival of the human species in the midst of the untold miseries of daily existence. The first is that of father and daughter: Richard Dalloway and beautiful Elizabeth. The second is defined by the absent presence of Peter Walsh in Clarissa's worlds, real and sub/un/conscious. She speaks to him in her mind; she imagines his responses to her life as she is experiencing it. But, the novel ends with his experience of "her":

> ".... She had influenced him more than any person he had ever known. And always in this way coming before him without his wishing it, cool, lady-like, critical; or ravishing, romantic.... What is it that fills me with extraordinary excitement? It is Clarissa, he said. For there she was."

Multiple levels are at work in *Mrs Dalloway*. Like the continuous sound of the waves on the shore, "the screaming pain of suppressed insanity, the numbing reality of a semi-dysfunctional marriage, the delight of youthful memories, the angst of ebbing energies, the despair of desires still throbbing and unfulfilled"[21] touch us and go all the time. When Clarissa goes on with her party after hearing of Septimus' suicide, she does so not out of callousness, but as a reaffirmation of life and creativity against power of death and disintegration. *Mrs Dalloway* can be read as Woolf's answer to those forces that lead civilization into chaos. These are also some of the many reasons that the novel speaks so coherently to us even today!

REFERENCES

Bell, A.O. (Ed.) (1981). "*The Diary of Virginia*", London: Woolf, Penguin, Vol. 2, 1920–24.

Bose, B. (Ed) (2001). "*Mrs. Dalloway*", New Delhi: Worldview Publications.

Gordon, L. (1986). "The Question of Madness" in "*Virginia Woolf: A Writer's Life*", Oxford: Oxford University Press.

Nicholson, N. (Ed) (1980). "*Woolf, Virginia*". *The Letters,* Vol. VI, London: Hogarth Press.

Poole, R. (1995). *The Unknown Virginia Woolf.* Cambridge: Cambridge University Press.

Rose, P. (1978). "*Woman of Letters: A life of Virginia Woolf*". London: Routledge & Kegan Paul.

Showalter, E. (1922). "*Introduction to Mrs Dalloway*". London: Penguin Twentieth Century Classics.

Woolf, V. (1922). *Jacob's Room* notebook 3, Berg Collection, New York Public Library.

Woolf, V. (1929). *A Room of One's Own.* London: Grafton.

---

[21] Bose, xxxiii.

About the Editors

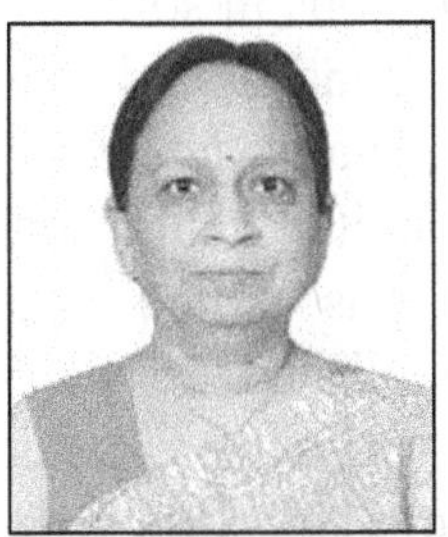

Professor Surila Agarwala is the Head, Department of Psychology and Dean of the Faculty of Social Science, Dayalbagh Educational Institute, Deemed University, Dayalbagh, Agra. She completed her post graduation from Allahabad University in 1970 and joined the Dayalbagh Educational Institute as lecturer in the same year. She did her Ph.D. in 1986 on Intuition. She has 40 published papers to her credit and has received many best paper awards in National and International Conferences and Seminars. Her area of research is Clinical Psychology, specially Behavior Modification and Organizational Behavior.

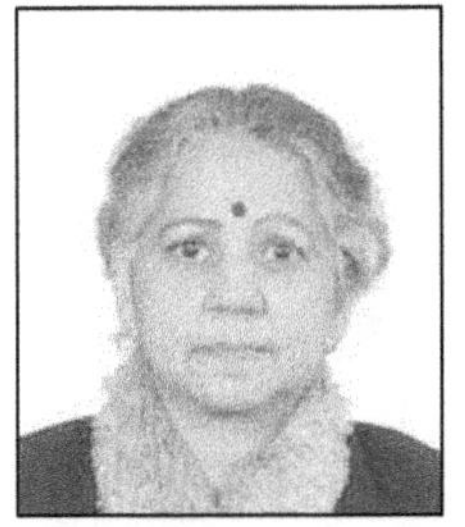

Dr Ira Das is Professor in the Department of Psychology, Dayalbagh Educational Institute, Deemed University, Dayalbagh, Agra, since 2000. Her areas of specialization include Psychometrics, Affective Psychology and Organizational Behavior. Presently she is working on Psycho-neuroimmunology.

She has constructed and standardized a number of psychological tests, presented more than hundred research papers in National and International Seminars and Conferences, published about 80 papers in reputed Journals and books. She has been the editor of the Journal of Psychological and Educational Research from 1978 to 1988.

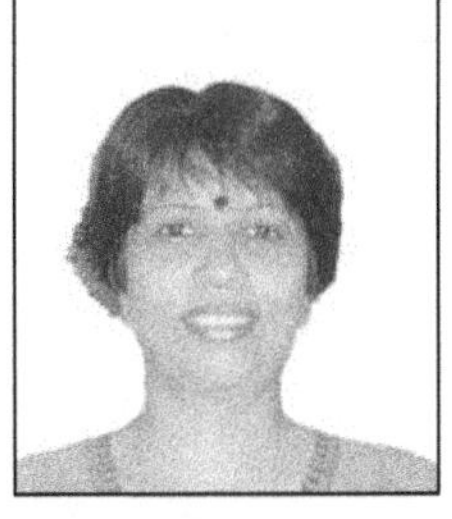

Dr. Kavita Kumar is Lecturer in the Department of Psychology at D.E.I., Deemed University, Dayalbagh, Agra. She is the recipient of Gold medals in both B.A. and M.A. (Psychology) from the same University. Before completing her Ph.D. in Organizational Psychology from B.R. Ambedkar University, Agra, she took several courses in Psychology from Wesleyan University, Middletown, CT, USA and Computer courses from Long Island University, Brooklyn, NY, USA. She has several research papers and book chapters to her credit. She has also attended and organized a number of National and International Conferences and won the best paper award in the International Conference on Health Psychology, 2008. Presently, she is teaching Undergraduate, Postgraduate and M.Phil. courses on Organizational Behavior, Psychopathology and Health Psychology etc.

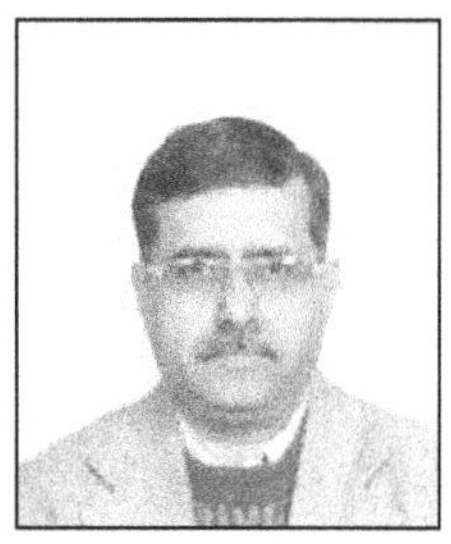

Dr Surat Kumar is Head, Applied Sciences, Faculty of Engineering, Dayalbagh Educational Institute, Dayalbagh Agra since January 2000. He obtained his Ph.D. degree from Central Drug Research Institute, Lucknow in Medicinal Chemistry. He has served in various research and academic positions in some of the most renowned institutions in Germany, Canada and the United States of America for about 14 years. He has extensively travelled abroad and delivered plenary and invited talks and chaired in various international and national conferences. He has edited one proceeding and contributed monographs in 4 books. He has published 25 peer reviewed papers in high impact factor journals. He has organized various international and national conferences. He is working in the area of Structural Biology and Genetic Engineering.

Author Index

www.ingramcontent.com/pod-product-compliance
Lightning Source LLC
Chambersburg PA
CBHW080227270326
41926CB00020B/4168

9788184244762